Allergy and Clinical Immunology

T0201353

Allergy and Clinical Immunology

EDITED BY

Hugh A. Sampson, MD

Kurt Hirschhorn Professor of Pediatrics
Dean for Translational Biomedical Sciences
Director, Elliot and Roslyn Jaffe Food Allergy Institute
Division of Allergy/Immunology; Department of Pediatrics
Icahn School of Medicine at Mount Sinai
New York, NY, USA

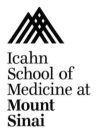

Icahn
School of
Medicine at
**Mount
Sinai**

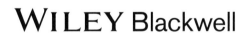

This edition first published 2015 © 2015 by John Wiley & Sons, Ltd.

Registered Office
John Wiley & Sons, Ltd, The Atrium, Southern Gate, Chichester, West Sussex, PO19 8SQ, UK

Editorial Offices
9600 Garsington Road, Oxford, OX4 2DQ, UK
The Atrium, Southern Gate, Chichester, West Sussex, PO19 8SQ, UK
111 River Street, Hoboken, NJ 07030-5774, USA

For details of our global editorial offices, for customer services and for information about how to apply for permission to reuse the copyright material in this book please see our website at www.wiley.com/wiley-blackwell

Library of Congress Cataloging-in-Publication Data

Mount Sinai expert guides. Allergy & clinical immunology / edited by Hugh A. Sampson.
       p. ; cm.
    Allergy & clinical immunology
    Includes bibliographical references and index.
    ISBN 978-1-118-60916-3 (pbk.)
I. Sampson, Hugh A., editor.   II. Title: Allergy & clinical immunology.
[DNLM: 1. Hypersensitivity.   2. Allergens.   3. Immune System Diseases.   4. Immune System Phenomena.
WD 300]
    RC584
    616.97–dc23
                                        2014049390

A catalogue record for this book is available from the British Library.

Wiley also publishes its books in a variety of electronic formats. Some content that appears in print may not be available in electronic books.

Cover image: Stock Photo File #6124416 © David Marchal
Cover design by Ruth Bateson

Set in 8.5/12pt Frutiger by SPi Publisher Services, Pondicherry, India
Printed and bound in Malaysia by Vivar Printing Sdn Bhd

1   2015

Contents

Part 2: CLINICAL IMMUNOLOGY

A color plate section appears between pages 206 and 207

Contributors

Shradha Agarwal MD
Assistant Professor of Medicine
Division of Allergy/Immunology
Icahn School of Medicine at Mount Sinai
New York, NY, USA

Supinda Bunyavanich MD, MPH
Assistant Professor
Elliot and Roslyn Jaffe Food Allergy Institute
Division of Allergy/Immunology
Department of Pediatrics
Department of Genetics and Genomic Sciences
Icahn School of Medicine at Mount Sinai
New York, NY, USA

Paula J. Busse MD
Associate Professor
Department of Medicine
Division of Clinical Immunology
Icahn School of Medicine at Mount Sinai
New York, NY, USA

Jean-Christoph Caubet MD
Chef de clinique
Division of Allergy
Department of Pediatrics
University Hospitals of Geneva
Geneva, Switzerland

Mirna Chehade MD, MPH
Associate Professor of Pediatrics and Medicine
Elliot and Roslyn Jaffe Food Allergy Institute
Division of Allergy/Immunology
Department of Pediatrics
Icahn School of Medicine at Mount Sinai
New York, NY, USA

Beth E. Corn MD
Assistant Professor of Medicine
Department of Clinical Immunology
Icahn School of Medicine at Mount Sinai
New York, NY, USA

Amanda L. Cox MD
Assistant Professor of Pediatrics
Elliot and Roslyn Jaffe Food Allergy Institute
Division of Allergy/Immunology
Department of Pediatrics
Icahn School of Medicine at Mount Sinai
New York, NY, USA

Charlotte Cunningham-Rundles MD, PhD
Professor of Medicine
Departments of Medicine and Pediatrics
The David S. Gottesman Professor
The Immunology Institute
Icahn School of Medicine at Mount Sinai
New York, NY, USA

Elizabeth J. Feuille MD
Clinical Fellow
Division of Allergy/Immunology
Icahn School of Medicine at Mount Sinai
New York, NY, USA

Satish Govindaraj MD
Associate Professor
Department of Otolaryngology–Head
   and Neck Surgery
Icahn School of Medicine at Mount Sinai
New York, NY, USA

Emma Guttman-Yassky MD, PhD
Associate Professor of Dermatology
   and Immunology
Departments of Dermatology and Immunology
Director, Center for Excellence in Eczema
Director, Occupational and Contact
   Dermatitis Clinic
Director, Laboratory for Investigation of
   Inflammatory Skin Diseases
Icahn School of Medicine at Mount Sinai
New York, NY, USA

Yan W. Ho MD
Resident of Otolaryngology Program
Department of Otolaryngology–Head
   and Neck Surgery
Icahn School of Medicine at Mount Sinai
New York, NY, USA

Jacob D. Kattan MD
Assistant Professor of Allergy and Immunology
Elliot and Roslyn Jaffe Food Allergy Institute
Division of Allergy/Immunology
Department of Pediatrics
Icahn School of Medicine at Mount Sinai
New York, NY, USA

Saakshi Khattri MD
Research Associate
Laboratory of Investigative Dermatology
Rockefeller University
New York, NY, USA

Jennifer S. Kim MD
Attending Physician
NorthShore University HealthSystem
Evanston, IL, USA;
Elliot and Roslyn Jaffe Food Allergy Institute
Division of Allergy/Immunology
Department of Pediatrics
Icahn School of Medicine at Mount Sinai
New York, NY, USA

Michael Mullen MD
Professor of Medicine
Director, Institute of Advanced Medicine
Icahn School of Medicine at Mount Sinai
New York, NY, USA

Anna Nowak-Węgrzyn MD
Associate Professor of Pediatrics
Elliot and Roslyn Jaffe Food Allergy Institute
Division of Allergy/Immunology
Department of Pediatrics
Icahn School of Medicine at Mount Sinai
New York, NY, USA

Roberto Posada MD
Associate Professor of Pediatrics (Infectious
   Diseases) and Medical Education
Director Pediatric, Adolescent and Young
   Adult HIV Program
Icahn School of Medicine at Mount Sinai
New York, NY, USA

Elena S. Resnick MD
Assistant Professor of Allergy and Clinical
   Immunology
Icahn School of Medicine at Mount Sinai
New York, NY

Mariya Rozenblit
Medical Student
Icahn School of Medicine at Mount Sinai
New York, NY, USA

Hugh A. Sampson MD
Kurt Hirschhorn Professor of Pediatrics
Dean for Translational Biomedical
   Sciences
Director, Elliot and Roslyn Jaffe Food
   Allergy Institute
Division of Allergy/Immunology
Department of Pediatrics
Icahn School of Medicine at Mount Sinai
New York, NY, USA

Gail F. Shust MD
Assistant Professor
Department of Pediatrics and Medical
   Education
Icahn School of Medicine at Mount Sinai
New York, NY, USA

Scott H. Sicherer MD
Elliot and Roslyn Jaffe Professor of Pediatrics,
   Allergy/Immunology
Jaffe Food Allergy Institute
Icahn School of Medicine at Mount Sinai
New York, NY, USA

Gwen S. Skloot MD
Associate Professor of Medicine
Division of Pulmonary,
   Critical Care and Sleep Medicine
Icahn School of Medicine at Mount Sinai
New York, NY, USA

Timothy Sullivan MD
Instructor
Division of Infectious Diseases
Icahn School of Medicine at Mount Sinai
New York, NY, USA

Julie Wang MD
Associate Professor of Pediatrics
Elliot and Roslyn Jaffe Food
   Allergy Institute
Division of Allergy/Immunology
Department of Pediatrics
Icahn School of Medicine at Mount Sinai
New York, NY, USA

Kate Welch MD
Clinical Fellow
Division of Allergy/Immunology
Icahn School of Medicine at Mount Sinai
New York, NY, USA

Series Foreword

Now more than ever, immediacy in obtaining accurate and practical information is the coin of the realm in providing high quality patient care. The Mount Sinai Expert Guides series addresses this vital need by providing accurate, up-to-date guidance, written by experts in formats that are accessible in the patient care setting: websites, smartphone apps and portable books. The Icahn School of Medicine, which was chartered in 1963, embodies a deep tradition of pre-eminence in clinical care and scholarship that was first shaped by the founding of the Mount Sinai Hospital in 1855. Today, the Mount Sinai Health System, comprised of seven hospitals anchored by the Icahn School of Medicine, is one of the largest health care systems in the United States, and is revolutionizing medicine through its embracing of transformative technologies for clinical diagnosis and treatment. The Mount Sinai Expert Guides series builds upon both this historical renown and contemporary excellence. Leading experts across a range of disciplines provide practical yet sage advice in a digestible format that is ideal for trainees, mid-level providers and practicing physicians. Few medical centers in the USA could offer this type of breadth while relying exclusively on its own physicians, yet here no compromises were required in offering a truly unique series that is sure to become embedded within the key resources of busy providers. In producing this series, the editors and authors are fortunate to have an equally dynamic and forward-viewing partner in Wiley Blackwell, which together ensures that health care professionals will benefit from a unique, first-class effort that will advance the care of their patients.

Scott Friedman MD
Series Editor
Dean for Therapeutic Discovery
Fishberg Professor and Chief, Division of Liver Diseases
Icahn School of Medicine at Mount Sinai
New York, NY, USA

Preface

In the past 60 years, allergic disorders have increased dramatically in "westernized" countries, especially in North America, Europe and Australia/New Zealand. In the last half of the twentieth century, increases in respiratory allergies, i.e. asthma and allergic rhinitis, largely accounted for the rise in prevalence. However, in the last 15 years the prevalence of food allergies/anaphylaxis and atopic dermatitis have increased over two- to three-fold while the prevalence of respiratory allergies have leveled-off. Allergic disorders now affect about one-third of the US population and cost the health care system several billions of dollars each year in medical expenses and lost wages. Drug allergy is estimated to affect about 10% of the world's population and 20% of hospitalized patients. Over the past two decades, scientists and clinicians have made great strides in the diagnosis and management of allergic disorders. The past several decades have also witnessed tremendous advances in our recognition of immunodeficiency disorders and our understanding of the human immune system. Advances in molecular genetic techniques and other technical advances have led to the identification and characterization of many new immunodeficiency disorders that have enabled clinicians to more appropriately treat patients afflicted with these disorders. Early recognition and initiation of therapy is key to preserving a more normal life for children afflicted with these disorders. In addition, investigators have now recognized that adults also develop various forms of primary and secondary immunodeficiency diseases and require timely evaluation and management of their disorder.

In this book, members of the pediatric and adult Divisions of Allergy and Immunology at the Icahn School of Medicine at Mount Sinai have teamed-up to provide a clinician-friendly manual outlining the diagnosis and management of a wide variety of allergic and immunodeficient disorders. Members of the Allergy/Immunology group have provided a brief outlines on the etiology and pathogenesis of various disorders, succinct guidelines on the relevant historical and laboratory information necessary for establishing a timely and accurate diagnosis, guidelines on the most current forms of therapy to manage the various disorders, and a brief discussion of anticipated natural history and outcomes. Each chapter author provides her/his perspective on evaluating and managing various allergic and immunologic disorders based on years of experience dealing with allergic and immunodeficient patients. This book is not meant to be an exhaustive discussion of allergic/immunologic conditions (although references are provided to satisfy the most inquisitive reader), but a useful guidebook enabling the busy clinician to recognize patients afflicted with allergic or immunologic disorders and provide them with the most current management strategies.

Hugh A. Sampson, MD
Kurt Hirschhorn Professor of Pediatrics
Dean for Translational Biomedical Sciences
Director, Elliot and Roslyn Jaffe Food Allergy Institute
Division of Allergy/Immunology; Department of Pediatrics
Icahn School of Medicine at Mount Sinai
New York, NY, USA

List of Abbreviations

ABG	arterial blood gas
ACD	allergic contact dermatitis
ACE-I	angiotensin-converting enzyme inhibitor
AD	atopic dermatitis
ADA	adenosine deaminase
AD-HIES	autosomal dominant hyper IgE syndrome
AGEP	acute generalized exanthematous pustulosis
AHR	airway hyper-responsiveness
AKC	atopic keratoconjunctivitis
ALPS	autoimmune lymphoproliferative syndrome
APECED	autoimmune polyendocrinopathy, candidiasis, and ectodermal dystrophy (syndrome)
APT	atopy patch test
ASM	aggressive systemic mastocytosis
BMP	basic metabolic panel
BP	blood pressure
cART	combination antiretroviral therapy
CBC	complete blood count
CD	celiac disease
CDC	Centers for Disease Control and Prevention
CGD	chronic granulomatous disease
CLL	chronic lymphocytic leukemia
CM	cow's milk
CM	cutaneous mastocytosis
CMC	chronic mucocutaneous candidiasis
CMV	cytomegalovirus
COPD	chronic obstructive pulmonary disease
CRP	C-reactive protein
CSF	cerebrospinal fluid
CT	computed tomography
CU	chronic urticaria
CVID	common variable immunodeficiency
DAF	decay accelerating factor
DBPCFC	double-blind, placebo-controlled oral food challenge
DCM	diffuse cutaneous mastocytosis
DGP	deamidated gliadin peptide
DLCO	diffusion capacity for carbon monoxide
DRESS	drug reaction or rash with eosinophilia and systemic symptom
EASI	Eczema Area and Severity Index
EG	eosinophilic gastroenteritis
EGD	esophagogastroduodenoscopy

EIA	enzyme immunoassay
EoE	eosinophilic esophagitis
ESR	erythrocyte sedimentation rate
FDA	Food and Drug Administration
FDEIA	food-dependent, exercised-induced anaphylaxis
FeNO	fractional exhaled nitric oxide
FESS	functional endoscopic sinus surgery
FEV_1	forced expiratory volume in 1 second
FISH	fluoroescence in situ hybridization
FPIES	food protein-induced enterocolitis syndrome
FPIP	food protein-induced proctocolitis
FVC	forced vital capacity
G-CSF	granulocyte colony-stimulating factor
GERD	gastroesophageal reflux disease
GI	gastrointestinal
GM-CSF	granulocyte macrophage colony-stimulating factor
GPC	giant papillary conjunctivitis
HAE	hereditary angioedema
H&E	hematoxylin and eosin
HEENT	head, eyes, ears, nose, and throat
HEPA	high-efficiency particulate air
HES	hypereosinophilic syndrome
5-HIAA	5-hydroxyindoleacetic acid
HIES	hyper IgE syndrome
HLA	human leukocyte antigen
HMW	high molecular weight
HPF	high power field
HSCT	hematopoietic stem cell transplantation
HUS	hemolytic uremic syndrome
HVAC	heating, ventilating, and air conditioning
IFA	immunofluorescent antibody
IFN	interferon
Ig	immunoglobulin
IL	interleukin
IPEX	immune dysregulation, polyendocrinopathy, X-linked
ISM	indolent systemic mastocytosis
ITP	immune thrombocytopenia
IVIg	intravenous immunoglobulin
LAD	leukocyte adhesion deficiency
LFT	liver function test
LMW	low molecular weight
LTC4	leukotriene C4
LTP	lipid transfer protein
MAC	membrane attack complex
MASP	mannan-binding lectin-associated protease
MBL	mannose-binding lectin
MBP	mannose-binding protein
MCAS	mast cell activation syndrome

MCL	mast cell leukemia
MHC	major histocompatibility complex
MMAS	monoclonal mast cell activation syndrome
MRI	magnetic resonance imaging
MRSA	methicillin-resistant *Staphylococcus aureus*
MSG	monosodium glutamate
NARES	non-allergic rhinitis with eosinophilia
NIH	National Institutes of Health
NRTI	nucleoside reverse-transcriptase inhibitor
NSAID	non-steroidal anti-inflammatory drug
OA	occupational asthma
OAS	oral allergy syndrome
OFC	oral food challenge
OMC	osteomeatal complex
PAC	perennial allergic conjunctivitis
pd	plasma-derived
PE	pulmonary embolism
PEFR	peak expiratory flow rate
PEP	post-exposure prophylaxis
PGD2	prostaglandin D2
PLE	protein-losing enteropathy
PMTCT	prevention of mother-to-child transmission
PNH	paroxysmal nocturnal hemoglobinuria
ppb	parts per billion
PPI	proton pump inhibitor
PrEP	pre-exposure prophylaxis
RADS	reactive airway dysfunction syndrome
RAST	radioallergosorbent test
RSV	respiratory syncytial virus
SAC	seasonal allergic conjunctivitis
SCF	stem cell factor
SCID	severe combined immunodeficiency
SCIT	subcutaneous immunotherapy
SCORAD	Severity Scoring of Atopic Dermatitis
SJS	Stevens–Johnson syndrome
SLE	systemic lupus erythematosus
SLIT	sublingual immunotherapy
SM	systemic mastocytosis
SM-AHNMD	systemic mastocytosis with an associated hematologic non-mast cell lineage disorder
SNOT	sinonasal outcome test
TEN	toxic epidermal necrolysis
TMEP	telangiectasia macularis eruptiva perstans
TNF	tumor necrosis factor
TREC	T-cell receptor excision circle
Treg	regulatory T-cell
TSH	thyroid stimulating hormone
TTG	tissue transglutaminase

UACS	upper airway cough syndrome
UP	urticaria pigmentosa
URI	upper respiratory infection
URTI	upper respiratory tract infection
VIP	vasoactive intestinal peptide
VIT	venom immunotherapy
VKC	vernal keratoconjunctivitis
VL	viral load
WAS	Wiskott–Aldrich syndrome
WASp	Wiskott–Aldrich syndrome protein
WB	Western blot
WHIM	warts, hypogammaglobulinemia, infections, and myelokathexis (syndrome)
WHO	World Health Organization
WIP	WASp-interacting protein
XLN	X-linked neutropenia
XLT	X-linked thrombocytopenia

About the Companion Website

This series is accompanied by a companion website:

www.mountsinaiexpertguides.com

The website includes:
- Case studies
- ICD codes
- Interactive MCQs
- Patient advice

PART 1

Allergy

CHAPTER 1

Atopic Dermatitis in Infants and Young Children

Jean-Christoph Caubet[1] and Anna Nowak-Węgrzyn[2]
[1]Division of Allergy, Department of Pediatrics, University Hospitals of Geneva, Geneva, Switzerland
[2]Department of Pediatrics, Division of Allergy/Immunology, Jaffe Food Allergy Institute, Icahn School of Medicine at Mount Sinai, New York, NY, USA

OVERALL BOTTOM LINE

- Atopic dermatitis (AD) is a common, chronic, relapsing, inflammatory skin disorder and may be the initial step of the so-called atopic march.
- Pathogenesis is complex and not fully understood, but recent investigations have highlighted two cornerstone features of AD: defective epidermal barrier and cutaneous inflammation involving both IgE- and T-cell-mediated responses.
- Diagnosis of AD is based on clinical features.
- A complete allergy investigation is required in patients with moderate to severe AD or a history of exacerbation after food ingestion. The younger the age of onset and the more severe the rash, the more likely foods are to trigger AD in children.
- Although there is no cure for AD, the goals of treatment are to reduce symptoms, prevent exacerbations, minimize side effects, and provide adequate psychological support.

Section 1: Background

Definition of disease

- AD is a familial, common, inflammatory skin disorder characterized by chronically relapsing course and intensely pruritic eczematous flares. The term "eczema" alone generally refers to AD and these terms are often used interchangeably.

Disease classification

- Although clinically indistinguishable, AD has been categorized into an immunoglobulin E (IgE) associated form (true AD, formerly called extrinsic AD) and a non-IgE-associated form ("non-atopic" dermatitis, formerly called intrinsic AD). However, this classification is controversial as the absence of sensitization to common food allergens and aeroallergens may be only a transient factor.

Incidence/prevalence

- AD affects an estimated 18 million people in the United States.
- The estimated lifetime prevalence in children ranges from 10–30%.
- Wide variations in prevalence have been observed between countries, suggesting that environmental factors determine AD expression.

Mount Sinai Expert Guides: Allergy and Clinical Immunology, First Edition. Edited by Hugh A. Sampson.
© 2015 John Wiley & Sons, Ltd. Published 2015 by John Wiley & Sons, Ltd.
Companion website: www.mountsinaiexpertguides.com

Economic impact

- The economic impact of AD is important and will likely increase in proportion to increasing disease prevalence. The current estimates range widely, from $364 million to $3.8 billion dollars per year.

Etiology

- The exact etiologic factors leading to AD are not well defined.
- Genetically predisposed patients with AD have an epidermal barrier dysfunction, linked to decreased or impaired function of essential barrier proteins (i.e. filaggrin and ceramide).
- Common triggers in AD include food proteins, aeroallergens, stress, climate, irritants, and microbes.

Pathology/pathogenesis

- AD is mainly characterized by a defective epidermal barrier and cutaneous inflammation.
- Genetically predisposed patients with AD have an epidermal barrier dysfunction; contributing factors include decreased ceramide levels and loss of function of crucial protein (e.g. filaggrin). This can result in enhanced transepidermal water loss and facilitated penetration of environmental allergens, promoting allergic skin inflammation.
- The complex underlying immune response of AD involves both IgE-mediated and T-cell-mediated delayed immune responses. Acute skin lesions of AD are characterized by cells containing Th2 cytokines (i.e. IL-4, IL-5, IL-13 and IL-22), whereas Th1 cells expressing γ-interferon (IFN-γ) are most commonly found in more chronic lesions.
- Although elevated serum total IgE levels can be found in 80–85% of patients with AD, the clinical relevance of associated sensitizations has been difficult to ascertain.
- Foods can cause exacerbation in a subset of patients (i.e. approximately one-third of young children with a moderate or severe AD). Similarly, exacerbation of AD can occur with exposure to aeroallergens such as house dust mites, animal danders, and pollens.
- Most patients with AD have an inadequate innate immune response to epicutaneous microbes, in part responsible for increased susceptibility to infections (bacteria, yeast, viruses) and colonization with *Staphylococcus aureus*. These microbes contribute, at least partially, to the skin inflammation and can potentially lead to exacerbations of the disease.

Predictive/risk factors

Risk factor	Odds ratio
Genetic factors (filaggrin mutation)	3.73–7.1
Breastfeeding	Controversial
Tobacco	1.97
Familial history of atopy	2–6

Section 2: Prevention

BOTTOM LINE/CLINICAL PEARL
- For infants at high risk of atopy, exclusive breastfeeding for at least 4 months and/or feeding with extensively hydrolyzed formula decreases cumulative incidence of AD in the first 2 years of life. There is no prevention strategy proven to protect beyond the first few years of life.

Screening

Not applicable for this topic. Studies on screening for filaggrin mutations are ongoing.

Primary prevention

- Exclusive breastfeeding for at least 4 months and/or feeding with extensively hydrolyzed formula decreases cumulative incidence of AD in the first 2 years of life.
- Although several studies support a preventative effect of treating with probiotics during pregnancy or early infancy to delay the onset of AD, controversy persists and more studies are needed to confirm these data.

Secondary prevention

- Optimal skin care remains the cornerstone of the management of AD.
- Avoidance of common irritants and specific allergen triggers (foods and/or aeroallergens) in selected patients constitute a large part of secondary prevention of AD.
- Other important measures include control of household temperature and humidity; use of mild soaps for bathing (neutral pH and minimal defatting capabilities); bathing in warm water once a day for 15–20 minutes, pat dry and immediate application of emollients; nails trimming to decrease abrasion to skin; use of clothing made of cotton instead of synthetic fibers and wool.

Section 3: Diagnosis (Algorithm 1.1)

Algorithm 1.1 Diagnosis of atopic dermatitis

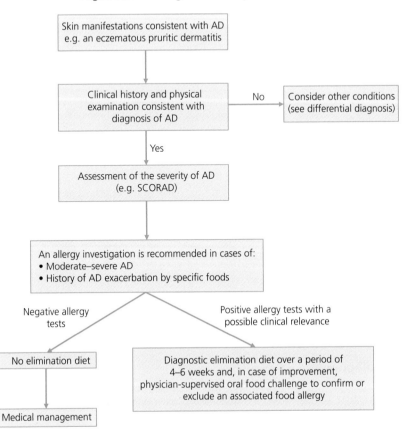

> **BOTTOM LINE/CLINICAL PEARLS**
> - The diagnosis of AD is based on a constellation of clinical features.
> - Recurrent pruritus is the only symptom of AD.
> - Physical examination reveals xerosis and typical eczematous lesions with different morphologic aspects and locations depending on the age of the patient. Eczematous rashes tend to be generalized and affect the face and extensor surfaces of the limbs in infants and toddlers, while in older children and adults rashes localize to the peri-orbital area, flexor surfaces of the joints, and about the wrists and ankles.
> - Allergic investigations are usually not indicated for patients with mild AD.
> - In patients with moderate–severe atopic dermatitis or with a positive history of exacerbation after exposure to a specific allergen, an allergy investigation including skin tests, specific IgE measurement, and/or an oral provocation test are indicated.

Differential diagnosis

Differential diagnosis	Features
Scabies	Papules, finger web involvement, positive scraping for scabies mite
Allergic contact dermatitis	Positive exposure history, rash in area of exposure, absence of family history
Seborrheic dermatitis	Greasy, scaly lesions, absence of family history
Zinc and biotin deficiency	Eczematous lesions localized in peri-oral area and rectum (oral, anal)
Psoriasis	Localized patches on extensor surfaces, scalp, buttocks, pitted nails
Ichthyosis	Usually non-pruritic, not the typical distribution pattern seen in AD, no inflammatory lesions (except in Netherton's syndrome)
Netherton's syndrome (severe, autosomal recessive form of ichthyosis associated with mutations in the SPINK5 gene)	Chronic skin inflammation, universal pruritus, severe dehydration and stunted growth, hair shaft defect (trichorrhexis invaginata), also known as "bamboo hair"
Immunodeficiency: severe combined immunodeficiency syndrome, hyper-IgE syndrome, Wiskott–Aldrich syndrome	Severe eczema, positive history of multiple infections, growth failure

Typical presentation
- Atopic dermatitis occurs in the first year of life in 60% of cases, and by the age of 5 years in nearly 85% of cases. Patients typically present with pruritus and chronically relapsing/remitting eczematous lesions having a typical morphology and distribution related to the age of the patient.

Clinical diagnosis
History
- The diagnosis of AD is based on a constellation of clinical features, pruritus being the cardinal symptom of this disorder.

- One of the major clinical features of AD is its chronicity, characterized by an intermittent course with flares and remission.
- A careful allergy history is of major importance to identify potential allergen triggers (e.g. aeroallergens and foods), particularly in patients with moderate–severe AD. Identification of common irritants is also an important part of the history.
- The clinician should evaluate the impact on quality of life, particularly sleeping and psychologic aspects.

Physical examination
- Characteristic skin findings in AD include primarily xerosis and eczematous lesions with different morphologic aspects and locations depending on the age of the patient.
- Acute and subacute eczematous skin lesions are typically found in infants and young children, with intensely pruritic, erythematous, papulo-vesicular lesions, excoriation, and serous exudate. The lesions are typically localized on the scalp, face (cheeks and chin), and extensor surfaces of the extremities. In older children, lesions are more commonly found in the flexor surfaces (antecubital and popliteal fossa), neck, wrists, and ankles.
- Lichenification is rarely seen in infancy but is characteristic of childhood AD.
- Of note, peri-orbital hyperpigmentation and Dennie–Morgan folds (prominent folds of skin under the lower eyelid) are common peri-ocular findings in patients with AD.

Useful clinical decision rules and calculators
- The UK diagnostic criteria are the most extensively validated for AD and are based on the classic diagnostic criteria of Hanifin and Rajka.
- The patient must have an itchy skin condition in the last 12 months plus three or more of the following criteria:
  - Onset below age 2 (not used in children under 4 years);
  - History of flexural involvement;
  - History of a generally dry skin;
  - Personal history of other atopic disease (in children aged under 4 years, history of atopic disease in a first degree relative may be included); and
  - Visible flexural dermatitis as per photographic protocol.

Disease severity classification
- There are many tools to evaluate the severity of AD, although they have been used mainly in clinical research trials. The most well known:
  - *Severity Scoring of Atopic Dermatitis (SCORAD):* uses the "rule of 9's" to assess disease extent and evaluates five clinical characteristics to determine disease severity; and
  - *Eczema Area and Severity Index (EASI):* assesses extent of diseases at four body sites and measures four clinical signs on a scale of 0–3.

Laboratory diagnosis
List of diagnostic tests
- Skin prick tests and/or specific IgE to common food allergens should be restricted to patients with moderate–severe AD or to patients having a positive history of exacerbation after specific food ingestion.
- The most common food allergens in childhood AD are hen's egg, cow's milk, peanut, soybean, wheat, tree nuts, fish, and shellfish. Hen's egg, cow's milk, and peanut account for about 80% of food allergy diagnosed by food challenge in children with AD.

- Skin prick tests and/or specific IgE to aeroallergens (i.e. pollens, animal danders, and dust mites) should be performed according to the history and the age of the patient.
- Atopy patch testing is an additional tool in selected cases in which skin prick tests or specific IgE fail to identify a suspected food. It is not recommended as a routine diagnostic test in AD.
- Oral food challenges are considered the gold standard to diagnose an associated food allergy.
- Scraping to exclude tinea corporis is occasionally helpful.
- A swab of infected skin may help with the isolation of a specific organism and antibiotic sensitivity assessment.
- Skin biopsy is usually not required to confirm the diagnosis of AD but in rare difficult cases it can be useful to exclude other causes.

Lists of imaging techniques

Not applicable for this topic.

Potential pitfalls/common errors made regarding diagnosis of disease

- Positive skin prick tests or specific IgE to food(s) should only lead to a restrictive elimination diet in selected patients with moderate–severe AD or a positive history of exacerbation after food ingestion. Elimination diets based on positive skin prick tests or food-specific IgE levels should be of limited duration unless there is clear evidence of clinical food allergy.
- Scabies should always be excluded in patients with severe pruritus.
- In patients with severe AD, poor growth, and/or frequent or severe infection, an immunodeficiency should be suspected.

Section 4: Treatment (Algorithm 1.2)
Treatment rationale

- The first line therapy is based on restoring skin hydration (e.g. hydrating baths and emollient creams) and reducing inflammation (e.g. topical corticosteroids and/or calcineurin inhibitors).
- Rarely, patients need systemic treatments with oral corticosteroids or immunosuppressive agents. These treatments should be re-evaluated and adapted regularly in order to minimize potential side effects.
- Antibacterial or antiviral drugs are indicated only in patients with clinical signs of active infection, particularly resulting from *Staphylococcus aureus* and herpes simplex virus infection. In addition, the role of allergens, irritants, physical environment, and emotional stressors need to be considered, as controlling these factors is of major importance in optimizing management.
- Food elimination diets should be restricted to selected patients with a positive allergy investigation and the potential benefits (decreased AD severity and improved quality of life) and potential disadvantages (decreased quality of life because of food avoidance and risk of anaphylactic reactions to a food) need to be discussed with the patient and his/her family.
- A 4–6 week trial of food elimination may be followed by food reintroduction (oral food challenge) under physician supervision to document reappearance of eczematous lesions. In a subset of children with persistent AD and no prior history of acute allergic reactions upon food ingestion, following food elimination, classic acute allergic symptoms may be observed following food reintroduction including hives or even anaphylaxis.
- Oral non-sedating antihistamines have a minor effect on the control of pruritus associated with AD. The first generation, sedating antihistamines (e.g. hydroxyzine) can be helpful when used at bedtime to facilitate falling asleep.

Algorithm 1.2 Management of atopic dermatitis

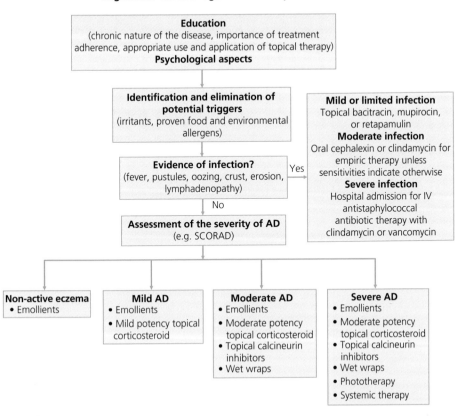

Step-up or step-down treatment according to the symptoms control

- Patients should understand that therapy is not curative but that avoidance of exacerbating factors together with proper daily skin care can result in control of symptoms and improve the long-term outcome. The clinician should take into account the impact of AD on quality of life and correctly manage the associated stress that can be responsible for acute exacerbations.

When to hospitalize
- Hospitalization is rarely required for patients with AD.
- Patients with severe AD who do not improve with correct outpatient therapy might require hospitalization.
- Patients with cellulitis or severe secondary infection (e.g. eczema herpeticum caused by primary infection with herpes simplex virus) may need intravenous antibiotics and sedation.
- Hospitalization is sometimes necessary to clear the patient's skin before skin testing and/or oral food challenge.

Managing the hospitalized patient
- Appropriate antimicrobial agent therapy.
- Intensive skin care may include soaking bath or wet wraps.
- Oral food challenges to the suspected food can be carried out during hospitalization.

- Hospitalization is beneficial in selected patients by removing the patient from environmental triggers (irritants, allergens) and by intensifying treatment.
- Adequate educational information should be provided to the patient and their family in order to improve adherence with the treatment regimen.
- Psychological issues are also more easily addressed during a hospitalization.

Table of treatment

Treatment	Comment
Identification and elimination of triggering factors	Avoidance of common irritants (e.g. soaps, toiletries, wool, and chemicals) are recommended as well as a correct control of temperature and humidity that may trigger the itch–scratch cycle Elimination diets should only be recommended in selected patients based on a positive allergy investigation
Emollients	An effective moisturizer constitutes the cornerstone of the treatment of AD as it helps to restore and preserve the skin barrier (e.g. CeraVe®, Vanicream®, Vaseline®)
Topical corticosteroids	Used primarily to control acute exacerbation of AD Seven classes ranked according to their potency. The choice and the duration will be based on the severity of the lesions and should be re-evaluated regularly. In general, the least potent steroid that is effective should be used
Topical calcineurin inhibitors	Currently indicated as second line treatment for intermittent use in children aged 2 years and older with moderate–severe AD (tacrolimus ointment 0.03%) and mild–moderate AD (pimecrolimus cream 1%). Of note, tacrolimus ointment 1% is indicated for patients 16 years and older
Systemic corticosteroids	Rarely indicated, but a short course of oral prednisone can be used in severe acute exacerbation of AD
Antistaphylococcal antibiotics	In patients with extensive skin infection, a course of systemic antibiotics is indicated: cephalosporin (e.g. cephalexin twice daily for 14–21 days) or penicillinase-resistant penicillins are usually beneficial Topical mupirocin is useful for the treatment of localized impetigo lesions
Antiviral therapy	In patients with disseminated herpes simplex virus infection, acyclovir is indicated, orally for less severe infection and intravenously for widely disseminated disease (30 mg/kg/day)
• Cyclosporine • Mycophenolate mofetil • Azathioprine • IFN-γ	These drugs have multiple potential severe side effects and should be used only in selected patients with persistent severe AD
Psychological	Psychological evaluation or counseling should be considered in patients with AD due to the main impact on their quality of life and as stress is a potential trigger
Phototherapy	UV therapy can be a useful treatment for recalcitrant AD. The most effective phototherapy option that is available in the United States is narrow band UVB
Wet dressing	This tool can be used in combination with topical corticoids

Prevention/management of complications

- Patients should be carefully instructed in the used of topical corticosteroids (i.e. avoidance of face, genital, and intertriginous areas). Although the systemic effects of topical corticosteroids

are minor, corticophobia is one of the main limiting factors in the treatment of patients with AD. The clinician should provide full explanations to achieve good adherence.
- Although there was a Food and Drug Administration (FDA) Black Box warning in 2005, it seems that the benefits of using calcineurin inhibitors in the appropriately selected patient population outweighs the theoretical risk of increased malignancy.
- Use of systemic immunosuppressive drugs may be associated with several, potentially severe, side effects and these drugs should be restricted to patients with severe and uncontrolled AD unresponsive to standard treatment.

CLINICAL PEARLS
- Clinicians should use a systematic approach that includes skin hydration, topical anti-inflammatory medications, antipruritic therapy, and antibacterial measures.
- Elimination of exacerbating factors, including allergens, is a cornerstone of AD management.
- The clinician should recognize that AD has a significant effect on the patient's and family's quality of life.

Section 5: Special populations
Not applicable for this topic.

Section 6: Prognosis

BOTTOM LINE/CLINICAL PEARLS
- AD typically manifests in early childhood, with onset before 5 years of age in approximately 90% of patients.
- Although it was initially reported that more than 80% of children outgrow their AD by adolescence, more recent studies present less optimistic outcomes with AD persisting into adulthood, even if the relapses are often less common and mild.
- Adults with a history of childhood AD are at an increased risk for occupational hand dermatoses.
- AD is usually considered as the first step of the so-called atopic march and it is estimated that 30–60% of patients with AD will develop allergic rhinitis or asthma.

Natural history of untreated disease
Not applicable for this topic.

Prognosis for treated patients
Not applicable for this topic.

Follow-up tests and monitoring
- The patients and/or parents should be instructed on the specific aspects of the disease (i.e. mainly its chronicity and exacerbating factors) and on appropriate treatment options to control the symptoms. A treatment plan for skin care should be provided and re-evaluated regularly during follow-up visits.
- As the diagnosis is only based on clinical criteria, it is important to reassess if the diagnosis is correct, particularly in patients with uncontrolled symptoms despite an optimal treatment.

Section 7: Reading list

Boguniewicz M, Leung DYM. Atopic dermatitis. In Adkinson NF, Busse WW, Bochner BS, et al. (eds) Middleton's Allergy: Principles and Practice, 8th edn. Saunders; 2013, 540–58

Brenninkmeijer EE, Schram ME, Leeflang MM, Bos JD, Spuls PI. Diagnostic criteria for atopic dermatitis: a systematic review. Br J Dermatol 2008;158:754–65

Caubet JC, Eigenmann PA. Allergic triggers in atopic dermatitis. Immunol Allergy Clin North Am 2010;30:289–307

Hanifin JM, Cooper KD, Ho VC, Kang S, Krafchik BR, Margolis DJ, et al. Guidelines of care for atopic dermatitis, developed in accordance with the American Academy of Dermatology (AAD)/American Academy of Dermatology Association. Administrative Regulations for Evidence-Based Clinical Practice Guidelines. J Am Acad Dermatol 2004;50:391–404

Leung DY, Bieber T. Atopic dermatitis. Lancet 2003;361:151–60

Mancini AJ, Kaulback K, Chamlin SL. The socioeconomic impact of atopic dermatitis in the United States: a systematic review. Pediatr Dermatol 2008;25:1–6

Schneider L, Tilles S, Lio P, Boguniewicz M, Beck L, LeBovidge J, et al. Atopic dermatitis: a practice parameter update 2012. J Allergy Clin Immunol 2013;131:295–9, e1–27

Suggested websites

A website to evaluate the SCORAD: http://adserver.sante.univ-nantes.fr/Scorad.html

Section 8: Guidelines
National society guidelines

Guideline title	Guideline source	Date
Atopic dermatitis: A practice parameter update 2012	J Allergy Clin Immunol	2013 (http://www.ncbi.nlm.nih.gov/pubmed/23374261)
Guidelines for the diagnosis and management of food allergy in the United States: Summary of the NIAID-Sponsored Expert Panel Report	J. Allergy Clin Immunol	2010 (http://www.ncbi.nlm.nih.gov/pubmed/21134568)

International society guidelines

Guideline title	Guideline source	Date
Eczematous reactions to food in atopic eczema: position paper of the EAACI and GA2LEN	European Academy of Allergy and Clinical Immunology (EAACI)	2007 (http://www.ncbi.nlm.nih.gov/pubmed/17573718)
Diagnosis and treatment of atopic dermatitis in children and adults: European Academy of Allergy and Clinical Immunology/American Academy of Allergy, Asthma and Immunology/PRACTALL Consensus Report	European Academy of Allergy and Clinical Immunology/ American Academy of Allergy, Asthma and Immunology/ PRACTALL Consensus Group	2006 (http://www.ncbi.nlm.nih.gov/pubmed/16867052)

Section 9: Evidence

Type of evidence	Title, comment	Date
Prospective study	Prevalence of IgE-mediated food allergy among children with atopic dermatitis **Comment:** This study demonstrates that approximately one-third of children with refractory, moderate–severe AD have IgE-mediated clinical reactivity to food proteins	1998 (http://www.ncbi.nlm.nih.gov/pubmed/9481027)
Prospective study	Common loss-of-function variants of the epidermal barrier protein filaggrin are a major predisposing factor for atopic dermatitis **Comment:** This work establishes a key role for impaired skin barrier function in the development of atopic disease	2006 (http://www.nature.com/ng/journal/v38/n4/abs/ng1767.html)
Prospective study	Loss-of-function variants in the filaggrin gene are a significant risk factor for peanut allergy **Comment:** Filaggrin mutations represent a significant risk factor for IgE-mediated peanut allergy, indicating a role for epithelial barrier dysfunction in the pathogenesis of this disease	2011 (http://www.ncbi.nlm.nih.gov/pubmed/21377035)

Section 10: Images

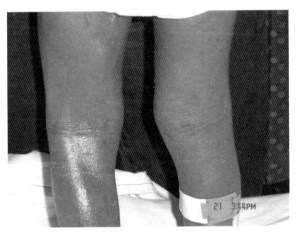

Figure 1.1 A child with multiple food allergies and severe persistent atopic dermatitis (AD) with acute exacerbation due to *Staphylococcus aureus* superinfection. Note the diffuse erythroderma and open sores. See color plate 1.1.

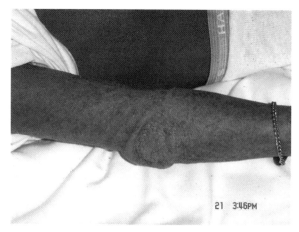

Figure 1.2 AD chronic lesions of skin hypertrophy, lichenification, hyperpigmentation, and xerosis. See color plate 1.2.

Additional material for this chapter can be found online at:
www.mountsinaiexpertguides.com
This includes a case study, multiple choice questions, advice for
patients, and ICD codes

CHAPTER 2

Atopic Dermatitis in Teenagers and Adults

Saakshi Khattri[1] and Emma Guttman-Yassky[2]
[1]Rockefeller University, New York, NY, USA
[2]Icahn School of Medicine at Mount Sinai, New York, NY, USA

OVERALL BOTTOM LINE
- Most common inflammatory skin disease affecting 15–25% children and 2–7% adults.
- Characterized by pruritic, erythematous plaques with oozing and crusting in the acute stages and lichenification in chronic stages.
- Characterized by remissions and exacerbations.
- Mild atopic dermatitis can be treated with emollients and topical medications such as corticosteroids and calcineurin inhibitors. Moderate to severe disease requires systemic treatment (UV therapy, systemic steroids, cyclosporine).
- Recent research suggests immune basis of disease with involvement of Th2, Th22, and some involvement of Th17 lymphocytes.

Section 1: Background
Definition of disease
- Atopic dermatitis (AD) is a chronic, erythematous, eczematous, pruritic rash that generally begins in childhood; however, late AD can occur in adults.
- It is characterized by remissions and exacerbations.

Disease classification
- *Acute atopic dermatitis:* characterized by erythematous, eczematous, weeping lesions in the acute stage. Secondary infection with *Staphylococcus aureus* can give rise to impetiginization.
- *Chronic atopic dermatitis:* lichenification (thickening of skin markings) is a prominent feature of the disease.
  Another classification is based on age at onset:
- *Childhood AD or early onset AD:* starts in children and is the most common form. Lesions are generally located in the antecubital and popliteal fossae, the face and neck. The lesions are typically exudative.
- *Adult onset AD or late onset AD:* distribution can be the same as that seen in the childhood type; however, lichenification and excoriations are more common and exudative lesions are less commonly seen.

Mount Sinai Expert Guides: Allergy and Clinical Immunology, First Edition. Edited by Hugh A. Sampson.
© 2015 John Wiley & Sons, Ltd. Published 2015 by John Wiley & Sons, Ltd.
Companion website: www.mountsinaiexpertguides.com

The third classification is based on level of the IgE:

- *Extrinsic AD:* 80% of AD patients and is characterized by high levels of IgE in the serum; these patients are more likely to have other atopic diseases. Activation of Th2 cytokines including IL-4, IL-5, and IL-13 resulting in increased production of IgE by B cells and increased levels of eosinophils.
- *Intrinsic AD:* remaining 20% cases of AD. These patients have normal levels of IgE. There is a mixed response with both Th2 and Th1 activation.

Incidence/prevalence

- 15–25% of children.
- 2–7% of adults.
- Approximately 75% of children will outgrow the disease by the age of 10 years.

Economic impact

Huge economic impact which includes:

- Co-payment for doctor's office visits;
- Cost of over-the-counter emollients and moisturizers;
- Cost of prescription medications;
- Incidental expenses such as buying air purifiers to remove aeroallergens, dietary changes;
- Cost incurred due to missing work (for adults with AD and of parents who need to take their children with AD for doctor visits).

Etiology

- Genetic factors may have a role such as mutations in the filaggrin (*FLG*) gene (a loss of function mutation). Filaggrin regulates epidermal terminal differentiation and helps create a cornified envelope.
- Environmental factors such as allergen exposure, changes in weather, and temperature changes.
- Some food allergies may have a role in disease flares, particularly in children.
- Stress exacerbates atopic dermatitis.

Pathology/pathogenesis

- Immune activation with up-regulation of T cells, dendritic cells, several cytokines, chemokines, and other inflammatory molecules produced by distinct T-cell subsets (primarily Th2, Th22).
- Disrupted skin barrier (decreased filaggrin, and other barrier proteins) and increased trans-epidermal water loss which may trigger abnormal keratinocyte hyperplasia and secondary inflammation.
- Th2 and Th22 cytokines are responsible for key disease features such as down-regulation of barrier proteins and epidermal hyperplasia.

Predictive/risk factors

Not applicable for this topic.

Section 2: Prevention

- No intervention has been demonstrated to prevent the development of disease. However, if trigger factors are determined, then avoidance of trigger factors can help prevent flares or relapses of the disease.

Screening

Not applicable for this topic.

Primary prevention

Not applicable for this topic.

Secondary prevention

- If trigger factors are determined then their avoidance can help prevent flares.
- Avoidance of stressful situations that trigger AD may be useful.
- Some infants and children have AD flares from ingestion of certain foods (e.g. eggs, milk, peanuts, and wheat). If these foods are found to exacerbate AD, then avoidance can help reduce flares of the disease.
- Some patients have flares of AD caused by aeroallergens such as dust mites, pollen, birch, and so on. Using an air purifier may help reduce flares.

Section 3: Diagnosis (Algorithm 2.1)

Algorithm 2.1 Diagnosis of atopic dermatitis

History: Erythematous, pruritic lesions that come and go. May or may not have history of asthma, hay fever, or allergic rhinitis. Any family history of atopy? Any secondary infection of skin lesions? Does the patient have any trigger factors (e.g. food, stress, humidity)?

Physical examination: Are the lesions around mouth and on cheeks in young children? Are the lesions on flexor surfaces (antecubital and popliteal fossae)? Are the lesions erythematous, papules, patches, or plaques? Any associated edema, dryness of surrounding skin? Any crusting? Any skin thickening or lichenification?

Tests:
Serum IgE
Eosinophil count
Skin biopsy is not required as diagnosis is clinical but can be carried out

Diagnosis – atopic dermatitis

> **BOTTOM LINE/CLINICAL PEARLS**
> - Relapsing, remitting pattern.
> - Typical morphology and distribution in flexural areas, acute cases begin with erythematous papules and erythema and in chronic forms there is lichenification. Impetiginization is seen in children with AD.
> - Associated with pruritus, dry skin.
> - Lichenification of antecubital and/or popliteal fossae seen in chronic cases.
> - History of atopy: asthma, allergic rhinitis, hay fever.
> - May or may not have elevated IgE (increased IgE in 80% of cases), eosinophilia.

Differential diagnosis

Differential diagnosis	Features
Acute irritant contact dermatitis	Confined to localized area exposed to irritant
	Lichenification is not seen
	Lasts days to weeks
	Not remitting or relapsing in nature unless irritant exposure occurs again
Allergic contact dermatitis	Systemic disease with a delayed cell-mediated hypersensitivity reaction to an allergen
	Constitutional symptoms including fever can be seen in severe cases
	Acute, subacute, and chronic forms

Typical presentation
- The disease presents with erythematous, pruritic papules, patches, and plaques with superficial erosions from scratching.
- There can be some associated edema.
- Dry skin is also a prominent feature.
- Lichenification is noted in chronic cases of AD. Sometimes, the lesions are secondarily infected with *S. aureus*, and appropriate treatment is mandated. The lesions are typically seen in flexural regions, as well as the face and neck; however, any part of the body can be involved.
- There could be a history of asthma, allergic rhinitis, or hay fever.

Clinical diagnosis
History
- Diagnosis is based on clinical features.
- A personal or family history of atopy should be sought.
- Any trigger factors such as changes in weather, stress, allergens such as food, aeroallergens (e.g. dust mite), or seasonal pollens that exacerbate the disease should be determined.
- Any history of superimposed infection by *S. aureus* should be sought.

Physical examination
- Since the diagnosis is clinical, it is important to look at the skin in its entirety including nape of neck and behind the ears. The physician should look for erythematous papules, patches, or plaques. Scaling and crusting is noted if the patient is a child. Look for typical distribution pattern (antecubital and popliteal fossae, face, and neck in children). Edema can also be seen and

dryness, especially of uninvolved skin, is commonly seen in adults. Due to the pruritic nature of the lesions, superficial erosions can be seen as a result of scratching. In chronic cases, lichenification is noted.

Useful clinical decision rules and calculators
Not applicable for this topic.

Disease severity classification
SCORAD (Scoring AD) is a useful scoring system to help calculate disease severity and monitor response (if any) to treatment. It has three components:
1. *Body surface area:* Rule of 9's (see Figure 2.1).
2. *Intensity:* choose a representative lesion and calculate intensity score ranging 0–3 (0 being none and 3 being severe). Dryness is scored on an area without active inflammation.
3. *Subjective symptoms:* average loss of sleep and degree of pruritus based on 0–10 scale over the last 72 hours (0 no itch or no loss of sleep and 10 being most severe itch and total loss of sleep).

Laboratory diagnosis
List of diagnostic tests
- Blood tests looking at eosinophil count, total and allergen-specific IgE levels.
- Diagnosis is usually clinical and skin biopsy is generally not required.
- In cases with superimposed infection, a skin swab should be carried out especially to rule out methicillin-resistant *S. aureus*.

Lists of imaging techniques
Not applicable for this topic.

Potential pitfalls/common errors made regarding diagnosis of disease
- Irritant contact dermatitis and allergic contact dermatitis are skin conditions that can be mistaken for AD.

Section 4: Treatment (Algorithm 2.2)
Treatment rationale
- First line treatment especially for milder cases is hydration of the skin. Baths with colloidal oatmeal or unscented soap are preferred. Following a bath, an unscented moisturizer should be applied to gently towel dried skin. Baths should be 15–20 minutes and the water should not be too hot. Bleach baths a few times per week can be beneficial in preventing infections and reducing flares.
- Topical steroids can be used in mild to moderate cases or when the first line treatment does not help. However, they should be applied only to lesional skin as there is concern of skin atrophy and adrenal suppression from prolonged use. Calcineurin inhibitors (e.g. tacrolimus and pimecrolimus) are newer agents that are increasingly being used.
- Symptomatic management in the form of antihistamines for itching should be carried out concurrently.
- In cases of superimposed *S. aureus* infection, oral or topical antibiotics are needed. Bleach baths can help prevent infection, and should be added to treatment regimens.
- UVB phototherapy is a good option for moderate to severe disease, but is not feasible for most patients.

- In severe cases of AD or when topical treatment fails, systemic therapy can be used.
- Tapering courses of oral prednisone (very short time) or cyclosporin (should not be used longer than 1–2 years because of concerns of irreversible kidney damage) are also used for severe disease. Other immunosuppressants like azathioprine and mycophenolate mofetil have also been tried.
- Research is underway to look at biologics such as ustekinumab/anti-p40/IL-23, dupilumab/anti-IL-4R, and other biologics for moderate to severe AD.

Algorithm 2.2 Treatment of atopic dermatitis

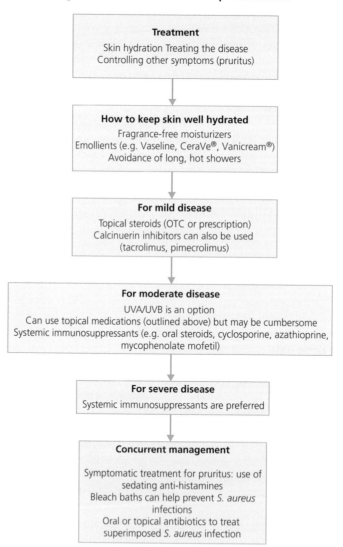

When to hospitalize

- *Eczema herpeticum:* viral infections such as herpes simplex can spread rapidly and cause a severe infection known as eczema herpeticum. This may present with fever, malaise, and a widespread, crusted, blistering rash. Treatment with oral antiviral agents such as acyclovir is indicated. Severe cases may need hospitalization.
- *Erythrodermic atopic dermatitis:* generalized redness of the skin. Inpatient hospital treatment is usually required for intravenous hydration and temperature control of the affected individual.

Managing the hospitalized patient

- Intravenous hydration and temperature regulation for erythrodermic eczema.

Table of treatment

Treatment	Comments
Conservative	Topical emollients, fragrance-free moisturizers for mild cases
Medical • Topical steroids • Topical calcineurin inhibitors • Oral steroids • Other immunosuppressants like cyclosporine, azathioprine, mycophenolate mofetil	• Monitor renal functions when using cyclosporine • Watch for steroid-related side effects (skin atrophy, adrenal insufficiency)
Complementary	• Stress reduction • Avoidance of triggers (if triggers are known)
Other	• UVA–UVB therapy • Bleach baths can help prevent *S. aureus* infection

Prevention/management of complications

- Skin atrophy and adrenal suppression can be seen with prolonged use of topical steroids, especially high potency steroids. Limit use to 2 weeks.
- Adrenal suppression, osteoporosis, striae, cataracts, elevated blood glucose, and psychosis can be seen with prolonged use of high dose oral steroids. Patients should be closely monitored when on oral steroids especially for long periods of time. Every effort must be made to taper a patient of oral steroids as quickly as possible and to use the lowest dose possible to prevent side effects.
- Renal impairment is a concern with long-term use of cyclosporine; hence should be avoided in patients with baseline impaired renal function. Blood tests to check renal function should be carried out at regular intervals when a patient is taking this medication.
- When using pimecrolimus, excessive exposure to sunlight should be avoided.
- Burning at the site of application is the most frequent adverse effect with tacrolimus. Again, sunlight exposure should be avoided when using this medication.

CLINICAL PEARLS
- Keeping skin hydrated is of primary importance; use moisturizers, emollients.
- Topical steroids can be used for mild to moderate disease.
- Severe disease may need systemic immunosuppressants, either oral steroids or medications like cyclosporine.
- Flares of disease may need short courses of oral corticosteroids.

Section 5: Special populations

Pregnancy

- Treatment is more focused on skin hydration and topical steroids. Oral steroids can be used if disease is severe or to treat flares.
- Avoid systemic immunosuppressive medications like cyclosporine or mycophenolate mofetil because of the possibility of teratogenicity.
- Avoid topical calcineurin inhibitors.

Children

- Skin hydration is essential.
- Topical steroids are most often used.
- Systemic steroids can be used for severe disease and for treating flares; however, watch closely for side effects.
- Oral cyclosporine can be used in children, but use should be for the shortest duration possible and renal function should be monitored.

Elderly

- Same management as for adults, be watchful for side effects.

Others

Not applicable for this topic.

Section 6: Prognosis

BOTTOM LINE/CLINICAL PEARLS
- AD is a chronic, remitting, relapsing disease.
- Emollients should be used to keep skin hydrated.
- Medications are used to control disease and preventing flares.
- Avoidance of any trigger factors can help prevent flares.
- Antihistamines can help with itching.

Natural history of untreated disease

- Without treatment patients continue to suffer and develop lesions of AD.

Prognosis for treated patients

- In successfully treated patients, there is a tremendous improvement in quality of life.
- Patients who do not respond to treatment continue to suffer.

Follow-up tests and monitoring

Not applicable for this topic.

Section 7: Reading list

Habif TP. Clinical Dermatology - A Colour Guide to Diagnosis and Therapy. 5th ed. Edinburgh, Mosby Elsevier. 2009

Wolff K, Johnson RA, Saavedra AP. Fitzpatricks Color Atlas and Synopsis of Clinical Dermatology. 7th ed. New York, McGraw-Hill. 2013

Suggested websites

www.nationaleczema.org

Section 8: Guidelines

Not applicable for this topic.

Section 9: Evidence

Not applicable for this topic.

Section 10: Images

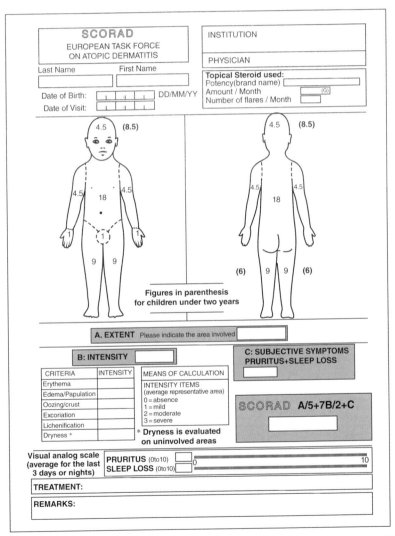

Figure 2.1 SCORAD: Scoring Atopic Dermatitis, is a scoring system for assessment of atopic dermatitis. Availalbe at http://www.fondation-dermatite-atopique.org/en/healthcare-professionals-space/scorad

Additional material for this chapter can be found online at:
www.mountsinaiexpertguides.com
This includes a case study, multiple choice questions, advice for
patients, and ICD codes

CHAPTER 3

Contact Dermatitis

Mariya Rozenblit and Emma Guttman-Yassky
Icahn School of Medicine at Mount Sinai, New York, NY, USA

OVERALL BOTTOM LINE
- Contact dermatitis is an inflammatory reaction of the skin caused by direct contact with a substance and it is classified as irritant or allergic.
- Allergic contact dermatitis occurs when an allergen induces a type IV hypersensitivity reaction, whereas in irritant contact dermatitis the chemical itself directly damages the skin.
- The most common agents that cause irritant contact dermatitis include cleaning agents, industrial solvents, acids or bases, and plants. The most common allergens are nickel sulfate (found in jewelry), neomycin sulfate (found in creams), and balsam of Peru and fragrances (found in topical medications and cosmetics).
- Diagnosis is based on history and findings on physical examination, and allergic contact dermatitis can be confirmed by patch testing.
- Treatment consists of removing the offending agent, wet dressings, and topical glucocorticoid creams.

Section 1: Background
Definition of disease
- Contact dermatitis is an inflammatory reaction of the skin caused by direct contact with a substance.

Disease classification
- Contact dermatitis can be classified as allergic or irritant. Allergic contact dermatitis occurs when an allergen induces a type IV hypersensitivity reaction, whereas in irritant contact dermatitis, the chemical or agent itself directly damages the skin.

Incidence/prevalence
- The prevalence of contact dermatitis in the United States is estimated at 136 cases per 10 000 individuals, with the highest rates among hairdressers, bakers, and florists.
- Contact dermatitis is the most common occupational disease, accounting for 30% of all occupational diseases.
- These statistics are gathered from an annual survey conducted by the National Bureau of Labor and Statistics, which may underestimate the prevalence of this disease by 10- to 50-fold because of underreporting for fear of job loss.

Mount Sinai Expert Guides: Allergy and Clinical Immunology, First Edition. Edited by Hugh A. Sampson.
© 2015 John Wiley & Sons, Ltd. Published 2015 by John Wiley & Sons, Ltd.
Companion website: www.mountsinaiexpertguides.com

Economic impact

- Direct costs associated with this condition are estimated to be $1.4 billion due to physician visits and prescriptions, and indirect costs are around $499 million due to lost work days and restricted activity days.

Etiology

- The most common agents that cause irritant contact dermatitis include cleaning agents, industrial solvents, acids and bases, and plants.
- There are more than 3700 allergens that can cause allergic contact dermatitis. The most common allergens are nickel sulfate (found in jewelry), neomycin sulfate (found in creams), and balsam of Peru and fragrances (found in topical medications and cosmetics).

Pathology/pathogenesis

- The pathogenesis of contact dermatitis is not yet fully understood.
- In irritant contact dermatitis, exposure to a chemical damages epidermal keratinocytes leading to activation of the innate immune system and release of cytokines such as IL-1α, IL-1β, tumor necrosis factor α (TNF-α), granulocyte macrophage colony-stimulating factor (GM-CSF), and IL-8.
- These cytokines activate Langerhans cells, dendritic cells, and endothelial cells, which recruit infiltrating cells such as neutrophils, lymphocytes, macrophages, and mast cells that further promote the inflammatory cascade.
- Allergic contact dermatitis consists of two phases: a sensitization phase and an elicitation phase.
- During the sensitization phase, similar to irritant contact dermatitis, allergens induce the epidermal keratinocytes to release cytokines and activate the innate immune system. Langerhans cells and dendritic cells that have encountered the antigen then migrate to the draining lymph nodes where they activate Th1, Th2, Th17, and regulatory T cells. These hapten-specific T cells then proliferate, circulate, and – along with mast cells and eosinophils – migrate to the site of the initial exposure to the allergen.
- On re-exposure to the allergen, the hapten-specific T cells, mast cells, and eosinophils release cytokines that stimulate the keratinocytes and induce an inflammatory cascade. This is referred to as the elicitation phase.

Predictive/risk factors

Risk factor	Odds ratio
History of atopic dermatitis	4.19
Occupation	4.00
Female	3.29

Section 2: Prevention

BOTTOM LINE/CLINICAL PEARLS

- Prevention strategies are aimed at decreasing the risk of exposure to the irritant or allergen. Industries are encouraged to replace dangerous substances with less toxic or less irritative chemicals. Workers are encouraged to change their environment, or their behavior (such as decreasing the frequency of hand washing). Individual protective measures such as gloves, barrier creams, and moisturizers are also recommended.

- Studies have shown that barrier creams decrease acute irritation and moisturizers can accelerate regeneration of the disrupted barrier in the skin.
- A Cochrane review in 2010 concluded that barrier creams, moisturizers, and educational interventions show a protective effect. However, larger studies are needed to reach statistical significance.

Screening

Not applicable for this topic.

Primary prevention

- Education regarding possible irritants and allergens is a very effective primary prevention strategy. National educational programs targeting high-risk professions to increase awareness and motivate workers to avoid exposure and to use skin protection have been shown to be highly effective in Europe and such programs should be instituted in the United States.
- Legislation to reduce exposure to certain chemicals is also a powerful method of primary prevention. Regulation of nickel exposure in Denmark was shown to decrease the incidence of nickel allergy.

Secondary prevention

- Patient education regarding avoidance of exposure, changing specific behaviors, and using personal protective equipment has been shown to be effective.

Section 3: Diagnosis (Algorithm 3.1)

BOTTOM LINE/CLINICAL PEARLS
- The patient's occupation, possible exposure to irritants or allergens in the environment, and any history of atopic dermatitis are key findings in the history.
- Patients with irritant contact dermatitis present with sharply demarcated erythema and superficial edema at the site of contact. In severe reactions, vesicles, blisters, or erosions can form within the erythematous lesions as well.
- In allergic contact dermatitis, the lesions are intensely pruritic and classically appear 2 days after exposure. The lesions can extend beyond the area of contact, and are erythematous, edematous, with superimposed vesicles and/or papules.
- Patch testing is negative in irritant contact dermatitis and positive in allergic contact dermatitis and can help to identify the offending allergen.

Differential diagnosis

Differential diagnosis	Features
Atopic dermatitis	Usually begins in infancy and is associated with a family history of the atopic triad: atopic dermatitis, allergic rhinitis, asthma. Lesions are pruritic, poorly defined, may be accompanied by lichenification and are often found in flexural areas
Seborrheic dermatitis	Lesions are distributed along the sebum glands on the face, scalp, and trunk. Lesions are scaly and intermittent with worsening in the winter and early spring

(Continued)

Differential diagnosis	Features
Psoriasis	Lesions are chronic, recurring, scaly plaques
Drug eruption	Can mimic any type of dermatologic lesion. Timing since drug administration and resolution after drug withdrawal are key. Eosinophilia >1000/μL, lymphocytosis with atypical lymphocytes, and abnormal liver function test results may be found

Algorithm 3.1 Diagnosis of contact dermatitis

History: Does the patient have a high-risk occupation such as a hairdresser, baker, florist, etc? Is the patient at risk of exposure to possible irritants or allergens? Does the patient have a history of atopic dermatitis? How soon did the lesions appear after exposure? Are the skin lesions pruritic?

Physical examination: Is the erythema sharply demarcated? Is it in the distribution (streaky or bizarre pattern) of exposure to an irritant or allergen? Is it in a common location for exposure (ear lobe, dorsum of foot, wrist, collar, lips)?

Allergic contact dermatitis	Irritant contact dermatitis
Lesions can exceed area of contact and can be ill-defined	Lesions are usually well demarcated
Pruritis is the main symptom	Symptoms after acute exposure include burning, stinging, or pain
Lesions classically apppear 24–72 hours after exposure	Lesions appear rapidly after exposure, usually within minutes to hours
The reaction is described as crescendo: it becomes more severe and takes longer to resolve	The reaction is described as "decrescendo": it reaches its peak quickly then begins to heal

Patch test: Positive in allergic contact dermatitis. Negative in irritant contact dermatitis. Irritant contact dermatitis is a diagnosis of exclusion.

Typical presentation

- In irritant contact dermatitis, patients may experience burning or stinging within seconds of exposure. Skin findings may occur within minutes or can be delayed up to 24 hours depending on which substance the patient is exposed to. Patients with acute irritant contact dermatitis present with sharply demarcated erythema and edema in the distribution of exposure to the substance, which may be linear or streaky. Repeated exposure results in chronic irritant contact dermatitis, which usually appears on the hands as scaling with fissures and crusting and lichenification.
- In allergic contact dermatitis, the lesions typically appear 48 hours after contact with the allergen and repeated exposure worsens the eruption. Patients with acute allergic contact dermatitis present with well-demarcated erythema and edema with superimposed closely

spaced non-umbilicated vesicles. Bullae, erosions, and crusts can also appear in severe reactions. Repeated exposure leads to chronic allergic contact dermatitis, which manifests as plaques of lichenification, scaling, excoriations, and hyperpigmentation. Typical locations include the earlobe, dorsum of the foot, wrist, collar area, and lips.

Clinical diagnosis
History
- Key findings in the history include age of onset, the patient's occupation, possible environmental exposures, and if there is any family history of atopic dermatitis.

Physical examination
- Key findings on physical examination include the appearance, the location, and the pattern of distribution of the skin lesions.

Useful clinical decision rules and calculators
Not applicable for this topic.

Disease severity classification
Not applicable for this topic.

Laboratory diagnosis
List of diagnostic tests
- A patch test consists of applying a small concentration of dilute known allergen to the upper back. The patches are then removed and evaluated at 48 and 96 hours.
- A positive patch test shows erythema at the site of contact. The intensity of the reaction is graded on a scale of 0–3.
- Patch tests are negative in irritative contact dermatitis and positive in allergic contact dermatitis.

Lists of imaging techniques
Not applicable for this topic.

Potential pitfalls/common errors made regarding diagnosis of disease
- It is often very difficult to identify the irritant or allergen, because exposure may occur in many different types of environments (e.g. home, workplace, hobbies, leisure activities) and to several irritants and allergens simultaneously. Identification of the allergen or irritant is especially difficult if the exposure is infrequent, if there is cross-reactivity with another substance, or if the source of the exposure is contact with another person.
- Contact dermatitis also frequently coexists with atopic dermatitis and it can be clinically difficult to distinguish between the two.

Section 4: Treatment (Algorithm 3.2)
Treatment rationale
- The offending agent should be identified and removed.

- Treatment for acute cases includes wet dressings with Burow's solution, antibiotic ointments (Mupirocin), followed by moderate to potent topical corticosteroids. First line treatment is topical glucocorticoids such as triamcinolone 0.1% or even clobetasol 0.05%.
- In severe cases, where more than 20% of body surface area is involved, a 5–7 day course of oral prednisone taper can be prescribed.
- In chronic cases, a potent topical glucocorticoid should be used such as betamethasone or triamcinolone 0.1%. The ointment should be preferred in cases of propylene glycol allergy.

When to hospitalize
Not applicable for this topic.

Managing the hospitalized patient
Not applicable for this topic.

Algorithm 3.2 Treatment of contact dermatitis

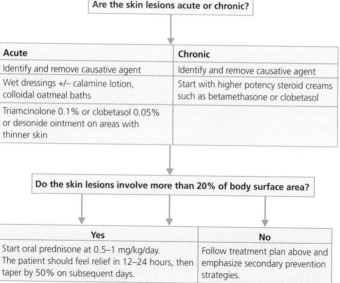

Are the skin lesions acute or chronic?	
Acute	**Chronic**
Identify and remove causative agent	Identify and remove causative agent
Wet dressings +/– calamine lotion, colloidal oatmeal baths	Start with higher potency steroid creams such as betamethasone or clobetasol
Triamcinolone 0.1% or clobetasol 0.05% or desonide ointment on areas with thinner skin	

Do the skin lesions involve more than 20% of body surface area?	
Yes	**No**
Start oral prednisone at 0.5–1 mg/kg/day. The patient should feel relief in 12–24 hours, then taper by 50% on subsequent days.	Follow treatment plan above and emphasize secondary prevention strategies.

Table of treatment

Treatment	Comments
Medical	Wet dressings *Mild:* desonide 0.05% *Moderate:* fluticasone propionate 0.05% or triamcinolone 0.1% *Severe:* clobetasol 0.05%
Educational	Avoidance of irritant or allergen Use of personal protective equipment

Prevention/management of complications

- Long-term use of topical glucocorticoids should be avoided to prevent possible complications such as skin thinning, atrophy, and increased risk of infection.

CLINICAL PEARL
- The most important predictor of treatment success is correct identification and removal of the irritant or allergen.

Section 5: Special populations

Not applicable for this topic.

Section 6: Prognosis

BOTTOM LINE/CLINICAL PEARL
- After removal of the offending agent, healing usually occurs within 2 weeks in acute cases, but can take as long as 6 weeks in chronic cases.

Natural history of untreated disease

- Chronic untreated contact dermatitis leads to hyperkeratoses, scaling, fissuring, and lichenification. The damage to the skin may limit the ability of the patient to perform activities at work or in the home, especially if the hands are affected, leading to decreased quality of life.

Prognosis for treated patients

- Excellent if the inciting agent is identified and removed.

Follow-up tests and monitoring

Not applicable for this topic.

Section 7: Reading list

Ale IS, Maibach HA. Diagnostic approach in allergic and irritant contact dermatitis. Expert Rev Clin Immunol 2010;6:291–310

Alikhan A, et al. Revised minimal baseline series of the International Contact Dermatitis Research Group: evidence-based approach. Dermatitis. 2011;22(2):121–2

Bauer A, Schmitt J, Bennett C, Coenraads PJ, Elsner P, English J, et al. Interventions for preventing occupational irritant hand dermatitis. Cochrane Database Syst Rev 2010;6:CD004414

Belsito DV. Occupational contact dermatitis: etiology, prevalence, and resultant impairment/disability. J Am Acad Dermatol 2005;53:303–13

Bourke J, Coulson I, English J; British Association of Dermatologists Therapy Guidelines and Audit Subcommittee. Guidelines for the management of contact dermatitis: an update. Br J Dermatol 2009; 160:946–54

Cashman MW. Contact dermatitis in the United States: epidemiology, economic impact, and workplace prevention. Dermatol Clin 2012;30:87–98

Larese Filon F, Bochdanovits L, Capuzzo C, Cerchi R, Rui F. Ten years incidence of natural rubber latex sensitization and symptoms in a prospective cohort of health care workers using non powdered latex gloves
2000–2009. Int Arch Occup Environ Health 2014;87:463–9

Smedley J, Williams S, Peel P, Pedersen K; Dermatitis Guideline Development Group. Management
of occupational dermatitis in healthcare workers: a systematic review. Occup Environ Med 2011;
69:276–9

van Gils RF, Boot CR, van Gils PF, Bruynzeel D, Coenraads PJ, van Mechelen W, et al. Effectiveness of
prevention programmes for hand dermatitis: a systematic review of the literature. Contact Dermatitis
2011;64:63–72

Suggested websites

Not applicable for this topic.

Section 8: Guidelines
National society guidelines

Guideline title	Guideline source	Date
Guidelines for the management of contact dermatitis: an update	Agency for Healthcare Research and Quality (AHQR)	Br J Dermatol 2009;160:946–54 (http://www.guideline.gov/ content.aspx?id=15881)
Contact dermatitis: a practice parameter	American Academy of Allergy Asthma and Immunology (AAAAI)	Ann Allergy Asthma Immunol 2006;97(Suppl 2):S1–38 (https://www.aaaai.org/Aaaai/ media/MediaLibrary/PDF%20 Documents/Practice%20 and%20Parameters/contact_ dermatitis_-2006.pdf)

International society guidelines

Guideline Title	Guideline source, summary	Date
Revised minimal baseline series	International Contact Dermatitis Group. Establishes an international standardized list of allergens to be included in patch testing	2013 (http://www.ncbi.nlm.nih.gov/ pubmed/21504701)

Section 9: Evidence

Type of evidence	Title, comment	Date
Randomized controlled trial	A prospective randomized clinical trial of 0.1% tacrolimus ointment in a model of chronic allergic contact dermatitis **Comment:** Demonstrated that an immunosuppressive agent is effective in treating allergic contact dermatitis	2006 (http://www.ncbi.nlm.nih.gov/pubmed/16781290)
Meta-analysis	Interventions for preventing occupational irritant hand dermatitis **Comment:** A Cochrane review of four randomized controlled trials that established that barrier creams and moisturizers have a positive effect in preventing contact dermatitis	2010 (http://www.ncbi.nlm.nih.gov/pubmed/20556758)
Systematic review	Evidence-based guidelines for the prevention, identification, and management of occupational contact dermatitis **Comment:** A systematic review of 786 papers that established guidelines for the prevention and treatment of occupational contact dermatitis	2010 (http://www.ncbi.nlm.nih.gov/pubmed/20831687)
Retrospective study	A survey of exposures related to recognized occupational contact dermatitis in Denmark in 2010 **Comment:** Identified common substances that cause contact dermatitis, which is important in planning preventative programs in the future	2014 (http://www.ncbi.nlm.nih.gov/pubmed/24102286)
Retrospective study	Allergic contact dermatitis in Danish children referred for patch testing – a nationwide multicenter study **Comment:** Raised the issue that contact dermatitis is prevalent in children as well and identified common allergens and risk factors	2014 (http://www.ncbi.nlm.nih.gov/pubmed/24102181)

Section 10: Images

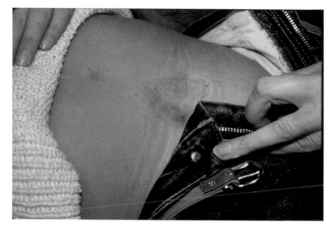

Figure 3.1 Contact dermatitis to nickel from belt buckle. See color plate 3.1.

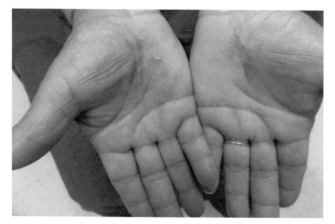

Figure 3.2 Contact dermatitis to propylene glycol, a preservative used in steroid creams. Consider this diagnosis if patient is not responding to treatment. See color plate 3.2.

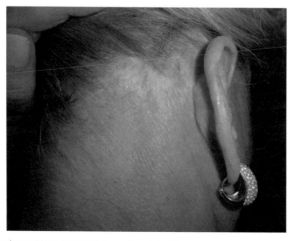

Figure 3.3 Contact dermatitis to Bronopol. See color plate 3.3.

Additional material for this chapter can be found online at:
www.mountsinaiexpertguides.com
This includes a case study, multiple choice questions, advice for
patients, and ICD codes

CHAPTER 4

Allergic Rhinitis

Supinda Bunyavanich

Department of Pediatrics, Department of Genetics and Genomic Sciences, Icahn School of Medicine at Mount Sinai, New York, NY, USA

OVERALL BOTTOM LINE

- Allergic rhinitis is a common disease, affecting 10–30% of adults and 40% of children.
- Common symptoms of allergic rhinitis include nasal congestion, rhinorrhea, sneezing, and itching of the nose, palate, and eyes.
- Symptoms of allergic rhinitis can be seasonal or perennial.
- Allergens that commonly cause allergic rhinitis include dust mites, animal danders, molds, and pollens from trees, grasses, and weeds.
- Treatment of allergic rhinitis can include allergen avoidance, pharmacotherapy, and immunotherapy.

Section 1: Background

Definition of disease

- Allergic rhinitis is an IgE-mediated inflammation of the naso-ocular region. Caused by seasonal and/or perennial aeroallergens, common symptoms include nasal congestion, rhinorrhea, sneezing, and itching of the nose, palate, and eyes.

Disease classification

- *Seasonal allergic rhinitis:* caused by an IgE-mediated reaction to seasonal allergens such as tree pollen, grass pollen, and weed pollen.
- *Perennial allergic rhinitis:* caused by an IgE-mediated reaction to perennial allergens such as dust mites, molds, and animal allergens.

Incidence/prevalence

- Allergic rhinitis is common, affecting 10–30% of adults and 40% of children in the United States.

Economic impact

- Allergic rhinitis accounts for 2.5% of all clinic visits.
- 2 million school days and 6 million work days are lost each year due to allergic rhinitis.

Etiology and pathology/pathogenesis

- Repeated exposure to aeroallergens can lead to allergic sensitization in susceptible individuals.
- Subsequent exposure to aeroallergens to which a person is sensitized elicits IgE-mediated inflammation of the naso-ocular region.
- Inflammation of the naso-ocular region leads to nasal congestion, rhinorrhea, sneezing, and itching.

Mount Sinai Expert Guides: Allergy and Clinical Immunology, First Edition. Edited by Hugh A. Sampson.
Companion website: www.mountsinaiexpertguides.com

Predictive/risk factors
- Family history of atopy.
- Male sex.
- Birth during pollen season.
- Firstborn status.
- Early use of antibiotics.
- Maternal smoking exposure during first year of life.
- Exposure to indoor allergens.
- Serum IgE >100 IU/mL before age 6 years.
- Presence of allergen-specific IgE.

Section 2: Prevention
No interventions have been demonstrated to prevent the development of the disease.

Screening
Not applicable for this topic.

Primary prevention
Not applicable for this topic.

Secondary prevention
- For allergic rhinitis caused by dust mite, physical barriers such as pillow and mattress encasements, humidity control, and reducing areas that harbor dust mites can reduce an individual's exposure to the triggering allergen.
- For allergic rhinitis caused by pet dander, pet removal followed by aggressive cleaning is most helpful. High-efficiency particulate air (HEPA) air filters may be helpful. "Hypoallergenic" breeds of cats or dogs have not been confirmed to be effective in scientific studies.
- For allergic rhinitis caused by molds, mold removal using bleach solutions and humidity control can be helpful.
- For allergic rhinitis caused by pollens, patients should avoid outdoor activities during high pollen count days, close windows, and use air conditioners to help filter air, and shower before bedtime to remove allergens from hair and skin and reduce contamination of bedding.
- For allergic rhinitis caused by pests such as rodents and cockroaches, pest control should be the focus of secondary prevention.

Section 3: Diagnosis

BOTTOM LINE/CLINICAL PEARLS
- The patient may report runny nose, nasal congestion, sneezing, post-nasal drip, cough, itchy eyes, and/or irritated eyes when he/she does not have an upper respiratory infection.
- Examination findings include congested voice, allergic shiners (infra-orbital edema and darkening), Dennie–Morgan lines (lines or folds below the lower eyelids), the allergic salute (constant upward rub of the nose causing a transverse nasal crease), mouth-breathing, enlarged inferior nasal turbinates, pale turbinates, clear mucus in the nares, post-nasal drip, and cobblestoning of the pharynx.
- Diagnosis of allergic rhinitis is often made on clinical grounds, but ideally, patients should demonstrate symptoms, signs, **and** evidence of allergen sensitization. Allergen-specific testing

(either allergen-specific serum IgE levels or allergen skin testing) can be performed to detect and identify allergen sensitization.
- Sinus computed tomography (CT) may show thickening and/or opacification of sinus spaces.
- Nasal cytology is possible but not typically used outside of research settings.

Differential diagnosis

Differential diagnosis	Features
Upper respiratory infection	Relatively short in duration, typically <2 weeks. Nasal obstruction, rhinorrhea, and sneezing are common, nasal mucosa is typically erythematous, but nasal and ocular itching are less prominent
Chronic non-allergic rhinitis	Perennial symptoms without nasal itching or sneezing. Symptoms often exacerbated by changes in temperature, humidity, odors, or alcohol. Negative allergen skin test to environmental allergens
Rhinitis medicamentosa	History of vasoconstrictor nasal spray use or cocaine abuse. Beefy red nasal membranes on examination
Rhinitis caused by systemic medications	Use of medications including oral contraceptive pills, antihypertensive drugs, erectile dysfunction drugs, NSAIDs, psychiatric medications, cyclosporine, mycophenolic acid. Symptoms resolve within weeks of discontinuation
Atrophic rhinitis	Elderly patients. Chronic congestion with perception of bad odor. Negative allergen skin tests
Rhinitis of pregnancy	Pregnant patient. Improvement after pregnancy
Nasal polyps	Polyps may be visible on clinical rhinoscopy examination, fiberoptic rhinoscopy, or on imaging. Anosmia is common

Typical presentation
- A male, young adult presents with nasal congestion, clear rhinorrhea, itchy nose, sneezing paroxysms, and red, itchy, watery eyes. He has difficulty breathing through his nose, so speaks with a congested voice and breathes through his mouth. He cannot sleep well because of these symptoms. He complains of feeling constantly tired and is unable to focus at work. He must carry a box of tissues with him all the time. His symptoms come every spring, usually as soon as he sees pollen starting to coat his car. They resolve by early summer. His symptoms have been getting worse each year.

Clinical diagnosis
History
- The clinician should ask the patient to describe specific symptoms, in what months they occur, and if there are specific environmental conditions or times of day when symptoms are better or worse (e.g. at girlfriend's house where there is a cat, or every August and September when running outside).
- Inquiring about past medical history will inform whether the patient comes from an atopic background (e.g. history of asthma and/or atopic dermatitis) and may thus be at higher risk of developing allergic rhinitis, and if they may have other conditions on the differential diagnosis for allergic rhinitis.

- The clinician should ask if they have tried any medications for their symptoms and if these had any effect on their symptoms.
- An environmental history should be taken, with questions about the home, work, and leisure environments with particular focus on pets, carpeting, heating, ventilation, and air conditioning (HVAC) system, and visible mold and pests.

Physical examination
- Physical examination should include measurement of temperature, as fever may be indicative of an alternate infectious etiology for the patient's symptoms.
- The clinician should observe if the patient is speaking with congested voice, mouth-breathing, or performing the allergic salute.
- Examine the face for allergic shiners, Dennie–Morgan lines, and transverse nasal crease.
- Examine the eyes for conjunctival injection, excess lacrimation, and discharge.
- Use the standard office otoscope with disposable speculum to perform anterior rhinoscopy and look for enlarged or pale inferior turbinates, mucous discharge, septal deviation, and perforations in the nasal septum.
- Percuss frontal and maxillary sinus areas for tenderness.
- Examine posterior oropharynx for post-nasal drip, cobblestoning, and tonsil size.
- Examine the lungs to assess for possible asthma and skin for signs of atopic dermatitis.

Useful clinical decision rules and calculators
Not applicable for this topic.

Disease severity classification
Not applicable for this topic.

Laboratory diagnosis
List of diagnostic tests
- Allergen skin testing is recommended as the most comfortable, most sensitive, and least expensive method to detect allergen sensitization. This is performed by an allergist, who will place selected allergen solutions on the patient's skin and examine for wheal and flare reactions within 20 minutes. The results are immediately available and often illustrative and educational for the patient.
- Serum tests for allergen-specific IgE antibodies are another way to detect allergen sensitization. They provide similar information as allergen skin tests, but are more expensive and less sensitive for diagnosing environmental allergies. Selection and interpretation are best carried out by an allergist, as ordering excessive or irrelevant allergens can lead to confusion.

Lists of imaging techniques
- A sinus CT scan may be considered for a patient with persistent symptoms refractory to therapy.

Potential pitfalls/common errors made regarding diagnosis of disease
- Under-diagnosis, particularly for patients with perennial allergic rhinitis, who may falsely believe that their year-round symptoms are their "normal" baseline.
- Misdiagnosis of non-allergic rhinitis as allergic rhinitis, leading to inappropriate anti-allergy treatment and misdirected environmental avoidance.

Section 4: Treatment

Treatment rationale

- There are three main treatment paths for allergic rhinitis: allergen avoidance, pharmacotherapy, and immunotherapy. Choice of which path(s) to pursue should be made with the patient's preferences forefront, as each requires patient commitment for efficacy.
- Allergen avoidance involves implementing changes to the patient's home and work environments, and to the patient's lifestyle, to avoid contact with allergens that elicit this patient's symptoms (see section on secondary prevention). For example, this may include removal of pets from the home, removing upholstery and fabric reservoirs of dust mites, and alteration of activities during high pollen count days.
- Pharmacotherapy choices include intranasal glucocorticoids, oral and intranasal antihistamines, intranasal cromolyn, leukotriene antagonists, ipratropium bromide, and nasal saline irrigation.
- Immunotherapy involves the administration of gradually increasing doses of allergen extracts to a patient has demonstrated sensitivity to the respective allergens. Over time, the attained dose alters the patient's immune response to the allergen and results in fewer symptoms with exposure. Immunotherapy typically require years of commitment for efficacy. Subcutaneous immunotherapy is administered by an allergist or immunologist with monitoring, because allergic reactions are possible with administration. Sublingual and oral immunotherapy are not yet Food and Drug Administration (FDA) approved.

When to hospitalize

Not applicable for this topic.

Managing the hospitalized patient

Not applicable for this topic.

Table of treatment

Treatment	Comment
Conservative • Allergen avoidance • Nasal saline irrigation	• Patient with mild symptoms • Patients who prefer non-pharmacologic methods
Medical • Intranasal glucocorticoids (1–2 sprays once to twice daily depending on specific agent and patient's age)	• Maximal effect requires several days or weeks • Direct spray laterally to avoid epistaxis • Particularly effective for patients whose primary complaint is congestion

• Oral antihistamines
  • Diphenhydramine (5 mg/kg/day in divided doses every 6–8 hours)
  • Loratadine (5 mg/day for children 2–5 years, 10 mg/day for children ≥6 years or adults)
  • Fexofenadine (30 mg twice daily for children 2–11 years, 60 mg twice daily or 180 mg once daily for children ≥12 years or adults)
  • Cetirizine (2.5 mg once daily for children 6–12 months, 2.5 mg once or twice daily for children 12 months to <2 years, 2.5 mg twice daily or 5 mg once daily for children 2–5 years, 5–10 mg once daily for children ≥6 years or adults)
	• First generation antihistamines (e.g. diphenhydramine) cause sedation and sometimes paradoxical agitation in children and the elderly
	• Second generation antihistamines (loratidine, fexofenadine, and cetirizine) cause less sedation and are similarly efficacious to one another
	• Antihistamines are effective for itchy nose, eyes, palate, and ears

Treatment	Comment
• Intranasal antihistamines • Azelastine (1–2 sprays to each nostril twice daily) • Cromolyn sodium (1–2 sprays to each nostril up to 4 times daily) • Montelukast • Ipratropium bromide (2 sprays to each nostril 3–4 times daily) Immunotherapy (subcutaneous injections of allergens to which the patient is sensitized, typically administered weekly during build-up to target dose and then monthly injections of target dose for 3–5 years)	• Bad taste often reduces patient adherence • Fast onset • Good for episodic symptoms, administer 30 minutes before exposure • Excellent safety profile • Consider for pregnant, breastfeeding, and pediatric patients • Less effective than intranasal steroids but may be a good choice for patients who do not tolerate other nasal sprays • Decreases rhinorrhea primarily • Requires patient adherence to present for regular injections at allergist's office • The only treatment option that changes the body's immune response to the allergen • Allergic reactions can be a side effect of injections, so administration should be done in an allergist's office • Patient can have minimal or no symptoms to allergens upon completion of immunotherapy course

Prevention/management of complications
- Systemic side effects from intranasal glucocorticoids appear to be minimal to none in studies conducted thus far.
- Immunotherapy can result in allergic reactions and should therefore be administered in an allergist's office equipped to monitor for and handle allergic reactions.

CLINICAL PEARLS
- Allergen avoidance should be encouraged in patients with allergic rhinitis, as reduction or removal of exposure to the inciting allergen can be effective.
- Choice of pharmacologic treatment should take into account patients' specific symptoms and their preferences regarding timing of use and route of administration.
- Immunotherapy is the only treatment path that changes the body's immunologic response to allergen such that a patient may have few or no symptoms with exposure to the allergen after completion of the immunotherapy course.

Section 5: Special populations
Pregnancy/breastfeeding
- Skin testing should be deferred until after delivery, as there is risk of systemic allergic reaction with skin testing.
- Non-pharmacologic therapies should be considered first. Cromolyn sodium nasal spray is first line for mild allergic rhinitis during pregnancy and breastfeeding given its excellent safety profile. Budesonide is the only intranasal glucocorticosteroid with pregnancy category B classification (other agents are category C). There are no intranasal glucocorticosteroids with pregnancy category A rating. Loratadine and cetirizine have reassuring human data for drug safety in pregnant patients.
- Immunotherapy should not be initiated during pregnancy. If a pregnant patient is already on immunotherapy, then doses should not be increased during pregnancy.

Children

- Cromolyn sodium nasal spray has an excellent safety profile and should be considered.
- Cetirizine and fexofenadine are approved for children ≥6 months of age.
- Intranasal glucocorticosteroids do not appear to affect growth based on studies conducted thus far.

Elderly

- Avoid first generation antihistamines.

Section 6: Prognosis

> **BOTTOM LINE/CLINICAL PEARLS**
> - Continued exposure to an allergen can lead to more severe symptoms over time, and to more severe symptoms with exposure to lower concentrations.
> - Relocation to a new environment where the allergen is not present can lead to resolution of symptoms.
> - Over time, patients with allergic rhinitis may also develop heightened sensitivity to non-allergen irritants such as tobacco smoke, particulate pollution, and strong scents.
> - The only treatment path that changes the body's immunologic response to an allergen is allergen immunotherapy. Completion of an immunotherapy course can lead to reduction or resolution upon exposure to the allergen.

Section 7: Reading list

deShazo RD, Kemp SF. Allergic rhinitis: Clinical manifestations, epidemiology, and diagnosis. In: UpToDate, Post TW (ed), UpToDate, Waltham, MA. (Accessed Dec 17, 2014)

deShazo RD, Kemp SF. Pharmacotherapy of allergic rhinitis. In: UpToDate, Post TW (ed), UpToDate, Waltham, MA. (Accessed Dec 17, 2014)

Orban NT, Saleh H, Durham SR. Allergic and non-allergic rhinitis. In Adkinson NF Jr, Bochner BS, Busse WW, et al. (eds) Middleton's Allergy: Principles and Practice, 7th edn. Philadelphia, PA: WB Saunders, 2009, 973–87

Scadding GK, Durham SR, Mirakian R, Jones NS, Leech SC, Farooque S, et al. BSACI guidelines for the management of allergic and non-allergic rhinitis. Clin Exp Allergy 2008;38:19–42

Wallace DV, Dykewicz MS, Bernstein DI, Blessing-Moore J, Cox L, Khan DA, et al. The diagnosis and management of rhinitis: an updated practice parameter. J Allergy Clin Immunol 2008;122:S1–84

Suggested websites

American Academic of Allergy, Asthma, and Immunology. http://www.aaaai.org/conditions-and-treatments/allergies/rhinitis.aspx

American College of Allergy, Asthma, and Immunology. http://www.acaai.org/ALLERGIST/ALLERGIES/TYPES/RHINITIS/Pages/default.aspx

Section 8: Guidelines
National society guidelines

Guideline title	Guideline source	Date
The diagnosis and management of rhinitis: an updated practice parameter	American Academy of Allergy, Asthma, and Immunology (AAAAI)	2008 (DOI: http://dx.doi.org/10.1016/j.jaci.2008.06.003)

Section 9: Evidence

Type of evidence	Title	Date
Scientific evidence and clinical consensus	AAAAI Practice Parameter	http://www.aaaai.org/

Section 10: Images
Not applicable for this topic.

Additional material for this chapter can be found online at:
www.mountsinaiexpertguides.com
This includes a case study, multiple choice questions, advice for patients, and ICD codes

CHAPTER 5

Non-Allergic Rhinitis

Beth E. Corn

Department of Clinical Immunology, Icahn School of Medicine at Mount Sinai, New York, NY, USA

> **OVERALL BOTTOM LINE**
> - Rhinitis without an IgE component and/or allergic source.
> - Far-reaching entity that affects up to 19% of the population of the United States.
> - Treatment is limited to topical modalities including nasal washes, topical nasal steroids, and topical antihistamines.

Section 1: Background

Definition of disease

- Non-allergic rhinitis can be defined as rhinitis without an identifiable etiology and in particular there is no IgE-dependent component.
- It is associated with at least one of the following: nasal congestion, post-nasal drainage, rhinorrhea, and sneezing.
- All forms are associated with some degree of autonomic dysregulation.

Disease classification

Not applicable for this topic.

Incidence/prevalence

- Allergic rhinitis affects up to 60 million Americans.
- Between 44 and 87% of these cases are mixed rhinitis, meaning a combined allergic and non-allergic component.
- Pure non-allergic rhinitis comprises approximately one-quarter of all rhinitis cases.

Economic impact

- There is a significant economic burden in missed productive revenue and cost of symptomatic treatments.
- Based on data from 2002, there is a $7.3 billion direct cost (e.g. doctor visits, cost of medications). The indirect cost, including loss of productivity, is estimated at $4.2 billion.

Etiology

- The unifying factor of the various types of non-allergic rhinitis is the lack of an association with an IgE-mediated event.

Mount Sinai Expert Guides: Allergy and Clinical Immunology, First Edition. Edited by Hugh A. Sampson.
© 2015 John Wiley & Sons, Ltd. Published 2015 by John Wiley & Sons, Ltd.
Companion website: www.mountsinaiexpertguides.com

- All forms are associated with some degree of autonomic dysregulation.
- The various types of non-allergic rhinitis include the following:
  - Vasomotor rhinitis (idiopathic rhinitis);
  - Gustatory rhinitis;
  - Infectious rhinitis;
  - Non-allergic rhinitis with eosinophilia (NARES);
  - Occupational rhinitis;
  - Hormonal rhinitis;
  - Drug-induced rhinitis;
  - Atrophic rhinitis; and
  - Rhinitis medicamentosa.

Pathology/pathogenesis
- Non-allergic rhinitis is a non-IgE-mediated condition comprised of many different subsets, all of which have a presumed non-allergic etiology.

Predictive/risk factors
There are no known genetic markers or hereditary risk factors.

Section 2: Prevention

> **BOTTOM LINE/CLINICAL PEARLS**
> In those with associated risk factors, prevention includes avoidance of trigger factors:
> - *Infectious:* immediate treatment of infectious process.
> - *Occupational:* avoidance of irritants.
> - *Rhinitis medicamentosa:* avoidance of topical and oral decongestants.
> - *Rhinitis secondary to other medications:* prompt discontinuation of medication in patients adversely affected by medication. Examples of offending agents include oral contraceptives, drugs for erectile dysfunction, aspirin/NSAIDs, some antihypertensives, and benzodiazepines.

Screening
- Non-allergic rhinitis is a group of conditions that must be distinguished from allergic rhinitis. This can only be done with skin testing for sensitivity to aeroallergens and in vitro allergen-specific IgE tests (radioallergosorbent test, RAST).

Primary prevention
Not applicable for this topic.

Secondary prevention
- Aggressive therapeutic control with topical steroids and antihistamine sprays prevents ongoing symptoms.

Section 3: Diagnosis (Algorithm 5.1)

> **BOTTOM LINE/CLINICAL PEARLS**
> - Symptoms of rhinitis based on exposure to an offending agent (i.e. the relationship to provocative exposure including medications, irritants, and response to pharmacologic intervention).
> - Lack of the characteristic physical examination of allergic rhinitis – enlarged turbinates that are often erythematous rather than pale and blue commonly seen in allergic rhinitis. Please note none of these findings are diagnostic and a normal appearance of nasal mucosa does not exclude the diagnosis of non-allergic rhinitis.
> - Negative skin test or RAST (in vitro test) to aeroallergens.

Differential diagnosis

Differential diagnosis	Features
Allergic rhinitis	Pale bluish hue or palor of the nasal turbinate, blepheral edema, and discharge. Positive skin test or RAST to aeroallergens
Anatomic abnormalities	
Tumors (benign/malignant)	Unilateral symptoms
Nasal polyps	Edematous semi-translucent, opalescent gelatinous mass in nasal passage. Confirmation by endoscopic examination
Septal deviation	Asymmetrical appearance on physical examination
Hypertrophy of the nasal turbinates	Appearance on physical examination
Functional abmormalities	
Laryngopharyngeal reflux	Isolated feeling of a posterior drip with or without dyspepsia Rhinoscopy
Ciliary dysfunction syndrome (primary or secondary)	History of respiratory disease in the newborn with chronic sinopulmonary infections (primary) Heterotropy (primary) Mucociliary clearance test
CSF leak	History of recent surgery or trauma Halo test
Foreign body (particularly in pediatrics)	Unilateral symptoms, purulent discharge

Typical presentation
- Patient presents with vague, non-specific complaints of intermittent or continuous nasal symptoms including at least one of the following: nasal congestion, post-nasal drip, rhinorrhea, and sneezing, with or without a cough. The nasal symptoms are isolated without associated ocular symptoms or eczematous complaints. The predominant presentation of pure non-allergic rhinitis occurs in females older than age 20. Most often there is no identifiable trigger.

Algorithm 5.1 Diagnosis of non-allergic rhinitis

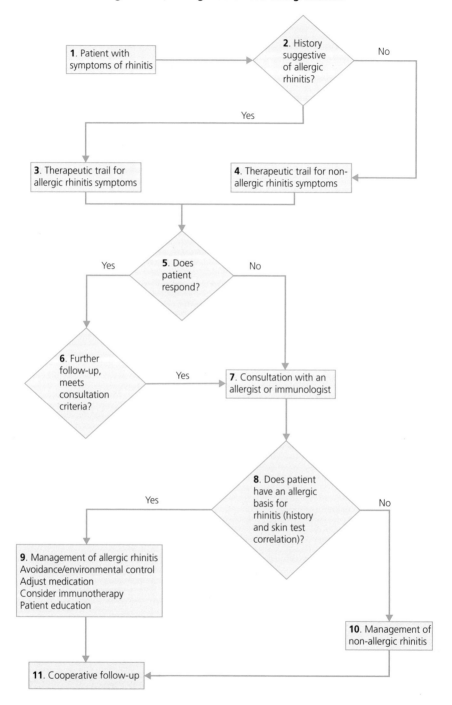

Clinical diagnosis

History

- Questions are intended to elucidate pattern, seasonality, chronicity, response to previous treatments, precipitating factors (triggers) as well as the presence of coexisting conditions. This information should be teased out for each symptom. As with any complaint or diagnosis, quality of life issues such as ability to work, socialize, and sleep through the night are factors that the patient may not bring up or associate with the primary complaint. It is therefore incumbent upon the physician to ask the appropriate questions and discuss relevant symptoms.
- Response to previous treatments including over-the-counter treatments and medications (antihistamines and nasal saline washes) and prescription medications (antihistamines and nasal steroids).
- Precipitating factors (triggers) including occupational exposure, domestic environmental exposure (pets, carpets, curtains), exercise, eating, medications, and weather changes.

Physical examination

- A detailed physical examination with particular emphasis on the head, eyes, ears, nose, and throat (HEENT), pulmonary and integumental systems.
- Signs and symptoms to be on the lookout for include nasal obstruction, deviation, enlarged turbinates, presence of a polyp, posterior pharyngeal drainage, presence of wheezing, presence of blephoral edema or allergic shiners, nasal crease, skin examination looking for evidence of atopy and eczema as well as dermatographism.

Useful clinical decision rules and calculators

- The patient who does not respond to initial treatment with topical nasal steroids or antihistamines warrants referral to an allergist.

Disease severity classification

Not applicable for this topic.

Laboratory diagnosis

List of diagnostic tests

- All patients presenting to an allergist with symptoms of rhinitis must undergo allergy testing and/or in vitro testing (serum allergen-specific IgE is a type of blood test used to diagnose allergies and determine what the patient is allergic to).
- Skin testing is often considered more sensitive and specific than in vitro tests and is the preferred test for ruling out allergic rhinitis. The particular agents tested are dependent on the history evoked including the particular region of the country, occupation, and activities.
- Nasal smears for eosinophilia, though not routinely performed, may identify eosinophilia in either allergic (expected) or non-allergic rhinitis to identify non-allergic rhinitis with eosinophilia (NARES).
- Beta 2 transferrin is diagnostic of cerebrospinal fluid (CSF) leak.

List of imaging techniques

- In certain cases, fiberoptic nasal endoscopy and/or rhinomanometry may be useful in determining etiology of the rhinitis including anatomic abnormality.

Potential pitfalls/common errors made regarding diagnosis of disease

- Once non-allergic rhinitis is diagnosed, the most common error is missing comorbid conditions, especially reflux, and to a lesser extent nasal polyps.

Section 4: Treatment
Treatment rationale
- Nasal steroids: familiarity and long-term successful history of use (until recently was the only therapeutic option).
- Topical nasal antihistamines approved in 2001.
- Combination of nasal steroids and topical nasal antihistamines, now available in a combined spray delivery system.
- Topical ipratropium bromide was specifically approved for rhinorrhea associated with non-allergic rhinitis.

When to hospitalize
Not applicable for this topic.

Managing the hospitalized patient
Not applicable for this topic.

Table of treatment

Treatment	Comments
Conservative	Topical nasal saline wash/rinse
Medical	• Topical nasal steroids • Topical antihistamine • Combination of above • Ipratropium bromide for isolated symptoms
Complementary	Topical capsaicin nasal spray

Prevention/management of complications
- Nasal steroids are contraindicated in patients with either increased intraocular pressure or cataracts. In addition, nasal steroids can lead to increased intraocular pressure and cataracts. If either of these occurs during treatment, the nasal steroids must be discontinued.

CLINICAL PEARLS
- Start with – topical nasal steroids.
- Then try – topical antihistamine.
- If more control needed – combination of above.
- For isolated symptoms of rhinorrhea – ipratropium bromide.

Section 5: Special populations
Pregnancy
- Only budesonide is approved in pregnancy (category B).
- All other nasal steroids as well as topical antihistamines and ipratropium are category C for pregnancy.

Children
Treated as above.

Elderly
Treated as above.

Others
Those with glaucoma or increased intraocular pressure are not candidates.

Section 6: Prognosis

> **BOTTOM LINE/CLINICAL PEARLS**
> * Non-allergic rhinitis is a chronic disease for which there is no cure.
> * Only continued treatment will control symptoms.

Natural history of untreated disease
* A subset of patients may develop allergic rhinitis or asthma.

Prognosis for treated patients
* Only continued treatment will control symptoms.

Follow-up tests and monitoring
* Monitor for any increase in intraocular pressure for those patients on nasal steroids.

Section 7: Reading list

Bhargava D, Bhargava K, Al-Abri A, Al-Bassam W, Al-Abri R. Non allergic rhinitis: prevalence, clinical profile and knowledge gaps in literature. Oman Med J 2011;26:416–20

Nozad CH, Michael LM, Betty Lew D, Michael CF. Non-allergic rhinitis: a case report and review. Clin Mol Allergy 2010;8:1

Salib RJ, Harries PG, Nair SB, Howarth PH. Mechanisms and mediators of nasal symptoms in non-allergic rhinitis. Clin Exp Allergy 2008;38:393–404

Van Gerven L, Boeckxstaens G, Hellings P. Up-date on neuro-immune mechanisms involved in allergic and non-allergic rhinitis. Rhinology 2012;50:227–35

Varghese M, Glaum MC, Lockey RF. Drug-induced rhinitis. Clin Exp Allergy 2010;40:381–4

Varricchio A, Capasso M, De Lucia A, Avvisati F, Varricchio AM, Bettoncelli G, et al. Intranasal flunisolide treatment in patients with non-allergic rhinitis. Int J Immunopathol Pharmacol 2011;24:401–9

Suggested websites
www.aaaai.org
www.acaai.org
www.eaaci.org

Section 8: Guidelines

Guideline title	Guideline source	Date
The diagnosis and management of rhinitis: an updated practice parameter	American Academy of Allergy, Asthma and Immunology (AAAAI); American College of Allergy, Asthma and Immunology (ACAAI); Joint Council of Allergy, Asthma and Immunology	2008 (http://www.jacionline.org/ article/S0091-6749(08)01123-8/ abstract)

Section 9: Evidence
Not applicable for this topic.

Section 10: Images
Not applicable for this topic.

Additional material for this chapter can be found online at:
www.mountsinaiexpertguides.com
This includes a case study, multiple choice questions, advice for
patients, and ICD codes

CHAPTER 6

Sinusitis

Yan W. Ho and Satish Govindaraj

Department of Otolaryngology–Head and Neck Surgery, Icahn School of Medicine at Mount Sinai, New York, NY, USA

OVERALL BOTTOM LINE

- Rhinosinusitis affects millions of people in the United States annually, or 15.2% of the population each year. The burden of disease includes lost workdays, increased health care costs, and increased doctor's visits.
- The accurate diagnosis of acute, recurrent acute, subacute, and chronic rhinosinusitis depends on symptoms, the duration of symptoms, and disease progression. There are many predisposing factors for rhinosinusitis: preceding viral infection, smoking, allergic rhinitis, asthma, anatomic obstruction, and immunodeficiency.
- The physical examination is helpful in detecting possible intracranial or ocular complications, and endoscopy is helpful for confirmation of diagnosis. Routine nasal cultures, laboratory testing, and imaging are not indicated unless disease is refractory to medical treatment or if there are complications.
- The preferred imaging of acute rhinosinusitis is CT of the sinus without contrast. However, CT with contrast can highlight abscesses and magnetic resonance imaging (MRI) can highlight soft tissue or nerve involvement.
- The mainstay of treatment of acute rhinosinusitis is supportive, with the addition of antibiotics, but for chronic rhinosinusitis treatment may require more adjunctive medications and possibly surgery.

Section 1: Background
Definition of disease

- Rhinosinusitis encompasses a broad range of diseases all characterized by inflammation of one or more paranasal sinuses. The diagnosis of rhinosinusitis is based on subjective and objective findings and depends on the duration of symptoms.

Disease classification

- *Acute rhinosinusitis:* up to 4 weeks of symptoms.
- *Recurrent acute rhinosinusitis:* four or more episodes of acute rhinosinusitis within 1 year with symptom-free periods in between.
- *Subacute rhinosinusitis:* 4–12 weeks of symptoms.
- *Chronic rhinosinusitis:* 12 weeks or more of symptoms.

Mount Sinai Expert Guides: Allergy and Clinical Immunology, First Edition. Edited by Hugh A. Sampson.
© 2015 John Wiley & Sons, Ltd. Published 2015 by John Wiley & Sons, Ltd.
Companion website: www.mountsinaiexpertguides.com

Incidence/prevalence

- According to data gathered through the National Health Interview Survey for calendar years 1997–2006, the annual disease prevalence of sinusitis was 15.2%.
- In the United States, it is estimated that approximately 20 million cases of acute bacterial rhinosinusitis occur annually.
- In the United States, 1999–2002, there were an estimated 3 116 142 visits annually due to acute rhinosinusitis, representing 0.30% of all ambulatory visits.
- Chronic rhinosinusitis has a period prevalence of 2% per decade, peaking between the ages of 20 and 59 years.

Economic impact

- In 1985–1992, sinusitis was the fifth most common diagnosis for prescribing antibiotics and, in 1996, sinusitis led to $3.5 billion dollars in health care expenditures.
- The burden of acute rhinosinusitis on patient quality of life is also substantial. Patients with sinusitis are significantly more likely to visit the emergency room, spend over $500 annually on health care, and see a medical specialist.
- Patients with sinusitis missed an average of 5.67 workdays annually versus 3.74 workdays for those without. Comparatively, health care expenditures due to sinusitis far exceeded those of ulcer disease, acute asthma, and hay fever.

Etiology

- The etiology of acute rhinosinusitis commonly involves predisposing factors that can be divided generally into three categories: environmental, anatomic, and systemic. They commonly occur at the same time, and can predispose patients to not only acute infections, but also contribute to development of chronic sinusitis.

Pathology/pathogenesis

- Acute bacterial rhinosinusitis is often preceded by an acute viral upper respiratory tract infection. After the first 10 days of a viral upper respiratory tract infection, approximately 0.5% of patients will go on to develop a bacterial acute rhinosinusitis. The most common bacterial organisms are *Streptococcus pneumoniae*, *Haemophilus influenzae*, and *Moraxella catarrhalis*. However, there is evidence that *Staphylococcus aureus* is becoming a major contributor to the development of acute rhinosinusitis. If these acute infections are not resolved or become recurrent, *S. aureus*, anaerobic and gram-negative organisms such as *Pseudomonas aeruginosa* become predominant.
- The transition between viral and bacterial acute rhinosinusitis has been studied extensively, and is thought to be secondary to altered mucociliary clearance and colonization of bacteria. The inflammation from the viral illness temporarily stuns the cilia, mucus remains trapped in the sinuses, and bacteria proliferate.
- Unlike acute rhinosinusitis, chronic rhinosinusitis or recurrent acute rhinosinusitis are more likely to be associated with the risk factors described.

Risk factors

- *Allergic rhinitis:* the association between allergic rhinitis and sinusitis has long been recognized, and has been attributed to decreased mucociliary clearance and mucus retention in the sinuses. The inflammation caused by the allergic response causes mucosal membranes to become edematous, thereby obstructing the outflow of mucus through sinus ostia. This leads to a buildup of mucus within sinus cavities, oxygen stores are depleted, and bacteria proliferate in this acidic environment. Most believe that the inflammation caused by allergic reaction causes obstruction of the sinus ostia but, in addition, some believe that the allergic response itself also causes an influx of eosinophils in the nasal cavity and the maxillary sinuses.

- *Cigarette smoke:* tobacco exposure in the form of smoking or second-hand smoke has been shown to increase bacterial and viral infections. A study on the microbiology of acute bacterial rhinosinusitis found that smokers were more likely to have cultures positive for *S. aureus*, methicillin-resistant *S. aureus* (MRSA), and beta-lactamase producing bacteria.
- *Pollution–exposures:* the link between pollution and other exposures to acute rhinosinusitis is less defined, but nonetheless, a correlation has been shown. In a study following rescue and recovery workers who were exposed to the 9/11 World Trade Center bombings, workers were found to have more frequent upper respiratory tract infections and rhinosinusitis in the short term. Long-term studies are currently being conducted.
- *Sinonasal anatomy:* abnormal sinonasal anatomy may contribute to the development of acute rhinosinusitis and, if left untreated, recurrent acute, subacute or chronic sinusitis. The presence of septal deviation, septal spurs, turbinate hypertrophy, Haller cells, agger nasi cells, or an obstructive mass, like a tumor or polyp, can pose as barriers to proper mucociliary clearance. Arguably, the impairment of mucociliary function due to local or systemic disease can also be considered as an anatomic predisposition to the development of rhinosinusitis. When comparing CT scans of patients with refractory acute rhinosinusitis and patients without sinonasal disease, patients in the first group were statistically more likely to have septal deviation towards the affected side. Patient with recurrent acute rhinosinusitis were significantly more likely to have Haller cells and smaller infundibular widths (mean of 0.591 mm versus 0.823 mm in unaffected individuals). They also were more likely to have concha bullosa and impinging septal spurs, although the difference was not statistically significant.
- *Dental anatomy:* particularly its relation to the maxillary sinus, dental anatomy can predispose patients to maxillary sinusitis. Depending on the development of the maxillary sinus, the maxillary teeth may be positioned very close to the inferior boundary of the sinus. Dental caries or gingivitis can easily spread into the maxillary sinuses and cause an acute maxillary sinusitis.
- *Ciliary dysfunction:* in many cases of rhinosinusitis, ciliary dysfunction is thought to have a role in the pathophysiology. Most often, it is caused by environmental, infectious, or inflammatory factors but, in rare cases, a congenital disorder including Kartagener syndrome or another type of primary ciliary dyskinesia is involved. Primary ciliary dyskinesia is a disorder with an autosomal recessive inheritance affecting the function of cilia. It is estimated to affect 1 in 7000–60 000 people. Manifestations include chronic otitis media, subfertility, and chronic rhinosinusitis. Usually, the investigation of these diseases is not indicated unless acute rhinosinusitis develops into recurrent acute or chronic rhinosinusitis.
- *Immunodeficiencies* (congenital or acquired): it is important to recognize the role of immunodeficiencies in patients who have recurrent or chronic rhinosinusitis. The investigation of acute rhinosinusitis should not routinely prompt an extensive immunologic investigation unless indicated by other signs and symptoms. The most common congenital immunodeficiencies that present with recurrent rhinosinusitis include selective IgA deficiency, common variable immunodeficiency, Wiskott–Aldrich syndrome, ataxia telangiectasia, hypogammaglobulinemia, myelokathexis syndrome, and caspase-8 deficiency. Common acquired and iatrogenic types of immunodeficiencies include HIV/AIDS, chemotherapy, transplantation, and the use of immunomodulating medications.
- *Gastroesophageal reflux disease (GERD)/laryngopharyngeal reflux:* reflux disease is increasingly being implicated as a contributor to chronic rhinosinusitis but its effects on the development of acute rhinosinusitis have yet to be studied.

- *Cystic fibrosis:* this disorder is caused by mutations in the cystic fibrosis transmembrane conductance regulator (*CFTR*) gene on chromosome 7. This results in the abnormal transport of chloride ions leading to altered viscosity of mucous secretions. Cystic fibrosis is not as relevant in isolated cases of acute sinusitis, but should be part of the investigation for chronic rhinosinusitis especially in patients with polyps.
- *Asthma:* the association between asthma and chronic rhinosinusitis has long been recognized, but a causal relationship has yet to be illuminated. Although the evidence is focused primarily on the effect of asthma on chronic rhinosinusitis, this phenomenon is also seen in acute rhinosinusitis. Patients who have viral upper respiratory tract infections are more likely to experience asthma exacerbations and have more severe attacks. Recently, multiple individuals also propose a "united airway disease" or "global airway disease" that links upper and lower airway diseases including allergy, sinusitis, and asthma.

Section 2: Prevention

> **BOTTOM LINE/CLINICAL PEARLS**
> - Practicing good hygiene and smoking cessation can help to minimize chances of an acute infection, while nasal irrigations and allergy and GERD control can help to lessen the burden of disease for those with chronic rhinosinusitis.

Screening
- Allergy testing.

Primary prevention
- Patients with chronic or recurrent acute rhinosinusitis cannot prevent infections from occurring, but can minimize the recurrence by practicing hand hygiene and avoiding other people who are ill.
- Smoking cessation can help to decrease the number and severity of sinus infections.

Secondary prevention
- The use of nasal saline irrigation has been shown to improve mucociliary function, decrease mucosal edema, and remove nasal debris and allergens. They have been shown to decrease rhinosinusitis symptoms and the need for antibiotics.
- Treating underlying GERD may also be helpful in decreasing chronic rhinosinusitis severity.
- Environmental control of allergens or initiation of immunotherapy are useful adjuncts for patients with chronic rhinosinusitis.

Section 3: Diagnosis

> **BOTTOM LINE/CLINICAL PEARLS**
> - The diagnosis of acute rhinosinusitis depends on a full, detailed history and physical examination, and does not require routine laboratory work or imaging. The cardinal symptoms of nasal obstruction, purulent drainage, and facial pain, along with physical examination finding of purulence from the OMC should be enough for a diagnosis.
> - When symptoms persist or recur despite proper medical therapy for acute rhinosinusitis, the clinician should investigate other causes for symptoms or other complications. If symptoms last for over 12 weeks, consider chronic rhinosinusitis or other diagnoses.

- If the disease is refractory to initial treatment or becomes recurrent or chronic, further investigation to rule out immunodeficiencies, cystic fibrosis, Wegener's granulomatosis, sarcoidosis, Churg–Strauss disease, or other autoimmune diseases may be necessary. Cultures may also help to guide antibiotic therapy and to detect drug-resistant organisms.
- Imaging is not indicated for acute rhinosinusitis unless there are signs of complications, but it is useful in persistent or chronic disease to detect anatomic anomalies and the extent of disease.

Differential diagnosis

Differential diagnosis	Features
Allergic rhinitis	It is difficult to distinguish rhinitis from rhinosinusitis by history alone. The physical examination helps to differentiate the two because in acute rhinosinusitis the nasal mucoca may be red and swollen and purulent drainage may be seen in the OMC, but in allergic rhinitis the turbinates are boggy and pale. The discharge in acute rhinosinusitis may turn gray, yellow, or green, whereas in allergic rhinitis it would be clear and watery
Non-allergic rhinitis	This group of rhinitis is by definition not an IgE-mediated sensitivity to allergen
Infectious rhinitis	Viral or fungal rhinosinusitis ex: rhinovirus, adenovirus
Vasomotor rhinitis	Vasomotor rhinitis is characterized by nasal obstruction, rhinorrhea, and congestion and symptoms are exacerbated by certain odors, alcohol, spicy foods, emotions, temperature, barometric pressure changes, and bright lights
Eosinophilic non-allergic rhinitis	This is characterized by the presence of many eosinophils in nasal secretions, a negative history for allergen exacerbation, and negative skin tests. It is sensitive to steroid therapy
Rhinitis medicamentosa	Rhinitis due to excessive use of systemic or more likely topical use of decongestants (i.e. Afrin®) The use over 3 days may predispose patients to the development of this
Rhinitis due to pregnancy, hypothyroidism, Horner's syndrome	Pregnancy can increase intravascular and extravascular volume. Estrogen also has cholinergic effects by increasing vessel dilatation and mucous production
Temporomandibular joint disease	The location of the facial pain tends to be pre-auricular, radiating to the temple or neck. It is reproducible by palpation or movement of the jaw. In addition, the pain is exacerbated by chewing. There may be an audible click on jaw opening
Headache (migraines)	Sinus headaches are a type of migraine headache, and can resemble rhinosinusitis due to symptoms of facial pressure, pain over the cheeks, forehead, and around the eyes, which may be accompanied by nasal congestion, lacrimation, rhinorrhea, or eyelid edema. The investigation of these patients reveals minimal to no sinus disease, and the severity of symptoms does not correlate with endoscopic or radiologic findings
Trigeminal neuralgia	Facial pain can be caused by trigeminal neuralgia, also called "tic douloureux." This disease is characterized by brief, repetitive, lancing, facial pain that is unilateral. The distribution of pain can be any one or more of the three distributions of the trigeminal nerve. These painful attacks can be triggered by a cutaneous stimulus, including chewing, shaving, and wind blowing on the face. Medical treatment, usually with carbamazepine, oxcarbazepine, or other anticonvulsants are the first line of treatment, followed by surgical therapy, which involves either transecting a branch of the trigeminal nerve or performing a microvascular decompression of the nerve

(Continued)

Differential diagnosis	Features
CSF rhinorrhea	The rhinorrhea from CSF would be positive for beta-transferrin, and would be greatly exacerbated by Valsalva maneuvers and leaning forward. Often the drainage is unilateral
Sinus neoplasms	When rhinosinusitis is refractory to medical treatment or when an abnormality is found on physical examination, the possibility of a sinus neoplasm should be considered. CT scans can give bony detail, but MRI is better at distinguishing inflammatory causes from neoplastic causes of rhinosinusitis. The most common neoplasms in the sinonasal tract are squamous cell carcinoma, adenoid cystic carcinoma, and adenocarcinoma. Others include neuroectodermal (melanoma, olfactory neuroblastoma), sinonasal undifferentiated carcinoma, and metastatic lesions
Nasal polyposis	Nasal polyps are visible on endoscopic examination. They are commonly seen in patients with cystic fibrosis
Autoimmune disease	Autoimmune diseases can also be associated with rhinitis or sinonasal lesions
Wegener's granulomatosis	This is an inflammatory disease of the blood vessels characterized by granulomas formed in the kidneys, lungs, and upper respiratory tract. Common symptoms in the upper respiratory tract include epistaxis, rhinitis, saddle nose, gingival hyperplasia, and subglottis stenosis due to granulomatous lesions
Sarcoidosis	This is an autoimmune disease that can also cause rhinosinusitis with additional features including nasal crusting, anosmia, and epistaxis. Patients may have hilar opacification on chest radiographs with elevated angiotensin-converting enzyme levels
Odontogenic diseases	Odontogenic causes of maxillary rhinosinusitis are relatively uncommon, although it causes an estimated 10–12% of all cases of maxillary rhinosinusitis. In the evaluation of a patient with acute rhinosinusitis, it is prudent to look for an odontogenic source for the infection. Any history of an infected tooth or recent dental surgery should trigger a detailed dental examination. On physical examination tenderness with palpation of an infected tooth may prove diagnostic of an odontogenic source

Typical presentation

- Patients typically present with a variable duration of symptoms that may include mucopurulent rhinorrhea, headache, facial pain, anosmia, and congestion. Other associated symptoms include fever, chills, cough, malaise, dental or ear pain. The time course of their symptoms will define the type of rhinosinusitis which will then guide treatment strategies.

Clinical diagnosis

History

- When diagnosing acute rhinosinusitis, it is also important to distinguish between viral and bacterial etiologies. According to the clinical practice guidelines, all acute rhinosinusitis symptoms should be diagnosed as viral if the duration of symptoms is less than 10 days and if they are not worsening. However, if the symptoms persist beyond 10 days or worsen after initial improvement, then the diagnosis of acute bacterial rhinosinusitis is applicable.
- Symptoms that are most sensitive and specific for acute rhinosinusitis include mucopurulent drainage (anterior or posterior), nasal obstruction/congestion, and facial pressure/pain/fullness.

Other symptoms include hyposmia or anosmia, headache, fever, cough, malaise, fatigue, dental pain (maxillary), ear fullness, or otalgia.

- The most recent clinical practice guidelines on adult sinusitis focus on the three cardinal symptoms of rhinosinusitis: mucopurulent drainage, nasal obstruction, and facial discomfort. Specifically, the diagnosis requires the presence of purulent nasal discharge *and* either nasal obstruction or facial pain/pressure/fullness.
- The diagnosis of chronic rhinosinusitis requires 12 weeks or longer of two of four cardinal symptoms including mucopurulent drainage, nasal obstruction, facial pain/pressure/fullness, or decreased sense of smell *and* inflammation as documented as purulent mucus or edema in middle meatus or ethmoid region, polyps in the nasal cavity, or radiographic evidence of inflammation in the paranasal sinuses.

Physical examination

- During the basic head and neck examination, the examiner should focus on the forehead, maxilla, and peri-orbital region to detect erythema, swelling, or tenderness to palpation in those areas overlying the sinuses. Facial cellulitis may be an indication that an acute rhinosinusitis has spread outside of the sinuses. A thorough ophthalmologic examination with extraocular movements and visual acuity should be performed to rule out subperiosteal or intraorbital abscess. Tenderness to palpation of the temporomandibular joint may guide the clinician towards an alternate cause for facial or ear pain. An intraoral examination might reveal oroantral fistulas or dental causes for sinusitis or facial pain. A complete neurologic examination may be necessary to detect or exclude complications such as meningitis, encephalitis, intracranial abscess, or nerve palsies.
- Perhaps the most relevant finding of all is the detection of purulent fluid in the nasal cavity or posterior nasopharynx. Clinicians who are equipped with nasal endoscopes have a particular advantage of visualizing the turbinates, nasal septum, osteomeatal complex, nasopharynx, and eustachian tube orifices. Any anatomic abnormalities may also be detected at this time. During acute rhinosinusitis, nasal mucosa may be edematous or erythematous, and purulent material may be draining from the sinus ostia or pooling within the nasal passages (Figure 6.2).

Useful clinical decision rules and calculators

- Surveys have been developed in order to objectively measure the burden of disease on patient's quality of life. These surveys, the sinonasal outcome tests (SNOT), help to score patient symptoms and give a reference for comparison after medical treatment or surgery. There are many surveys that have been developed including SNOT-20 and SNOT-22 used for chronic rhinosinusitis, and a modified SNOT-16 that assesses the impact of acute rhinosinusitis on quality of life of patients. This is a useful tool not only for initial evaluation, but also for subsequent monitoring of symptoms after treatment.

Disease severity classification

Not applicable for this topic.

Laboratory diagnosis

List of diagnostic tests

- Routine use of laboratory tests is deemed to be unnecessary in cases of acute rhinosinusitis. The diagnosis can be established solely by a good history and examination. However, if the disease is refractory to initial treatment or becomes recurrent or chronic, further investigation to rule out immunodeficiencies, cystic fibrosis, Wegener's granulomatosis, sarcoidosis, Churg–Strauss disease, or other autoimmunes diseases may be necessary.

- Obtaining nasal cultures can facilitate culture-directed antimicrobial treatment, but the routine use of nasal cultures has not been proven to be useful or cost effective for acute rhinosinusitis. If patients are immunocompromised or if there is concern of drug resistance, nasal cultures may be performed to help direct therapy. Traditionally, cultures from the OMC or middle meatus are preferred under direct vision. However, there is evidence that cultures of the nasopharynx correlate well with cultures of the middle meatus under direct endoscopic visualization, and may be useful in the primary care setting. Cultures may be particularly helpful in recurrent acute rhinosinusitis given the fact that these patients are similar to chronic rhinosinusitis but tend to require more antibiotic therapy.
- In patients with evidence of atopy or allergy, skin and laboratory testing can be conducted to investigate if allergy to environmental exposures may be contributing to the severity or frequency of rhinosinusitis. This may also lead to treatments that can help decrease the severity and frequency of sinus disease.

Lists of imaging techniques

- *Radiographs:* X-rays in the four traditional views (Waters', Caldwell's, lateral, and submental) may be useful in uncertain or recurrent cases of acute rhinosinusitis. Waters' view (Figure 6.3) with the occiput tipped down and patient's chin and nasal tip against the plate, has good visualization of the maxillary sinuses with a positive predictive value of 82.5% and negative predictive value of 76.9%. Caldwell's view, with the forehead and nasal tip against the plate, provides a good view of the ethmoid and frontal sinuses. The lateral and submental views allow visualization of the sphenoid and posterior ethmoid sinuses. A normal X-ray, especially in the frontal or maxillary sinuses, has a good negative predictive value (90–100%) but has a poor positive predictive value (as low as 80%).
- *Ultrasound:* the use of ultrasound in the diagnosis of acute rhinosinusitis is not mentioned as part of the clinical practice guidelines. However, in the setting of the primary care office, there is some preliminary evidence to support the use of an office ultrasound device that can be used to detect air–fluid levels in the maxillary sinus.
- *CT:* CT of the paranasal sinuses is not recommended as part of the routine investigation for acute rhinosinusitis. In cases with severe disease, immunocompromised state, or suspected complications, several guidelines including the rhinosinusitis initiative and the clinical practice guidelines advocate CT without IV contrast as the preferred imaging technique. The application of cone-beam CT has recently expanded to sinonasal disease and although this technique offers some advantages, like convenience of office-use and reduction of radiation dosage, its routine use has not been well studied for cost-effectiveness and efficacy. Common findings in a sinus CT include air–fluid levels in acute rhinosinusitis and mucosal thickening, periosteal thickening, and sclerosis in chronic rhinosinusitis.
- The most widely accepted radiographic staging system for chronic rhinosinusitis is the Lund–Mackay scale. This is an objective measure to grade the right and left sides independently, and it assesses the maxillary, anterior ethmoids, posterior ethmoids, sphenoids, frontal sinuses, and the ostiomeatal complex. Each sinus is scored 0 (no abnormality), 1 (partial opacification), or 2 (total opacification), while the ostiomeatal complex is scored either 0 or 2 (for absence or presence of disease). The highest score is 24.
- *MRI:* not used routinely for acute rhinosinusitis unless there are signs of aggressive disease or cases with complications. MRI provides better soft tissue information (useful for intracranial, intraorbital, and extrasinonasal manifestations of rhinosinusitis), especially when differentiating malignant from inflammatory causes of rhinosinusitis. In addition, it does not pose a radiation exposure concern.

Potential pitfalls/common errors made regarding diagnosis of disease

- It is important to distinguish between an acute viral and bacterial rhinosinusitis due to the pitfalls of over-prescribing antibiotics for a virally induced illness.
- Radiographic imaging is not routinely necessary in cases of simple rhinosinusitis.
- If patients present with persistent, recurrent, or chronic disease that fails medical management, a consultation with an otolaryngologist for further assessment with nasal endoscopy or a baseline CT scan of the sinuses would be indicated.

Section 4: Treatment

Treatment rationale

- Treatment of acute rhinosinusitis has to take into account the duration of disease, severity of symptoms, and patient compliance. If symptoms' duration is within 10 days and are not worsening, a viral rhinosinusitis is presumed and treatment is symptomatic with antipyretics and analgesics. Oral or topical decongestants may be used for nasal congestion, while mucolytics and expectorants may be used for cough. The utility of antihistamines and topical or systemic steroids in the treatment of viral rhinosinusitis is still under investigation.
- If symptoms last more than 10 days or if there is worsening or double worsening, then the presumptive diagnosis is a bacterial acute rhinosinusitis and this may be managed by watchful waiting for reliable patients or treated with antibiotics and other adjunctive therapies: analgesics and antipyretics, steroids, irrigations, decongestants, mucolytics, and allergy management.
- Most guidelines advocate the use of amoxicillin or amoxicillin-clavulanate as a first line of treatment based on its efficacy, low cost, and low side-effect profile. Those with an allergy to penicillin may be given macrolides or trimethoprim-sulfamethoxazole. The adequate duration of therapy is still debated, with most studies advocating 3–10 days of therapy.
- In patients with recurrent, subacute, or chronic rhinosinusitis, nasal cultures may help to guide antibiotic therapy, and there may be a role for nasal saline irrigations (with or without antibiotic and steroid additives). In those who fail medical therapy, surgical management with endoscopic sinus surgery, septoplasty, turbinate reduction, balloon sinuplasty, or even functional rhinoplasty may be necessary.

When to hospitalize

- After 7 days of treatment, if patients fail to improve or worsen, then the clinician should consider an otolaryngology evaluation for nasal endoscopy and culture. Intravenous antibiotic therapy may be indicated for severe symptoms or a culture that reveals only intravenous antibiotic options.
- Signs and symptoms that the disease has spread intracranially or intraorbitally include proptosis, visual changes (diplopia), severe headache and fever, abnormal extraocular movements, changes in mental status, peri-orbital inflammation, edema, or erythema. In addition, frontal sinus infections may spread to skin and soft tissue of the forehead leading to frontal osteomyelitis, an entity known as Pott's puffy tumor.
- If these signs are present, routine laboratory tests should be ordered such as complete blood count, BMP, and coagulation profile (in preparation for possible surgical intervention). Endoscopic examination should be performed in order to obtain nasal cultures or biopsies. Imaging such as CT head and sinus with or without contrast should be obtained. If abscess is suspected, contrast should be used.
- If there are signs of intracranial or intraorbital complications, the patient should be admitted for monitoring, intravenous antibiotics, and possible lumbar tap *after* imaging is performed.

Managing the hospitalized patient

- Intravenous antibiotics should be used in cases with intracranial or intraorbital complications and cases of failure of oral antibiotic treatment.
- The appropriate consultations should be made to other services, which include neurosurgery, ophthalmology, infectious disease, or medicine if there are other medical problems that may need to be addressed.
- If the imaging shows an abscess that necessitates surgical intervention, this should be coordinated expeditiously to avoid further sequelae of the infection.

Table of treatment

Treatment	Comment
Conservative	Watchful waiting is an acceptable management option for patients with uncomplicated acute rhinosinusitis (temperature <38.3°C, mild pain) and good follow-up
Medical • Antibiotics • Nasal saline irrigations/sprays • Intranasal steroid sprays • Mucolytics, decongestants, antihistamines	There are many combinations of antibiotics that can be used for treating acute rhinosinusitis. For chronic rhinosinusitis, antibiotic choice depends on the prevalent organisms and sensitivities. Chronic rhinosinusitis can also benefit from nasal irrigations and steroids Adjunctive therapies can be used to supplement antibiotic treatment
Surgical • Functional endoscopic sinus surgery (maxillary antrostomy, ethmoidectomy, sphenoidotomy, frontal sinusotomy • Balloon sinuplasty • Septoplasty • Turbinate reduction	When medical therapy has failed to resolve or improve symptoms, surgical intervention may be considered. This includes a variety of techniques (balloon or instrumentation) and can involve any location of the sinonasal tract that seems to be involved and seems to contribute to the disease

Prevention/management of complications

- Surgical complications include but are not limited to epistaxis, recurrent infections, damage to the orbit, CSF leak, nasolacrimal duct injury, and anosmia.

CLINICAL PEARLS
- Treatment for chronic rhinosinusitis is predominantly medical with surgery reserved for a small subset of patients who fail non-surgical therapy.
- Surgery for chronic rhinosinusitis does *not* replace medical therapy. Actually, medical therapy becomes more important after surgery is performed.
- In a patient with unilateral acute sinusitis, rule out a structural problem of drainage or an odontogenic source of infection.
- In patients with recurrent acute sinusitis, consider a CT scan at the time of an infection to help determine which sinuses are the problem. Classically, the patient with recurrent acute sinusitis has a normal CT scan between infections.

Section 5: Special populations
Pregnancy
- During pregnancy, increasing blood volume, shifts to the extravascular space, and increased estrogen all contribute to vascular dilatation and increased mucus production.
- Approximately 10–30% of women of childbearing age report worsening of rhinitis or sinusitis symptoms during pregnancy.
- It is of utmost importance to understand the risk : benefit ratio of rhinosinusitis and its management options when deciding how to counsel, diagnose, and treat patients during pregnancy.
- If a CT is necessary, performing one without contrast and after 17 weeks' gestation is best.
- Antimicrobials within category B such as penicillins, cephalosporins, clindamycin, erythromycin, and azithromycin are safer than those in category C such as clarithromycin, fluoroquinolones, aminoglycosides, sulfonamides, tetracycline, and vancomycin.
- Antihistamines such as chlorpheniramine, loratadine, and cetirizine are within category B.
- The only intranasal steroid spray in category B is budesonide.
- Surgery should only be considered as a last resort after other medical modalities have failed because of the risks of general anesthesia, which include preterm labor and effects on the fetus.

Children
- Systematic review of the literature has shown that rhinosinusitis is a major cause of morbidity to children who suffer from this disease.
- Although medical therapy is the mainstay of treatment for the pediatric population for rhinosinusitis of all categories, FESS may be beneficial in cases resistant to medical treatment (failing 2–6 weeks of antibiotic treatment).
- However, pediatric FESS seems to have less benefit in patients with underlying systemic diseases such as cystic fibrosis.
- Absolute indications for surgical intervention include complete nasal obstruction due to polyps in cystic fibrosis, orbital abscess, intracranial complications, antrochoanal polyp, mucocele and mucopyocele, and fungal sinosinusitis.

Elderly
- There are studies that show chronic sinusitis can affect cognitive functioning in the elderly population.
- It is important to treat rhinosinusitis in the aging population, but considerations need to be made when prescribing antibiotics in the setting of other comorbidities including renal and hepatic insufficiency.

Others
Not applicable for this topic.

Section 6: Prognosis

> **BOTTOM LINE/CLINICAL PEARLS**
> - Chronic rhinosinusitis is a chronic disease that requires ongoing medical therapy and management of underlying triggers such as allergies.
> - This condition is not a curable disease, but a chronic illness that requires ongoing medical therapy and possible lifestyle modification.
> - Surgery is used as an adjunct of treatment in those that have failed medical management. However, surgery does not alleviate the need for ongoing medical management.

Natural history of untreated disease
- Untreated chronic rhinosinusitis results in significant loss of quality of life as well as exacerbations of asthma.
- Patients will vary in the progression of their disease and this is due to underlying etiology of their chronic rhinosinusitis.

Prognosis for treated patients
- Medical treatment is ongoing and controls symptoms in the majority of cases.
- Surgery has an 80–90% success rate with complete or moderate improvement in symptoms and disease severity.

Follow-up tests and monitoring
- There is no consensus on frequency of monitoring of patients with chronic rhinosinusitis .
- In general, an evaluation every 3 months is recommended until the condition has stabilized. In patients with polyps, examination and endoscopy will detect early polyp growth before symptoms develop.
- Hyposmia or anosmia is the first symptom seen in polyp regrowth. This occurs before nasal obstruction, headaches, or posterior rhinorrhea.

Section 7: Reading list

Brook I. Microbiology and antimicrobial management of sinusitis. J Laryngol Otol 2005;119:251–8.

Cornelius RS, Martin J, Wippold FJ 2nd, Aiken AH, Angtuaco EJ, Berger KL, et al. ACR appropriateness criteria sinonasal disease. J Am Coll Radiol 2013;10:241–6

Desrosiers M, Evans GA, Keith PK, Wright ED, Kaplan A, Bouchard J, et al. Canadian clinical practice guidelines for acute and chronic rhinosinusitis. J Otolaryngol Head Neck Surg 2011;40(Suppl 2):S99–193

Meltzer EO, Hamilos DL. Rhinosinusitis diagnosis and management for the clinician: a synopsis of recent consensus guidelines. Mayo Clin Proc 2011;86:427–43

Meltzer EO, Hamilos DL, Hadley JA, Lanza DC, Marple BF, Nicklas RA, et al. Rhinosinusitis: establishing definitions for clinical research and patient care. J Allergy Clin Immunol 2004;114(Suppl):155–212

Rosenfeld RM, Andes D, Bhattacharyya N, Cheung D, Eisenberg S, Ganiats TG, et al. Clinical practice guideline: adult sinusitis. Otolaryngol Head Neck Surg 2007;137(Suppl):S1–31

Slavin RG, Spector SL, Bernstein IL, Kaliner MA, Kennedy DW, Virant FS, et al. The diagnosis and management of sinusitis: a practice parameter update. J Allergy Clin Immunol 2005;116(Suppl):S13–47

Section 8: Guidelines
National society guidelines

Guideline title	Guideline source	Date
Clinical Practice Guideline: Adult Sinusitis	Otolaryngology–Head and Neck Surgery	2007 (http://www.ncbi.nlm.nih.gov/pubmed/17761281)

International society guidelines

Guideline title	Guideline source	Date
Canadian clinical practice guidelines for acute and chronic rhinosinusitis	Allergy, Asthma and Clinical Immunology (AACI)	2011 (http://www.aacijournal.com/content/7/1/2)

Section 9: Evidence

Not applicable for this topic.

Section 10: Images

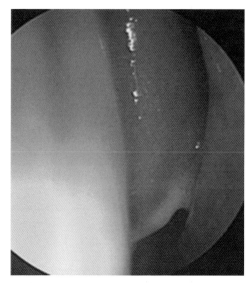

Figure 6.1 Nasal endoscopy of left middle meatus with purulent drainage noted in infundibulum. Patient had an acute maxillary sinusitis. See color plate 6.1.

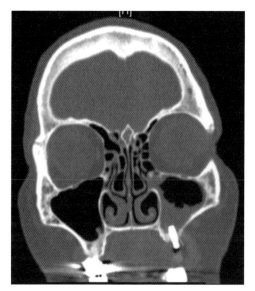

Figure 6.2 Acute sinusitis. Non-contrast CT scan of the sinuses with an acute left odontogenic maxillary sinusitis. Patient has an air–fluid level in the left maxillary sinusitis with a dental implant placed into the floor of the maxillary sinus. Patient required maxillary antrostomy to clear the infection.

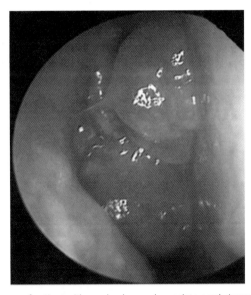

Figure 6.3 Nasal endoscopy of patient with nasal polyps and complete nasal airway obstruction. This patient had complaints of anosmia and nasal congestion. See color plate 6.2.

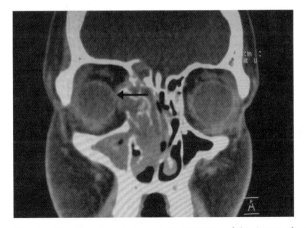

Figure 6.4 Chronic rhinosinusitis with polyposis. Non-contrast CT scan of the sinuses of patient in Figure 6.3 demonstrates expansile polyposis of the right sinonasal cavity. The arrow points to area of polyp extension from ethmoid cavity into the orbit. In these cases the periorbita of the eye is usually not violated; however, caution is needed during surgical clearance of polyps in this area to avoid risk of intraorbital injury. See color plate 6.3.

Additional material for this chapter can be found online at:
www.mountsinaiexpertguides.com
This includes a case study, multiple choice questions, advice for patients, and ICD codes

CHAPTER 7

Allergic Diseases of the Eye

Amanda L. Cox

Division of Pediatric Allergy/Immunology, Icahn School of Medicine at Mount Sinai, New York, NY, USA

OVERALL BOTTOM LINE

- Ocular allergy includes allergic conjunctivitis, atopic keratoconjunctivitis (AKC), and vernal keratoconjunctivitis (VKC).
- Both seasonal and perennial subtypes of allergic conjunctivitis are self-limited disorders of the conjunctiva, and occur upon exposure to environmental allergens.
- AKC and VKC are chronic inflammatory ocular disorders, exacerbated by environmental allergens and other factors, and affect the conjunctiva, cornea, and eyelids.
- AKC and VKC are associated with potentially sight-threatening corneal fibrosis.
- Giant papillary conjunctivitis (GPC), an inflammatory reaction to a foreign substance in the eye, is not a true allergic disease, but mimics features of ocular hypersensitivity, and so is sometimes categorized as an allergic eye disease.
- These conditions result from primarily type I and IV hypersensitivity responses and involve similar inflammatory mediators and cell populations.

Section 1: Background
Definition of disease

Ocular allergic diseases are multifactorial allergic inflammatory disorders of the ocular surface that affect the conjunctiva (the mucous membrane lining the anterior sclera and inner eyelid surfaces), eyelids, and, in some conditions, the cornea.

Disease classification

Allergic conjunctivitis disorders include acute, seasonal, and perennial forms, which are associated with discomfort, but are generally self-limited. VKC and AKC are more severe chronic allergic inflammatory eye diseases that can threaten sight. Giant papillary conjunctivitis (GPC) results from chronic mechanical trauma due to a foreign substance on the ocular surface.

Incidence/prevalence

- Allergic conjunctivitis is the most common form of ocular allergy and affects up to 20% of the population, including 60% of allergic rhinitis sufferers.
- AKC occurs most often in adults 30–50 years of age, with a history of atopic dermatitis, but the exact prevalence is unknown.
- VKC occurs most commonly in atopic males <20 years of age, in warm, dry, subtropical climates and is rare in cooler climates. Only 50% will show positive IgE testing.

Mount Sinai Expert Guides: Allergy and Clinical Immunology, First Edition. Edited by Hugh A. Sampson.
© 2015 John Wiley & Sons, Ltd. Published 2015 by John Wiley & Sons, Ltd.
Companion website: www.mountsinaiexpertguides.com

- GPC affects 1–5% of non-disposable soft contact lens wearers but 10-fold fewer rigid contact lens wearers. GPC predominantly affects young adults, and may be more common in individuals with asthma or allergic rhinitis.

Economic impact
Not applicable for this topic.

Etiology
- Allergic conjunctivitis has a similar etiology to that of other atopic diseases, with multiple environmental factors and genes involved, leading to an over-expression of Th2 cytokine expression and an allergic phenotype. Seasonal allergic conjunctivitis is a hypersensitivity response to seasonal pollen (tree, grass, ragweed) exposures, while chronic allergic conjunctivitis occurs with perennial allergen exposures, such as indoor mold, pets and dust mites.
- In AKC, environmental risk factors, such as chronic exposure to animals and winter months have been identified, while VKC is exacerbated often in the spring but can be triggered by non-specific stimuli. The genetic risk factors for AKC and VKC are the same as those for allergy in general with multiple genetic loci implicated.
- GPC is a non-infectious inflammatory process that is a reaction to repetitive and chronic lid movement over a foreign substance such as a contact lens.

Pathology/pathogenesis
- Acute, seasonal and perennial allergic conjunctivitis disorders are manifestations of type I IgE-mediated hypersensitivity in which antigen cross-links with IgE-antibody bound to the high-affinity IgE receptor on mast cells. Mast cells and eosinophils are increased in the conjunctival epithelium and substantia propria of individuals with allergic conjunctivitis. Phase I of the allergic response is mediated primarily by chemical mediators, including histamine, released immediately by mast cells. Histamine results in vasodilatation, vasopermeability, and ocular itching. Other cytokines and chemokines released by mast cells cause a late phase of the allergic reaction with influx of inflammatory cells including eosinophils, basophils, and neutrophils, followed by lymphocytes and monocytes.
- AKC results primarily from a type IV (delayed-type Th1 and Th2 lymphocyte) hypersensitivity reaction as well as some type I hypersensitivity reaction to environmental allergen exposures. AKC occurs in sensitized individuals who have atopic dermatitis, but the exact mechanisms are not known. CD4+ T cells, eosinophils, monocytes, mast cells, and fibroblasts contribute to the disease process. Elevated IgE is found in the tears and serum of AKC patients. Tears also contain CD4+ T cells and activated B cells, as well as increased cytokines IFN-γ, TNF-α, IL-4, IL-5, IL-10, and the chemokine eotaxin. Dysfunction of cell-mediated and aberrant innate immunity have been demonstrated in some patients with AKC. Lower tarsal conjunctivae and cornea can be involved.
- VKC involves some type I (IgE-mediated) but primarily type II (Th2)-mediated responses, as well as IgG-mediated responses, basophil hypersensitivity, and cellular delayed-type hypersensitivity. Conjunctival accumulation of CD4+ T cells may result in hyper-reactivity against substances that come in contact with the conjunctiva, such as allergens (pollen, dust mites, mold, animal dander) and other non-specific stimuli. Mast cells are induced to release mediators that stimulate fibroblast activity, production of collagen, and formation of giant papillae. IgE, histamine, tryptase and multiple inflammatory mediators are found in elevated levels in the tears, increased expression of histamine receptors is found in conjunctival tissue, and capillaries proliferate. The upper tarsal conjunctival surface is involved. Eosinophil infiltration and activation can cause corneal complications.

- GPC involves mechanical and immunologic processes. Debris that builds up on a contact lens surface over time may be recognized as foreign to mucous membranes of the conjunctiva and may trigger type I and IV hypersensitivity reactions. Blinking over a foreign substance may cause mechanical trauma to the eyelid and thereby provide an entry point for antigens to induce an immune response, release of inflammatory mediators, and infiltration of lymphocytes. Papillary formation, fibroblast proliferation, and collagen deposition leads to formation of giant papillae.

Predictive/risk factors

Atopy is a risk factor for SAC, PAC, AKC, and VKC.

Section 2: Prevention

No interventions have been demonstrated to prevent the development of ocular allergic disorders.

Screening

Not applicable for this topic.

Primary prevention

Not applicable for this topic.

Secondary prevention

- *Seasonal allergic conjunctivitis:* allergen avoidance measures including avoidance of outdoor exposure, use of air conditioning, keeping windows closed during peak seasons.
- *Perennial allergic conjunctivitis:* allergen avoidance measures for dust mites, indoor mold, and pets.
- *Atopic and vernal keratoconjunctivitis:* avoidance of non-specific triggers, eye-rubbing, and known allergens.
- *Giant papillary conjunctivitis:* avoidance of specific ocular irritant or stimuli, temporary discontinuation of contact lens use

Section 3: Diagnosis (Algorithm 7.1)

BOTTOM LINE/CLINICAL PEARLS
- Ocular allergy almost always presents with a history of pruritus.
- Diagnosis of acute, seasonal, and perennial allergic conjunctivitis is made clinically based on suggestive signs, pattern of symptoms, and demonstration of IgE-mediated sensitization (by epicutaneous skin prick tests or serum IgE levels) to specific allergens.
- Diagnosis of AKC is based on typical epidemiology and clinical features. Suspect AKC in adults with a history of atopic dermatitis who have ocular pruritus, eyelid dermatitis, and giant papillae on the conjunctival lining of the lower tarsus and inferior fornix.
- Diagnosis of VKC is based on typical epidemiology (primarily affects pre-pubertal boys living in warm climates) and clinical features (ocular pruritus, giant papillae on the conjunctival lining of the upper eyelid).
- While tears in all conditions have characteristic findings, tear evaluation is not typically part of the evaluation of patients for ocular allergy disorders. Eyelid tissue scrapings may be performed in some conditions, but are not routine.

Algorithm 7.1 Diagnosis of allergic diseases of the eye

Presentation of itchy eye, conjunctival hyperemia, tearing, ± eyelid swelling

Non-allergic, non-infectious
Dry eye
acne
rosacea
foreign body
chemical
medication

Itching of conjunctiva, clear mucoid discharge, allergic sensitization, no corneal involvement
Allergic conjunctivitis

Seasonal pattern with sensitization to seasonal allergens, (i.e. pollen)
Seasonal allergic conjunctivitis

Chronic pattern with sensitization to perennial allergens (dust mites, pets, indoor mold)
Perennial allergic conjunctivitis

Chemosis, stringy mucoid discharge, cobblestoning of eyelid

Chronic symptoms, patients with history of atopic dermatitis, presence of eyelid eczema, giant conjunctival papillae on lower tarsal conjunctiva, blepharospasm, frequent corneal involvement
Atopic keratoconjunctivitis

Giant papillae on upper tarsal conjunctiva, blepharospasm, possible corneal keratitis, patient <20 years of age with seasonal pattern of symptoms
Vernal keratoconjunctivitis

Mucopurulent discharge
Infectious conjunctivitis

Presence of foreign materials on ocular surface, no corneal involvement
Giant papillary conjunctivitis

Differential diagnosis

Differential diagnosis	Features
Allergic conjunctivitis (SAC or PAC)	Sensitized individual with seasonal allergies or year-round allergies Bilateral involvement Associated with allergic rhinitis No ocular surface damage Self-limiting Not sight-threatening
Atopic keratoconjunctivitis (AKC)	Sensitized individual Peak incidence 20–50 years of age Bilateral involvement Seasonal or perennial allergies Chronic symptoms, but may have seasonal exacerbations History of atopic dermatitis, and presence of eyelid dermatitis Photophobia Potential for cataracts and loss of sight
Vernal keratoconjunctivitis (VKC)	Sensitized individual Peak incidence 3–20 years of age Males predominate 3 : 1 Bilateral involvement Warm, dry climate Seasonal or perennial allergies Severe photophobia Potential for loss of sight
Giant papillary conjunctivitis (GPC)	Allergic sensitization not necessarily present Bilateral involvement Prosthetic or contact lens ocular exposure Contact lens intolerance Not sight-threatening

Note: Also consider other non-allergic causes of conjunctivitis: preservative toxicity, conjunctivitis medicamentosa, dry eye, contact dermatitis, blepharitis, pemphigoid, and infectious conjunctivitis.

Typical presentation

- Allergic disorders of the conjunctiva present with symptoms of conjunctival erythema, significant ocular pruritus, tearing, discharge, discomfort, and eye pain. Without pruritus, allergic conjunctivitis is unlikely. Mucus discharge is usually serous, clear or watery, but often stringy. Visual disturbance may occur in severe AKC or VKC but does not occur in allergic conjunctivitis. Patients may have eyelid or conjunctival membrane swelling (chemosis). Some of these disorders have seasonal patterns of onset or exacerbation, or are associated with an allergen exposure. Presentation of AKC or VKC may include thickening and erythema of the tarsal conjunctiva with pinprick size to >1 mm giant papillae, resulting in "cobblestoning" under the eyelid (Figure 7.1). Eyelid dermatitis and inflammation of the eyelid margin (blepharitis) may be seen. These more severe disorders may also present with conjunctival scarring and corneal involvement. GPC presents initially with mild irritation, itching, and mucous production that progresses to more intense itching and foreign body sensation, blurry vision, and intolerance to wearing contact lenses.

Clinical diagnosis

History

- Presence of additional atopic conditions (e.g. asthma, atopic dermatitis, urticaria, allergic rhinitis) or symptoms.
- Family history of atopy.
- Indoor and outdoor environmental exposures.
- Onset of allergic eye symptoms in relation to development of nasal allergies.
- Seasonal exacerbations versus chronic unremitting symptoms.
- Bilateral involvement.
- Presence of itching (primary complaint) and eye rubbing.
- Use of soft contact lenses, prosthetics, or presence of other foreign substance on eye surface.
- Complaints of mucus, glassy appearing eyes, or blepharospasm.
- Complaints of foreign body sensation, pain, photophobia.
- Change in vision or visual acuity.

Physical examination

- It is important to inspect the eyelid, conjunctiva and cornea, as well as assess any discharge. Ocular mobility and visual acuity should also be evaluated. Signs of allergic rhinosinusitis should be considered. Ophthalmologists may conduct a slit-lamp examination.
- Allergic conjunctivitis findings include bilateral tearing, conjunctival edema, hyperemia, watery discharge, chemosis, and eyelid edema.
- AKC is bilateral but severity may be asymmetric, and findings include thickened eyelids, intermittent eyelid swelling, scaly and indurated periocular skin, and flaking peri-ocular dermatitis on a reddened base. Eyelids can become lichenified and may develop cicatricial ectropion (lower eyelid eversion). Eyelid fissures, loss of eyelashes, lateral canthal ulceration and ptosis can develop. Lid margins may show meibomian gland inflammation, keratinization, and punctual ectropion (lid eversion). Blepharitis may be present. Conjunctival chemosis, hyperemia, and tarsal papillary hypertrophy of upper lids may develop.
- VKC is bilateral and findings include giant cobblestone-like papillae on the conjunctival lining of the upper eyelids (Figure 7.1). Other findings may include conjunctival and episcleral hyperemia, superficial keratopathy, non-purulent mucus discharge, yellow–gray infiltrates (Horner–Trantas dots), corneal shield ulcers, ptosis, and blepharospasm. The upper tarsal (palpebral) form of VKC involves the conjunctiva that covers the inside of the eyelid. The limbal form of VKC involves the thin border between the cornea and sclera.
- GPC findings include enlarged papillae on the upper tarsus, mucus production, conjunctival hyperemia, eyelid thickening, and occasionally ptosis. Papules are <0.3 mm in early stages but can progress to 1–2 mm in size. Protein deposits are often visible on contact lens surface.

Useful clinical decision rules and calculators

Not applicable for this topic.

Disease severity classification

- Allergic conjunctivitis is generally mild but may have significant effects on quality of life.
- VKC and AKC can progress to severe forms and be sight-threatening.
- GPC includes four stages of severity:
    i. mild mucus discharge, mild itching without papillae;
    ii. increased mucus production and itching, awareness of contact lens, blurred vision, upper tarsal papillae;

iii. severe mucus production and intense itching; contact lens coated with debris; increased size and number of papillae;

iv. all signs and symptoms severe, and contact lenses can only be worn briefly.

Laboratory diagnosis

List of diagnostic tests

- Diagnosis of all forms of ocular allergic disease is generally made clinically and by physical examination. Tests that can be done are generally limited to academic or confirmatory purposes but include:
  - For allergic conjunctivitis confirmation:
    - ➤ conjunctival scrapings for presence of eosinophils, tear film IgE levels, serum IgE levels, tear tryptase immunoassay.
    - ➤ Conjunctival provocation tests with allergen.
    - ➤ Demonstration of IgE-mediated hypersensitivity to aeroallergens via allergy skin prick testing or measurement of serum IgE levels to aeroallergens.
  - AKC: increased specific IgE in tears, increased serum IgE and blood eosinophils, eosinophils in conjunctival scrapings.
  - VKC: increased IgE and/or IgG, histamine, tryptase in tears.
  - GPC may be associated with elevated tear levels of IgE, IgM, and IgG, and tryptase but no increased tear histamine levels.
- Tear or conjunctival cytology may also be evaluated to rule out neoplastic processes and confirm an allergic condition.
- Conjunctival or eyelid cultures may be needed to rule out infectious processes.

Lists of imaging techniques

Not applicable for this topic.

Potential pitfalls/common errors made regarding diagnosis of disease

- Allergic conjunctivitis is under-reported as patients often do not seek medical evaluation and self-medicate with over-the-counter topical medications.
- Milder or initial stages of all allergic eye diseases have similar, overlapping features.
- It is important to exclude infectious conjunctivitis as treatment differs from that of allergic eye diseases.

Section 4: Treatment (Algorithm 7.2)

Treatment rationale

- First line treatment for all ocular allergic diseases involves avoidance of antigen or allergen where possible and, in the case of GPC, discontinuation of use of contact lenses. Cold compresses may alleviate some symptoms. Artificial tear substitutes act as a barrier for conjunctival mucosa, dilute allergens and inflammatory mediators, and flush ocular surface to provide relief of symptoms.
- Recurrence of GPC due to contact lenses can be prevented by use of preservative-free lens solution, changing lens type, frequent replacement of contact lenses, and reduced lens wearing time.
- Antiallergic therapeutic agents include systemic or topical antihistamine, and combination topical antiallergic+mast cell stabilizing agents. These medications relieve symptomatic itching and redness in the short term.
- Topical decongestants act as vasoconstrictors and reduce erythema but are for short-term use only.

Algorithm 7.2 Management of allergic diseases of the eye

1. Basic eye care: allergen avoidance, prevention of eye rubbing.
2. Treatment of dry eyes: cold compress, artificial tears
3. Topical decongestant/vasoconstrictor for transient symptom relief only
4. Topical antihistamine, topical mast cell stabilizer, topical NSAID or combination anti-allergy + mast cell stabilizer agent.
5. Topical calcineurin inhibitor (cyclosporine)
6. Topical corticosteroid + ophthalmology evaluation for more severe disease
7. Consider allergen-specific immunotherapy where there is a known allergenic trigger to reduce the severity of chronic disease and prevent exacerbations of seasonal diseases

- Mast cell stabilizers reduce mast cell degranulation and histamine release. They do not relieve existing symptoms but prevent degranulation with subsequent exposure to allergens.
- Multimodal topical agents act as histamine receptor antagonists, mast cell stabilizers, and suppressors of eosinophil infiltration and activation.
- Topical non-steroidal anti-inflammatory drugs (NSAIDs) can be used as an additive drug to reduce conjunctival hyperemia and pruritus.
- Corticosteroids are immunosuppressive and the most potent agents for more severe variants of ocular allergy but should be used with care because of the potential for adverse effects.
- Aggressive treatment should be considered for AKC and VKC, both of which can be sight-threatening in the most severe forms.
- Allergen-specific immunotherapy can induce clinical tolerance to specific allergens that trigger exacerbations, and may be an adjunct to treatment for allergic conjunctivitis (seasonal and perennial), AKC, and VKC.

When to hospitalize
Not applicable for this topic.

Managing the hospitalized patient
Not applicable for this topic.

Table of treatment

Treatment	Comment
Conservative • Allergen avoidance • Cold compresses • Prevention of eye rubbing • Desensitization • Topical lubricants/artificial tears • Cessation of contact lens use or removal of source of mechanical irritation	These measures may reduce the need for pharmacotherapy, relieve symptoms and may be sufficient in mild cases of ocular allergy

(Continued)

Treatment	Comment

Medical
Oral sedating or non-sedating antihistamines
• Topical antihistamines
  • Levacobastine
  • Emedastine
  • Pheniramine
  • Antazoline
• Topical decongestants/vasoconstrictors
  • Phenylephrine
  • Naphazoline
  • Oxymetazoline
• Topical mast cell inhibitors
  • Cromolyn
  • Lodoxamide
  • Pemirolast
  • Nedocromil
• Topical NSAIDs
  • Ketorolac
  • Diclofenac
  • Flurbiprofen
• Combination antihistamine + mast cell stabilizers
  • Olopatadine
  • Bepotastine besilate
  • Azelastine
  • Ketotifen
• Topical calcineurin inhibitors (AKC, VKC)
  • Tacrolimus
  • Cyclosporine
• Topical antibiotics
• Topical corticosteroids
  • Loteprednol
  • Rimexolone
• Oral immunomodulatory agents
  • Corticosteroid
  • Calcineurin inhibitors (severe AKC, VKC)
	Treatment should be tailored to severity of signs and symptoms
	
	Topical agents are more effective than systemic agents in most cases
	
	Mast cell stabilizers are not useful for acute symptoms but are helpful on a prophylactic basis
	
	Immunomodulatory agents should be reserved for more severe disease, as in VKC and AKC
	
	The use of topical steroids should be initiated in conjunction with an ophthalmologist. It is the last choice for allergic conjunctivitis, but may be necessary for VKC and AKC
	
	Allergen-specific immunotherapy is effective when the allergen triggering allergic ocular disease is well known and should be considered in patients who do not respond to medications or who experience side effects from medications

Surgical • Punctal plugs • Debridement of inflammatory debris • Surgical or laser removal of corneal plaques • Keratoplasty or cyanoacrylate glue application	Surgery is reserved for treatment of sight-reducing corneal disease in AKC and VKC Keratoplasty or cyanoacrylate glue application is indicated for corneal scarring and for extensive corneal thinning or perforation
Other • Topical immunomodulator (corticosteroid or tacrolimus) ointment • Intranasal topical corticosteroids	Treatment of peri-ocular atopic dermatitis in patients with AKC For patients with allergic rhinitis in conjunction with allergic eye symptoms

Prevention/management of complications
- Frequent eye examinations may be necessary in patients with severe or chronic ocular allergy.
- Vasoconstrictors can cause rebound conjunctival hyperemia and are not effective for severe or chronic ocular allergy.
- Oral or systemic antihistamines can cause decreased tearing and ocular dryness, which may exacerbate ocular allergy symptoms.

- Complications of topical steroid use include cataracts, glaucoma, and viral super-infection. Treatment with corticosteroids needs to be monitored carefully so cataracts or increased intraocular pressure can be detected early. Any suspected eye infection should be treated promptly.

CLINICAL PEARLS
- For all ocular allergic diseases, avoidance of known allergenic triggers is recommended.
- Medical agents may be used for any ocular allergic disease and should be tailored to the type and severity of disease, extent of ocular involvement, and risk for permanent sight impairment.
- VKC and AKC are severe, potentially sight-threatening due to corneal involvement, and require more aggressive treatment with stronger agents including topical immunomodulators. Treatment of these diseases requires close surveillance and monitoring.
- In AKC, it is important to control the facial and eyelid eczema.
- GPC once identified is treated with removal of the offending foreign substance, and generally self-resolves within 1–4 weeks.
- Consider ophthalmology referral for any patient who requires topical immunomodulator or who has refractory symptoms.

Section 5: Special populations
Not applicable for this topic.

Section 6: Prognosis

BOTTOM LINE/CLINICAL PEARLS
- Seasonal and perennial allergic conjunctivitis usually affect children and young adults and severity tends to lessen, or conjunctivitis resolves altogether, with increasing age. Most patients do experience relief with medical therapies.
- AKC management is difficult and patients are not cured. AKC has the highest association with corneal involvement and can lead to significant vision loss.
- VKC can cause severe damage to the ocular surface, corneal scarring, and vision loss if not properly treated. VKC may be recurrent (seasonally) or chronic, but usually resolves after adolescence.
- GPC symptoms and clinical findings resolve within days to weeks of removal of the source of mechanical irritation, and most patients can resume use of contact lenses if they comply with treatment and contact lens care.

Natural history of untreated disease
Not applicable for this topic (no published information).

Prognosis for treated patients
Not applicable for this topic (no published information).

Follow-up tests and monitoring
- For patients diagnosed with VKC or AKC, visual acuity should be monitored, and eyes examined for corneal involvement.
- For patients on topical corticosteroids, intraocular pressure must be measured periodically and eyes examined for development of cataracts.

Section 7: Reading list

Abelson MB, Smith L, Chapin M. Ocular allergic disease: mechanisms, disease sub-types, treatment. Ocul Surf 2003;1:127–49

Berdy GJ, Berdy SS. Ocular allergic disorders: disease entities and differential diagnoses. Curr Allergy Asthma Rep 2009;9:297–303

Bielory L. Ocular allergy overview. Immunol Allergy Clin North Am 2008;28:1–23

Kumar S. Vernal keratoconjunctivitis: a major review. Acta Ophthalmol. 2009 Mar;87(2):133-47.

Leonardi A. The central role of conjunctival mast cells in the pathogenesis of ocular allergy. Curr Allergy Asthma Rep 2002;2:325–31

Mantelli F, Lambiase A, Bonini S. A simple and rapid diagnostic algorithm for the detection of ocular allergic diseases. Curr Opin Allergy Clin Immunol 2009;9: 471

Suggested websites

American Academy of Allergy, Asthma and Immunology. www.aaaai.org

American Academy of Ophthalmology. www.aao.org

Section 8: Guidelines

Not applicable for this topic.

Section 9: Evidence

Not applicable for this topic.

Section 10: Images

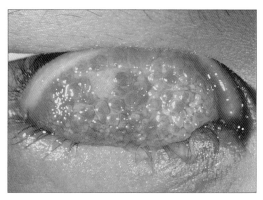

Figure 7.1 Vernal conjunctivitis – cobblestone papillae cover the superior tarsal conjunctiva. See color plate 7.1. From Rubenstein JB, Tannan A. Conjunctivitis: infectious and noninfectious. In Yanoff M, Duker JS, eds. Ophthalmology. 4th ed. St. Louis, MO, Mosby Elsevier; 2013:chap 4.6. Reproduced with permission.

Additional material for this chapter can be found online at: www.mountsinaiexpertguides.com
This includes a case study, multiple choice questions, advice for patients, and ICD codes

CHAPTER 8

Tests for Assessing Asthma

Gwen S. Skloot

Division of Pulmonary, Critical Care and Sleep Medicine, Icahn School of Medicine at Mount Sinai, New York, NY, USA

OVERALL BOTTOM LINE

- Spirometry before and after inhalation of a short-acting bronchodilator is the main test to diagnose and monitor asthma.
- Spirometry should be performed at initial evaluation and repeated after the patient is considered "stabilized" on therapy, during periods of loss of asthma control, or at a minimum of every 1–2 years.
- Measurement of peak expiratory flow at home is a helpful adjunct to monitor asthma.
- Other tests to consider when the diagnosis of asthma is in question include lung volume and gas exchange measurements, bronchoprovocation, allergy skin testing, and chest radiograph.
- Biomarkers of inflammation should be considered both for diagnostic and monitoring purposes.

Section 1: Background

- Tests for assessing asthma are important in the diagnosis and ongoing monitoring of the asthmatic patient. Understanding the tests that are available, when they should be performed, and the information that can be gleaned from them is crucial to the clinician.
- Asthma is a chronic inflammatory disorder of the airways characterized by airway obstruction that is generally reversible and by hyperresponsiveness to a variety of stimuli.
- Tests such as spirometry pre- and post-bronchodilator can provide information about a patient that is both diagnostic and prognostic over time.
- Bronchoprovocation tests are most useful in excluding a diagnosis of asthma.
- At times, it is necessary to obtain full pulmonary function testing to exclude entities such as emphysema, other obstructive lung diseases, diseases that may present with obstruction or restriction (e.g. sarcoidosis), or vocal cord dysfunction.
- Chest radiographs and allergy skin tests can be helpful adjuncts to testing when assessing a difficult patient.
- Biomarkers of inflammation are the newest tests to be introduced and while they are being used more often to both diagnose asthma and monitor response to therapy, they have not yet been fully implemented in clinical practice.
- Home peak flow monitoring can be part of a patient's asthma action plan and a useful adjunct to care.

Mount Sinai Expert Guides: Allergy and Clinical Immunology, First Edition. Edited by Hugh A. Sampson.
© 2015 John Wiley & Sons, Ltd. Published 2015 by John Wiley & Sons, Ltd.
Companion website: www.mountsinaiexpertguides.com

Section 2: Prevention

- Although current asthma therapy initiated early in life can impact symptoms and even reduce airflow limitation, there is no evidence that it can prevent accelerated loss of lung function in those who are destined to have severe disease.

Section 3: Diagnosis

- Spirometry is an important test in the diagnosis of asthma as well as for ongoing monitoring of asthma patients. Typical spirometry measurements include the maximal volume of air forcibly exhaled after a deep inspiration to total lung capacity (i.e. the forced vital capacity, FVC), the volume of air exhaled during the first second of the maneuver (i.e. forced expiratory volume in 1 second, FEV_1) and the ratio of these two parameters (i.e. FEV_1/FVC). In asthma, a reduction in the FEV_1/FVC is the hallmark of an obstructive pattern (Figure 8.1A).
- Patients with asthma generally demonstrate reversible airways obstruction following administration of a short-acting bronchodilator (e.g. albuterol) (Figure 8.1B) with an increase in either the FEV_1 or FVC of ≥200 mL and ≥12% from baseline. It is important to recognize that the bronchodilator response may vary from day to day or in response to therapy so that a single test result should never be used to exclude the diagnosis. Also, reversible airways obstruction is not specific for asthma so that the finding should be interpreted in the context of the clinical presentation. Spirometry should be performed at initial evaluation and repeated after the patient is considered "stabilized" on therapy, during periods of loss of asthma control, or at a minimum of every 1–2 years.
- When the diagnosis of asthma is uncertain, additional testing may be necessary. Bronchoprovocation, most commonly with methacholine (i.e. an agent that directly causes airway smooth muscle constriction by stimulation of acetylcholine receptors), should be considered mainly when the diagnosis of asthma is questionable and spirometry is normal. The test is conducted by administering serially increasing concentrations of inhaled methacholine until there is at least a 20% decrease in FEV_1 from baseline or the patient has received the highest concentration of methacholine permitted. A negative methacholine test rules out asthma with a high degree of certainty. A positive test, while not specific for the diagnosis of asthma, can quantify the degree of airway hyper-responsiveness.
- Other important diagnostic testing includes complete lung function assessment such as lung volume measurements (i.e. to assess for concurrent "restriction" or hyperinflation and/or air trapping), diffusing capacity (i.e. generally reduced in emphysema), and inspiratory flow volume loops (i.e. may be abnormal in cases of vocal cord dysfunction). A chest radiograph can help eliminate other pulmonary diseases that can present with obstruction on spirometry (e.g. bronchiectasis, sarcoidosis).
- The use of biomarkers of inflammation is gaining increasing interest as an adjunct to asthma assessment. Fractional exhaled nitric oxide (i.e. FeNO) is a simple test believed to reflect the degree of eosinophilic inflammation of the bronchial mucosa. Along with measurements of eosinophils in the sputum, the FeNO test can assist in asthma diagnosis.

Section 4: Treatment

- Treatment recommendations for asthma are based, in part, on objective testing results in conjunction with frequency of symptoms, exacerbations, and rescue inhaler use. The degree of spirometric impairment (i.e. assessment of FEV_1 and FEV_1/FVC) is one important determinant of

Table 8.1 Classifying asthma severity and initiating treatment in youths ≥12 years of age and adults. Assessing severity and initiating treatment for patients who are not currently taking long-term medications. The table demonstrates that spirometric impairment is an important determinant of asthma severity.

Components of Severity		Classification of asthma severity ≥12 years of a age			
		Intermittent	Persistent		
			Mild	Moderate	Severe
Impairment Normal FEV₁/FVS: 8–19yr 85% 20–39yr 80% 40–59yr 75% 60–80yr 70%	Symptoms	≤2 days/week	>2 days/week but not daily	Daily	Throughout the day
	Nighttime awakenings	≤2×/month	3–4×/month	>1×/week but not nightly	Often 7×/week
	Short-acting beta₂-agonist (not prevention of EIB)	≤2 days/week	>2 days/week but not daily, and not more than 1× on any day	Daily	Several times per day
	Interference with normal activity	None	Minor limitation	Some limitation	Extremely limited
	Lung function	• Normal FEV₁ between exacerbations • FEV₁ >80% predicted • FEV₁/FVC normal	• FEV₁ >80% predicted • FEV₁/FVC normal	• FEV₁ >60% but <80% predicted • FEV₁/FVC reduced >5%	• FEV₁ <60% predicted • FEV₁/FVC reduced >5%
Risk	Exacerbations requiring oral systemic corticosteroids	0–1/year (see note)	≥2/year (see note) ← Consider severity and interval since last exacerbation. →		
		Note: Frequency and severity may fluctuate over time for patients in any severity category. Relative annual risk of exacerbations may be related to FEV₁.			
Recommended Step for Initiating Treatment		Step 1	Step 2	Step 3	Step 4 or 5
				and consider short course of oral systemic corticosteroids	
		Note: In 2–6 weeks, evaluate level of asthma control that is achieved and adjust therapy accordingly.			

Source: The National Heart Lung and Blood Institute (NHLBI), National Asthma Education and Prevention Program, Expert Panel Report 3: Guidelines for the Diagnosis and Management of Asthma, 2007, p. 344.

asthma severity (Table 8.1). Asthma severity, in turn, is the foundation for the stepwise approach to asthma management and choice of specific therapy.

- Peak flow monitoring can be helpful as a home tool for ongoing monitoring. Daily peak flow monitoring is recommended for patients with moderate–severe persistent asthma and/or a history of severe exacerbations. Peak flow monitoring comprises an important part of an action plan that can alert the patient and physician to early changes in lung function that require treatment or a change in treatment.
- FeNO should be considered, in addition to standard testing, to assess response to asthma therapy and to assist in decisions regarding titration of inhaled corticosteroid dose.

Section 5: Special populations
Not applicable for this topic.

Section 6: Prognosis
- The degree of severity of spirometric obstruction portends the risk of future asthma exacerbations and is important in determining prognosis. The severity of spirometric abnormality is assessed by comparing the patient's results to reference values based on demographic factors such as age, height, gender, and race.
- Patients with the greatest degree of reversibility in terms of response to bronchodilator may be at the greatest risk for developing fixed airflow obstruction and accelerated loss of lung function.
- Although lung function declines in all adults as a result of aging, adults with asthma demonstrate greater declines, on average, than non-smoking, non-asthmatic adults.

Section 7: Reading list

Crapo RO, Casaburi R, Coates AL, Enright PL, Hankinson JL, Irvin CG, et al. Guidelines for methacholine and exercise challenge testing 1999. Am J Respir Crit Care Med 2000;161:309–29

Dweik RA, Boggs PB, Erzurum SC, Irvin CG, Leigh MW, Lundberg JO, et al. An official ATS Clinical Practice Guideline: interpretation of exhaled nitric oxide levels (FENO) for clinical applications. Am J Respir Crit Care Med 2011;184:602–15

Miller MR, Hankinson J, Brusasco V, Burgos F, Casaburi R, Coates A, et al. Standardisation of spirometry. Eur Respir J 2005;26:319–38

National Heart Lung and Blood Institute (NHLBI). National Asthma Education and Prevention Program, Expert Panel Report 3: Guidelines for the Diagnosis and Management of Asthma, 2007

Pellegrino R, Viegi G, Brusasco V, Crapo RO, Burgos F, Casaburi R, et. al. Interpretative strategies for lung function tests. Eur Respir J 2005;26:948–68

Suggested websites
This is the official site of the American Thoracic Society that provides a link to all pertinent consensus statements. www.thoracic.org

This is the official site of the National Heart, Lung and Blood Institute. The site provides access to the guidelines for the diagnosis and management of asthma including updates on selected topics. http://www.nhlbi.nih.gov/guidelines/asthma/index.htm

Section 8: Guidelines
International society guidelines

Guideline title	Guideline source, comment	Date
Global Initiative for Asthma: Global Strategy for Asthma Management and Prevention, revised 2014	Global Initiative for Asthma Report **Comment:** The report includes clinical practice guidelines for the diagnosis and management of asthma.	2014 (http://www.ginasthma.org/ documents/4)
Expert Panel Report 3: Guidelines for the Diagnosis and Management of Asthma	The National Heart, Lung and Blood Institute (NHLBI), National Asthma Education and Prevention Program **Comment:** The guidelines include sections on recommended testing for asthma diagnosis and management	2007 (http://www.nhlbi.nih.gov/files/ docs/guidelines/asthgdln.pdf)

Section 9: Evidence
Not applicable for this topic.

Section 10: Images

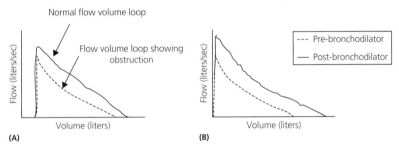

Figure 8.1 (A) shows the exhalation portion of a flow volume loop and demonstrates an obstructive pattern in contrast to normal spirometry. In obstruction, there is "scooping" of the descending limb of the flow volume loop attributable to a decrease in the FEV_1/FVC ratio. (B) demonstrates that in asthma, obstruction is generally reversible in response to bronchodilator. In the figure, there is less "scooping" post-bronchodilator and increase in flows. The increase in volume noted corresponds to an increase in forced vital capacity (FVC).

Additional material for this chapter can be found online at: www.mountsinaiexpertguides.com
This includes a case study, multiple choice questions, advice for patients, and ICD codes

CHAPTER 9

Asthma in Infants and Children

Kate Welch[1] and Jennifer S. Kim[2]
[1]Icahn School of Medicine at Mount Sinai, New York, NY, USA
[2]NorthShore University HealthSystem, Evanston, IL, USA

OVERALL BOTTOM LINE
- One of the most common chronic illnesses of childhood, asthma is an airway disorder characterized by reversible airway obstruction, bronchial hyper-responsiveness, and underlying inflammation.
- A careful history and physical examination must be undertaken, given the broad differential diagnosis of wheezing in an infant or young child and their inability to participate in formal testing.
- Multiple trigger factors exist and range from irritants and specific allergens to exercise or viral infections.
- Treatment of asthma is based on assessment of disease severity and on routine and periodic assessment of asthma control.

Section 1: Background

Definition of disease
- Asthma is a chronic inflammatory disease of the airways that is characterized by variable symptoms of airflow obstruction and bronchial hyper-responsiveness.
- The hallmark symptoms of cough and wheeze fluctuate but can be managed with anti-inflammatory drugs such as inhaled corticosteroids.

Disease classification
- Asthma is generally classified by the degree of severity, which is assessed by measurement of asthma control and the need to step-up or step-down therapies.
- Alternatively, asthma can be classified based on symptom triggers, and whether they fall into the broad categories of irritant, allergen, viral, or exercise-induced.

Incidence/prevalence
- The prevalence of childhood asthma varies in different countries and ranges from 1 to 18%; asthma affects more than 7 million children in the United States.
- Of children who have asthma, 50–80% develop symptoms before their fifth birthday.
- In early life, asthma is more prevalent in boys; after puberty, asthma affects more women.

Mount Sinai Expert Guides: Allergy and Clinical Immunology, First Edition. Edited by Hugh A. Sampson.
© 2015 John Wiley & Sons, Ltd. Published 2015 by John Wiley & Sons, Ltd.
Companion website: www.mountsinaiexpertguides.com

Economic impact

- According to the Centers for Disease Control and Prevention (CDC), the total economic impact of asthma in school-age children is roughly $2 billion per year, which includes direct medical expenditures, such as medications, inpatient hospitalizations, outpatient care, and emergency room visits, as well as parents' loss of productivity from asthma-related school absenteeism.

Etiology

- Asthma results from a complex interplay between genetic and environmental factors leading to an altered immune response.

Pathology/pathogenesis

- Asthma in patients of all ages is an inflammatory process. There is a characteristic interplay between inflammatory cells and mediators, as well as with IgE production in allergy-related disease.
- In asthmatics, a shift toward the Th2-cytokine profile results in eosinophilic inflammation and production of Th2 cytokines (IL-4, IL-5, and IL-13). Mast cells also have a role in bronchoconstriction via release of histamine, prostaglandins, and other mediators. Increased numbers of eosinophils in asthmatic airways induce inflammatory enzymes and cytokines. Macrophages can be activated by allergens to release inflammatory mediators and cytokines. Mast cells, lymphocytes, basophils, and dendritic cells have high-affinity IgE receptors which, when activated, initiate bronchospasm and promote airway inflammation.
- The "hygiene hypothesis" has gained much attention as a means to explain the shift toward a Th2 phenotypic profile and away from a Th1 profile. Several factors are thought to influence this shift: widespread use of antibiotics, Western lifestyle, urban environment, diet, and sensitization to dust mite and cockroach.
- The genetics of asthma are not clearly understood, although there is clearly a heritable component to the disease, as family history is the strongest risk factor.

Predictive/risk factors

- *Environmental factors* have a key role in the development and persistence of allergic symptoms.
- *Respiratory tract infections* are a classic trigger, especially in young children. Respiratory syncytial virus (RSV), influenza virus, and rhinovirus are common triggers, particularly in children younger than 3 years. Approximately 40% of children admitted with RSV will develop asthma later in childhood.
- *Allergens,* both indoor and outdoor, are important triggers of childhood asthma. Roughly 80% of children with asthma have concurrent allergies.
- *Other irritant exposures* include tobacco smoke, air pollution, perfumes, and propellant cleaning products.
- *Exercise-induced bronchospasm* occurs in up of 90% of children with asthma.

Section 2: Prevention

- There are no clear interventions to prevent the development of the disease.

Screening

Not applicable for this topic.

Primary prevention

Not applicable for this topic.

Secondary prevention
- Inhaled corticosteroids are the treatment of choice, adherence to which can prevent or reduce exacerbation rates.
- Allergens and irritants that worsen asthma should be controlled or eliminated from the environment.
- Written asthma management plans can help ensure proper and timely management of symptoms.

Section 3: Diagnosis

BOTTOM LINE/CLINICAL PEARLS
- A history of coughing or wheezing in an infant or child should prompt an investigation for asthma carefully considering a broad list of differential diagnoses.
- Examination findings during an exacerbation classically include wheezing and prolonged expiratory phase on auscultation, as well as a dry cough or tachypnea. Signs of associated atopic conditions may be present.
- Spirometry can be used to diagnose airflow obstruction in older children.

Differential diagnosis
- The differential diagnosis for both cough and wheeze must be considered in the infant or child presenting with asthma-like symptoms.
- In addition to a lack of response to asthma medications, the features in the differential diagnosis box may be seen.

Typical presentation
- As many as 80% of children with asthma will develop symptoms before their fifth birthday. Parents may note an increase in respiratory symptoms at night-time or a variation in symptoms with relatively quiet periods interspersed with exacerbations triggered by upper respiratory infections (URIs), exercise, weather or allergens.

Differential diagnosis	Features
Viral bronchiolitis	Viral prodrome, rhinitis
Foreign body aspiration	Acute onset
Cystic fibrosis	Failure to thrive and evidence of malabsorption
Swallowing dysfunction or gastroesophageal reflux	Symptoms usually exacerbated by eating
Vascular ring	May have persistent wheeze; usually exaggerated by position
Immunodeficiency	Recurrent infections
Vocal cord dysfunction	Inspiratory stridor, no nocturnal symptoms

Clinical diagnosis
History
- According to Expert Panel recommendations, the clinician should determine that:
  - Episodic symptoms of airflow obstruction are present;
  - Airflow obstruction is at least partially reversible; and
  - Alternative diagnoses are excluded.
- The clinician should enquire about cough, wheeze, difficulty breathing, and complaints of chest tightness.

- Identification of exacerbating factors should be elicited, including URIs, environmental allergens (animal dander, dust mites, cockroaches, pollen, mold), exercise, smoke or other airborne chemical irritants, changes in weather, or emotional expression (such as crying or laughing).
- The clinician should also ask whether symptoms occur nocturnally (while asleep).

Physical examination
- Physical examination is normal when the patient is not experiencing an exacerbation.
- During an acute exacerbation, tachypnea, coughing, wheezing, accessory muscle use, retractions, and a prolonged expiratory phase may be present.
- Associated atopic conditions may be present on examination and include atopic dermatitis or evidence of allergic rhinitis.

Disease severity classification
- *Asthma severity* is based on impairment as well as risk.
- *Impairment* takes into account frequency of symptoms, night-time awakenings, short-acting beta-2-agonist use, interference with normal activity, as well as baseline lung function, if known.
- *Risk* is based on the number of exacerbations requiring oral steroids.
- Severity is assigned based on the most severe category in which any feature occurs and is categorized as intermittent and persistent, with subcategories of persistent ranging from mild to moderate to severe.

Useful clinical decision rules and calculators
- Standard algorithms exist for assessing asthma severity (see Table 9.1).

Laboratory diagnosis
List of diagnostic tests
- There is no laboratory test to diagnose asthma. However, there are studies that can be considered in ruling out other conditions or in establishing comorbid disease.
  - Allergy testing, via skin prick testing or serum-specific IgE levels, is helpful in identifying environmental triggers, such as cockroach, dust mite, animal dander, and mold.
  - Pollens, while possible triggers for older children, are unusual triggers for infants and very young children.
  - Sweat, chloride testing for cystic fibrosis should be performed in children with frequent respiratory complaints, recurrent pneumonias, or nasal polyps.

Lists of imaging techniques
- Spirometry is recommended by the National Asthma Education and Prevention Program in patients 5 years of age and older if a diagnosis of asthma is suspected.
  - Airflow obstruction is defined as forced expiratory volume in 1 second (FEV_1) below 80% predicted and an FEV_1/FVC ratio of less than 85% for 8–19 year olds.
  - Reference values are based on age, height, sex, and race.
  - Pre- and post-bronchodilator administration should be performed to assess for reversibility (defined as an increase in FEV_1 greater than 12% from baseline).
- Spirometry cannot reliably be performed in children under 5 years of age. In this population, a trial of asthma medications may help to establish the diagnosis.
- A chest radiograph is recommended only in children who do not respond to initial therapy in order to identify an alternative diagnosis. Typical findings of asthma include hyperinflation, peri-bronchial thickening, and atelectasis.
- If swallowing dysfunction or aspiration are of concern, a video-fluoroscopic swallow study and/or barium swallow study may be considered.

Table 9.1 Classifying asthma severity and initiating treatment in children 5–11 years of age, who are not currently taking long-term control medication.

Components of Severity		Classification of asthma severity (5–11 years of age)			
		Intermittent	Persistent		
			Mild	Moderate	Severe
Impairment	Symptoms	≤2 days/week	>2 days/week but not daily	Daily	Throughout the day
	Nighttime awakenings	≤2 days/week	>2 days/week but not daily	>1×/week but not nightly	Throughout the day
	Nighttime awakenings	≤2×/month	3–4×/month	>1×/week but not nightly	Often 7×/week
	Short-acting beta$_2$-agonist use for symptom control (not prevention of EIB)	≤2 days/week	>2 days/week but not daily	Daily	Several times per day
	Interference with normal activity	None	Minor limitation	Some limitation	Extremely limited
	Lung function	• Normal FEV$_1$ between exacerbations • FEV$_1$ >80% predicted • FEV$_1$/FVC >85%	• FEV$_1$ = >80% predicted • FEV$_1$/FVC >80%	• FEV$_1$ =60–80% predicted • FEV$_1$/FVC =75–80%	• FEV$_1$ <60% predicted • FEV$_1$/FVC <75%
Risk	Exacerbations requiring oral systemic corticosteroids	0–1/year (see note)	≥2/year (see note) ─────────────────────────────────→ ←────── Consider severity and interval since last exacerbation. ──────→ Frequency and severity may fluctuate over time for patients in any severity category. Relative annual risk of exacerbations may be related to FEV$_1$.		
Recommended step for initiating therapy		Step 1	Step 2	Step 3, medium-dose ICS option	Step 3, medium-dose ICS option, or step 4 and consider short course of oral systemic corticosteroids
		In 2–6 weeks, evaluate level of asthma control that is achieved, and adjust therapy accordingly.			

Key: EIP, exercise-induced bronchospasm; FEV$_1$, forced expiratory volume in 1 second; FVC, forced vital capacity; ICS, inhaled corticosteroids.

Notes:
- The stepwise approach is meant to assist, not replace, the clinical decision-making required to meet individual patient needs.
- Level of severity is determined by both impairment and risk. Assess impairment domain by patient's/caregiver's recall of previous 2–4 weeks and spirometry. Assign severity to the most severe category in which any feature occurs.
- At present, there are inadequate data to correspond frequencies of exacerbations with different levels of asthma severity. In general, more frequent and intense exacerbations (e.g., requiring urgent, unscheduled care, hospitalization, or ICU admission) indicate greater underlying disease severity. For treatment purpose, patients who had ≥2 exacerbations requiring oral systemic corticosteroids in the past year may be considered the same as patients who have persistent asthma, even in the absence of impairment levels consistent with persistent asthma.

Source: Expert Panel Report 3: Guidelines for the Diagnosis and Management of Asthma Full Report 2007. National Heart, Lung, and Blood Institute. National Asthma Education and Prevention Program.

Potential pitfalls/common errors made regarding diagnosis of disease

- Classifying asthma in infants and young children poses a dilemma. Some babies and toddlers may have virus-induced wheezing but lack other atopic conditions often seen in children with asthma. These children may be labeled as having "reactive airway disease" and often outgrow the condition by 5 years of age. The diagnosis of asthma implies a chronic condition often associated with atopy, which is less likely to spontaneously resolve with age.

Section 4: Treatment

Treatment rationale

- The cornerstones of asthma treatment include inhaled corticosteroids and short- and long-acting beta-2-agonists. Short courses of systemic corticosteroids may be used for moderate to severe exacerbations.
- The goal of asthma therapy is to maintain long-term control of symptoms with the least amount of medication possible. As with the assessment of asthma severity, asthma control falls into two domains: reducing impairment and reducing risk.
  - Reducing impairment involves preventing chronic symptoms, minimizing use of short-acting rescue inhalers, and maintaining normal physical activity levels.
  - Reducing risk involves preventing recurrent exacerbations and minimizing medication side effects.
- According to Expert Panel guidelines, initiating daily long-term controller therapy in children 0–4 years of age is recommended in patients having four or more episodes of wheezing in the past year that lasted more than 1 day and affected sleep *and* who have risk factors for developing persistent asthma defined as either:
  - One of the following: parental history of asthma, a physician-diagnosis of atopic dermatitis, or evidence of sensitization to aeroallergens; *or*
  - Two of the following: evidence of sensitization to foods, >4% peripheral blood eosinophilia, or wheezing apart from colds.
- Initiating daily long-term control therapy in children 5–11 years of age is recommended for children who have persistent asthma as defined in Figure 9.1.
- Long-term control is best maintained through a well-established step-wise approach, by which the type and frequency of medications is increased when necessary and decreased when possible. Figure 9.1 shows management for children aged 5–11 years.
- Proper use and technique for medication delivery is crucial for effective and efficient treatment. Several delivery devices are available for infants and young children including an MDI plus valved holding chamber (VHC) with a face mask or a nebulizer with a face mask. Using the "blow by" technique, holding the mask or open tube near the infant's nose and mouth, is not effective. Crying decreases delivery to the lungs.

When to hospitalize

- Assessment of asthma exacerbations in infants will depend on physical examination rather than objective measurements. Use of accessory muscles, paradoxical breathing, inspiratory and expiratory wheezing, or tachypnea are signs of serious distress and should prompt emergent evaluation and likely hospitalization if response to treatment is inadequate.

Managing the hospitalized patient

- A patient who does not respond to emergency room treatments should be admitted to the hospital for administration of scheduled bronchodilators, steroids, and close monitoring. Serial physical examinations as well as peak flow monitoring can help determine when a child is back to baseline.
- Those children with severe acute exacerbations (status asthmaticus) require admission to an ICU and consideration of positive pressure and/or mechanical ventilation.

Table of treatment

The following long-term control medications are approved by the FDA for young children:
- ICS budesonide nebulizer solution (approved for children 1–8 years of age).
- ICS fluticasone DPI (approved for children 4 years of age and older).
- Combination product of long-acting inhaled beta2-agonist (LABA) salmeterol and fluticasone DPI (approved for children 4 years of age and older).
- LTRA montelukast, based on safety data rather than efficacy data, in a 4 mg chewable tablet (approved for children 2–6 years of age) and in 4 mg granules (approved down to 1 year of age).
- Cromolyn nebulizer (approved for children ≥2 years of age).

Prevention/management of complications

- The prevention of asthma complications relies on prevention of exacerbations. This is accomplished with regular use of controller medications and avoidance of known triggers, such as allergens and irritants.
- Use of rescue medications prior to exercise is advised for children with exercise-induced asthma.
- Use of scheduled bronchodilators or inhaled steroids during URIs may be effective in preventing or ameliorating asthma exacerbations during acute respiratory illnesses.
- Regular follow-up and assessment of asthma control is essential in determining the need to step-up or the ability to step-down therapy. Office visits are usually made at 1- to 6-month intervals, depending on the degree of control.
- Once asthma symptoms are well-controlled for at least 3 months, a reduction in pharmacologic therapy ("step-down") may be attempted. If asthma is not well-controlled, a "step-up" in therapy can be undertaken, and if it is very poorly controlled, therapy can be stepped up 1–2 steps along with a possible course of oral corticosteroids.

CLINICAL PEARLS
- Remember a broad differential when assessing a child for cough or wheeze.
- Frequent monitoring is necessary to maintain a child on the lowest efficacious regimen of asthma therapy.
- Consider allergic and environmental triggers of disease.

Section 5: Special populations
Risk factors for fatal asthma

Asthma history
- Previous severe exacerbation (e.g., intubation or ICU admission for asthma).
- Two or more hospitalizations for asthma in the past year.
- Three or more ED visits for asthma in the past year.
- Hospitalization or ED visit for asthma in the past month.
- Using >2 canisters of SABA per month.
- Difficulty perceiving asthma symptoms or severity of exacerbations.
- Other risk factors: lack of a written asthma action plan, sensitivity to Alternaria.

Social history
- Low socioeconomic status or inner-city residence.
- Illicit drug use.
- Major psychosocial problems.

Comorbidities
- Cardiovascular disease.
- Other chronic lung disease.
- Chronic psychiatric disease.

Section 6: Prognosis
Natural history of untreated disease
- Without treatment, asthma can lead to complications of exacerbations that can even result in death. Even when treated, long-term studies reveal that adults with a history of severe childhood asthma have diminished pulmonary function when compared with non-asthmatic controls. However, many children with mild to moderate asthma have no residual pulmonary effects.

BOTTOM LINE/CLINICAL PEARLS
- No markers are available to predict prognosis although severe persistent asthma is less likely to resolve or be "outgrown."
- Young children with recurrent, significant episodes of wheezing who also have eczema, aeroallergen sensitivity, or a parental history of asthma are more likely to have persistent asthma after age 5 years.

Prognosis for treated patients
- Whether childhood asthma is ever completely outgrown remains controversial but remission of symptoms occurs often although the potential for airway hyper-reactivity may persist. If asthma persists into adulthood and is treated appropriately, asthma does not typically affect life expectancy in the absence of other pulmonary comorbidities.

Follow-up tests and monitoring
- Physician evaluation should occur at 1- to 6-month intervals depending on the level of control. Three-month follow-ups are generally recommended if step-down therapy is anticipated.

Section 7: Reading list

Bacharier LB, Guilbert TW. Diagnosis and management of early asthma in preschool-aged children. J Allergy Clin Immunol 2012;130:287–96

Bousquet J, Mantzouranis E, Cruz AA, Aït-Khaled N, Baena-Cagnani CE, Bleecker ER, et al. Uniform definition of asthma severity, control, and exacerbations: document presented for the World Health Organization Consultation on Severe Asthma. J Allergy Clin Immunol 2010;126:926–38

Gruchalla RS, Pongracic J, Plaut M, Evans R 3rd, Visness CM, Walter M, et al. Inner City Asthma Study: relationships among sensitivity, allergen exposure, and asthma morbidity. J Allergy Clin Immunol 2005;115:478–85

Jenkins HA, Cherniack R, Szefler SJ, Covar R, Gelfand EW, Spahn JD. A comparison of the clinical characteristics of children and adults with severe asthma. Chest 2003;124:1318–24

Michelson PH, Williams LW, Benjamin DK, Barnato AE. Obesity, inflammation, and asthma severity in childhood: data from the National Health and Nutrition Examination Survey 2001–2004. Ann Allergy Asthma Immunol 2009;103:381

Suggested websites
http://www.nhlbi.nih.gov/health-pro/guidelines/current/asthma-guidelines
http://www.cdc.gov/asthma/
www.uptodate.com

Section 8: Guidelines
National society guidelines

Guideline title	Guideline source	Date
National Asthma Education and Prevention Program: Expert Panel Report 3 (EPR3)	NIH, National Heart, Lung and Blood Institute	2007 (http://www.nhlbi.nih.gov/files/docs/guidelines/asthsumm.pdf)

Section 9: Evidence

See NIH guidelines.

Section 10: Images

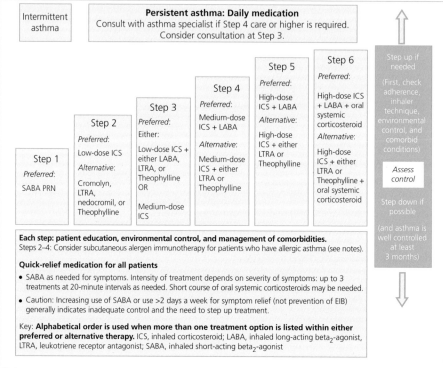

Figure 9.1 Stepwise approach for managing asthma in children 5–11 years of age. Source: Expert Panel Report 3: Guidelines for the Diagnosis and Management of Asthma Full Report 2007. National Heart, Lung, and Blood Institute. National Asthma Education and Prevention Program.

Additional material for this chapter can be found online at: www.mountsinaiexpertguides.com
This includes a case study, multiple choice questions, advice for patients, and ICD codes

CHAPTER 10

Asthma in Teenagers and Adults

Supinda Bunyavanich

Department of Pediatrics, Department of Genetics and Genomic Sciences, Icahn School of Medicine at Mount Sinai, New York, NY, USA

OVERALL BOTTOM LINE

- Asthma is a common, chronic disorder of the airways that causes wheezing, chest tightness, shortness of breath, and/or cough.
- Although much of asthma develops and occurs in childhood, a substantial number of teenagers and adults also have asthma.
- Asthma can be classified as mild intermittent, mild persistent, moderate persistent, and severe persistent asthma depending on frequency of symptoms.
- Treatment of asthma follows a stepwise approach according to severity and can include short-acting and long-acting beta-2-agonists, inhaled and oral glucocorticosteroids, mast cell stabilizers, leukotriene modifying agents, and omalizumab.
- Asthma action plans should be reviewed with patients on a regular basis, and periodic clinic visits are helpful for treatment adjustments as appropriate.

Section 1: Background

Definition of disease

- Asthma is a common, chronic disorder of the airways that is complex and characterized by variable and recurring symptoms, airflow obstruction, bronchial hyper-responsiveness, and underlying inflammation.

Disease classification

- Asthma can be classified as mild intermittent, mild persistent, moderate persistent, and severe persistent asthma depending on frequency of symptoms. Asthma may also be classified as intrinsic and extrinsic.

Incidence/prevalence

- The overall prevalence of asthma is about 8% of the US population.
- 50% of asthmatics are <5 years old.
- 33% of asthmatics are aged 15–44 years, and late-onset asthma comprises about 15% of asthmatics.

Economic impact

- Asthma costs the United States more than $30 billion every year in direct expenditure for treating asthma.

Mount Sinai Expert Guides: Allergy and Clinical Immunology, First Edition. Edited by Hugh A. Sampson.
© 2015 John Wiley & Sons, Ltd. Published 2015 by John Wiley & Sons, Ltd.
Companion website: www.mountsinaiexpertguides.com

Etiology and pathology/pathogenesis

- Much of asthma in teenagers and adults is continued childhood asthma or a relapse of earlier childhood asthma (see Chapter 9).
- New-onset asthma during adolescence or adulthood is possible.
- The complete causes of asthma are unknown.
- Genetic studies have identified genes associated with asthma, but the roles of these genes are not completely understood.

Predictive/risk factors

- Overweight.
- History of atopic dermatitis, allergic rhinitis, food allergy.
- Family history of atopy.
- Lower socioeconomic status.
- Male sex is a risk factor for asthma in childhood but there is no difference between males and females after age 30 years.
- Environmental allergen sensitization.
- Exposure to tobacco smoke.
- Exposure to pollution.
- Occupational exposure to chemicals.
- Maternal tobacco use while pregnant.
- Low birth weight.

Section 2: Prevention

- No interventions have been demonstrated to prevent the development of the disease.

Screening

Not applicable for this topic.

Primary prevention

Not applicable for this topic.

Secondary prevention

- Smoking cession by patient and household members.
- Exercise improves lung function.
- Avoidance of pollution and aeroallergens.
- Avoidance of beta-blockers, aspirin, and NSAIDs that may provoke asthma.
- Immunization for influenza reduces morbidity.

Section 3: Diagnosis

> **BOTTOM LINE/CLINICAL PEARLS**
> - Patient may report wheezing, shortness of breath, chest tightness, and/or coughing. Symptoms are often elicited by exercise, exposure to cold air or allergens, and upper respiratory infections.
> - Physical examination may show decreased breath sounds and expiratory wheezing. If the patient is not symptomatic at the time of examination, physical examination may be unremarkable.
> - Reversible obstruction on pulmonary function testing supports a diagnosis of asthma.

Differential diagnosis

Differential diagnosis	Features
Central airway obstruction	
Vocal cord dysfunction	Exercise-induced dyspnea and *inspiratory* stridor, with throat tightness during maximal exercise that resolves within 5 minutes of stopping. Common among young adult female patients. Vocal cord adduction may be observed by laryngoscopy when patient is symptomatic. Unresponsive to beta-agonist
Chronic obstructive pulmonary disease (COPD)	Chronic cough and sputum production. There is often a history of tobacco use. Daytime symptoms often worse than night-time. Chest X-ray findings. Airway obstruction not reversible on spirometry
Congestive heart failure	Exertional dyspnea, orthopnea, paroxysmal nocturnal dyspnea, productive cough. Pulmonary venous congestion, peripheral edema, improvement with heart failure therapy
Gastroesophageal reflux	Chronic cough can be an extra-esophageal symptom of GERD. Arytenoid and inter-arytenoid edema may be visible on laryngoscopy
Coronary artery disease	Patients are typically older and may demonstrate other risk factors such as hyperlipidemia and diabetes

Typical presentation

- An adult with a history of wheezing and eczema as an infant and current allergic rhinitis describes wheezing, chest tightness, and coughing during upper respiratory infections, exercise, and the spring pollen season. The cough is dry and typically worse at night. She wakes up coughing and feeling short of breath. She has poor exercise tolerance during these times. Her symptoms are better during the summer when it is warmer, the tree pollen season is over, and she has less frequent respiratory infections. Acute symptoms are improved following short-acting beta-2-agonist use.

Clinical diagnosis

History

- The clinician should take a detailed history of wheezing and previous asthma, including age of onset, past and current treatment, previous emergency department visits and hospitalizations for respiratory complaints, number of oral steroid courses previously taken for respiratory issues, and current symptoms and control (e.g. asthma control test).
- The clinician should also ask if there are respiratory symptoms that change with exertion, temperature, or time of day. The clinician should enquire whether there are any nocturnal awakenings due to cough or shortness of breath.

Physical examination

- Physical examination should include detailed examination of the ears, nose, throat, chest, heart, and extremities.
- Chest examination may reveal expiratory wheezing, prolonged expiration, and diminished breath sounds. During asthma exacerbations, the patient may be tachypneic, tachycardic, use accessory respiratory muscles, and have intercostal retraction.
- There may be no findings on examination when the patient is asymptomatic.

Useful clinical decision rules and calculators
Not applicable for this topic.

Disease severity classification
- *Mild intermittent asthma:* symptoms present for 2 days/week or less, or 2 nights/month or less.
- *Mild persistent asthma:* symptoms present for >2 days/week but less than daily, or >2 nights/month.
- *Moderate persistent asthma:* symptoms daily or more than once per night.
- *Severe persistent asthma:* symptoms throughout the day and frequent at night.

Laboratory diagnosis
List of diagnostic tests
- Peak flow rate and spirometry to assess lung function at baseline and during exacerbations.
- Exhaled nitric oxide.
- Impulse oscillometry.
- Bronchial provocation testing can be useful for difficult cases.
- Pulse oximetry may be used to assess oxygenation.
- Arterial blood gas during severe exacerbations to evaluate acid–base status and oxygenation.

Lists of imaging techniques
- Chest X-ray is helpful to assess other or additional pulmonary pathology.

Potential pitfalls/common errors made regarding diagnosis of disease
- Unremarkable physical examination, peak flow, and spirometry do not mean that the patient does not have asthma. These can all be normal when the patient is asymptomatic.

Section 4: Treatment
Treatment rationale
- The goal of treatment is to reduce impairment and reduce risk so that the patient can pursue normal activities, including regular exercise and normal work.
- Treatment follows a stepwise approach depending on asthma severity. Short-acting beta-2-agonist as needed is recommended for intermittent asthma. For more persistent disease, inhaled corticosteroids, long-acting beta-2-agonists, leukotriene-modifying agents, omalizumab, and oral corticosteroids may be considered in stepwise fashion.
- Monitoring and follow-up are essential.
- When initiating therapy, monitoring at 2–6 week intervals is recommended to ensure that asthma control is achieved. Depending on the level of control, subsequent follow-up can be at 1–6 month intervals for adjustments in therapy as needed. Step-up or step-down in treatment may occur.
- The patient should be given a written asthma action plan that details daily management as well as recommendations for therapeutic adjustments during exacerbations.

When to hospitalize
- Persistent respiratory distress unresponsive to short-acting beta-2-agonist is an indication for immediate evaluation by a health care provider. This is particularly important if the patient demonstrates ominous signs such as inability to speak or drink, use of accessory muscles of the chest, retractions, fatigue, drowsiness, confusion, cyanosis, and paradoxical abdominal movement with respiration.

Managing the hospitalized patient

- Intubation, mechanical ventilation, IV corticosteroids, and continuous albuterol nebulization should be implemented for impending or actual respiratory arrest.
- In the non-intubated patient with severe asthma exacerbation, nebulized albuterol, oxygen, systemic corticosteroids, and frequent assessments are recommended.

Table of treatment

Treatment	Comment
Conservative • Smoke-free home and workplace • Reduce allergen exposure • Regular exercise	Cigarette smoke exacerbates asthma Patients who are allergic to environmental allergens Improves lung function
Medical • Oxygen (2–4 L/min) • Short-acting beta-2-agonists • Albuterol (1.25–5 mg or 2+ puffs inhaled every 20 min–6 hours as needed)	Caution if comorbid COPD Fast-acting and relieves symptoms quickly Tachyphylaxis possible

• Long-acting beta-2-agonists:
  • Formoterol (12 µg inhaled every 12 hours)
  • Salmeterol (42–50 µg inhaled every 12 hours)
• Ipratropium (250–500 µg inhaled every 30 min–6 hours as needed)
	Often used in combination with inhaled corticosteroid as maintenance treatment
	Should not be used for acute symptoms
	Acts rapidly with minimal systemic adverse effects
	Not as effective as short-acting beta-2-agonist for acute systems

• Inhaled glucocorticosteroids (many varieties and dosing varies by specific type)	Effective for control of chronic asthma as a maintenance inhaler Minimal systemic absorption occurs Check inhaler technique to ensure drug delivery Rinse mouth after use

• Systemic glucocorticosteroids:
  • Prednisone (0.5–1 mg/kg/day PO)
  • Methylprednisolone (1.5 mg/kg IV every 8 hours)
• Mast-cell stabilizers:
  • Cromolyn sodium (2–4 puffs 4 times a day)
  • Nedocromil (2 puffs 4 times a day)
	Dose should be tailored to patient's requirements and can be tapered as patient improves
	
	Excellent safety profile
	Frequent administration may limit adherence

• Leukotriene modifying agents:
  • Montelukast (10 mg/day)
  • Zafirlukast (20 mg twice daily)
• Theophylline (dosing based on body weight and serum levels)
• Omalizumab (SC injection weight and IgE level based)
	Oral formulation, which may be preferable to patients who do not like inhalers
	
	Close monitoring of serum levels is needed to avoid toxicity
	FDA approved for individuals ≥12 years with serum IgE level 30–700 IU/mL, sensitization to a perennial aeroallergen, and symptoms inadequately controlled with inhaled steroids

• Magnesium sulfate (2 g IV over 10–15 min)	For status asthmaticus in inpatient setting

Prevention/management of complications

- Patients should be counseled on appropriate use of maintenance versus fast-acting medications for asthma control, and symptoms and signs of asthma exacerbation that necessitate urgent medical evaluation.
- Patients should review asthma action plan with their provider on a regular basis, as adherence to maintenance therapy and appropriate response to exacerbations is key to asthma control.

> **CLINICAL PEARLS**
> - The main goal of treatment is to allow patients to pursue normal activities and exercise.
> - Treatment should be stepwise according to asthma severity.
> - Patient education and adherence are key to control, and regular monitoring and asthma action plans help with this.

Section 5: Special populations

Pregnancy
- Shortness of breath during pregnancy may be due to restrictive physiology and not asthma.
- It is safer for pregnant women to be treated with asthma medications than to have asthma symptoms and exacerbations.
- Cromolyn sodium inhaler has an excellent safety profile and should be considered for prophylactic treatment before exercise.
- Budesonide is the preferred inhaled glucocorticosteroid during pregnancy.

Children
See Chapter 9.

Elderly
- Consider heart failure, coronary artery disease, COPD, parenchymal pulmonary disease in the differential diagnosis.

Section 6: Prognosis

> **BOTTOM LINE/CLINICAL PEARLS**
> - Remission from asthma is common in adolescents and young adults, but less common in older adults.
> - Patients with more severe symptoms and spirometry changes are less likely to have remission.
> - Asthmatics who smoke have the greatest decline in lung function compared to non-asthmatics and non-smoking asthmatics.

Section 7: Reading list

Bateman ED, Hurd SS, Barnes PJ, Bousquet J, Drazen JM, FitzGerald M, et al. Global strategy for asthma management and prevention: GINA executive summary. Eur Respir J 2008;31:143–78

British Thoracic Society and Scottish Intercollegiate Guidelines Network. British Guideline on the Management of Asthma. 2012. Available at: http://sign.ac.uk/guidelines/fulltext/101/

Li JT, Oppenheimer J, Bersnetin IL, Nicklas RA. Attaining optimal asthma control: a practice parameter. J Allergy Clin Immunol 2005;116: S3–11

National Heart, Lung, and Blood Institute, National Asthma Education and Prevention Program. Expert panel report 3: guidelines for the diagnosis and management of asthma. NIH publication no. 07-4051. Bethesda, Md.: National Heart, Lung, and Blood Institute; 2007:363–372. Available from: http://www.nhlbi.nih.gov/guidelines/asthma/asthgdln.pdf (accessed October 9, 2014).

Boulet LP. Diagnosis of Asthma in Adults. In Middleton's Allergy: Principles and Practice, Adkinson NF, Bochner BS, Burks AW, et al. (eds)., 8th ed. Saunders, Elsevier 2013;892–900.

Suggested websites

American Academy of Allergy, Asthma, and Immunology. http://www.aaaai.org

National Heart, Lung and Blood Institute. http://www.nhlbi.nih.gov/health/prof/lung/asthma/naci/asthma-info/asthma-guidelines.htm

Section 8: Guidelines
National society guidelines

Guideline title	Guideline source	Date
Guidelines for the Diagnosis and Management of Asthma (EPR-3)	National Heart, Lung, and Blood Institute	2007 (https://www.nhlbi.nih.gov/health-pro/guidelines/current/asthma-guidelines/index.htm)
Global strategy for asthma management and prevention	Global Initiative for Asthma (GINA) and National Heart, Lung, and Blood Institute	2008 (http://www.ginasthma.org/documents/4)
British Guideline on the Management of Asthma.	British Thoracic Society and Scottish Intercollegiate Guidelines Network	2012 (http://sign.ac.uk/guidelines/fulltext/101/)

Section 9: Evidence

See guidelines listed in Section 8.

Section 10: Images

Not applicable for this topic.

Additional material for this chapter can be found online at:
www.mountsinaiexpertguides.com
This includes a case study, multiple choice questions, advice for patients, and ICD codes

CHAPTER 11

Evaluation of Cough

Paula J. Busse

Department of Medicine, Division of Clinical Immunology, Icahn School of Medicine at Mount Sinai, New York, NY, USA

OVERALL BOTTOM LINE

- Patient history is critical to determine the etiology of cough and should address recent respiratory infections, smoking history, use of angiotension-converting enzyme inhibitors (ACE-I), history of childhood or present asthma, history of symptoms of allergic rhinitis, and whether the patient is immunocompromised.
- The most common causes of cough are due to upper airway syndrome (i.e. post-nasal drip), asthma, and gastroesophageal reflux disease (GERD).
- For patients with subacute and chronic cough, without a recent history of infection or identifiable etiology of cough, an empiric trial to treat upper airway syndrome is the initial step for diagnosis and management.
- If there is no improvement in cough after treatment for upper airway syndrome, spirometry should be obtained.
- A chest radiograph should be obtained in adults whose cough persists for longer than 8 weeks.

Section 1: Background

Definition of disease

- Cough is one of the most common presenting complaints for adults in the primary care setting and is associated with significant impact on quality of life. There are several disorders that can produce cough, and it is a diagnostic challenge that often requires a multidisciplinary approach.

Disease classification

- *Acute cough:* lasting <3 weeks.
- *Subacute cough:* 3–8 weeks' duration.
- *Chronic cough:* >8 weeks' duration.

Incidence/prevalence

- Cough is a frequent reason for seeking medical advice. Evaluation of cough is frequent: over 30 million outpatient visits occur per year in the United States for evaluation of cough.

Mount Sinai Expert Guides: Allergy and Clinical Immunology, First Edition. Edited by Hugh A. Sampson.
© 2015 John Wiley & Sons, Ltd. Published 2015 by John Wiley & Sons, Ltd.
Companion website: www.mountsinaiexpertguides.com

Economic impact
- Cost of treating cough exceeds several billion dollars annually on a global basis.

Etiology
- Upper airway cough syndrome (UACS; e.g. allergic rhinitis, irritant rhinitis).
- Airway disease (e.g. asthma, chronic bronchitis, bronchiectasis).
- GERD and laryngopharyngeal reflux.
- Current or recent respiratory tract infections.
- Medication side effects (ACE-I).
- Disease of pulmonary parenchyma (e.g. interstitial lung disease).
- Rare causes (recurrent aspiration, tracheobronchomalacia, laryngeal sensory neuropathy, tonsillar enlargement, irritation of external auditory canal, premature ventricular contractions).
- Psychogenic.

Pathology/pathogenesis
- Cough is produced via stimulation of the cough reflex arc.
- Irritation of cough receptors by chemical irritants (i.e. acid, cold, capasaicin-like compounds) or mechanical factors (i.e. touch or displacement) trigger activation of transient receptor potential vanilloid type 1 and transient receptor potential ankyrin type 1 receptors.
- Activation of these receptors travel via an afferent pathway to the "cough center" in the medulla, which stimulates an efferent signal to the vagus, phrenic, and spinal motor nerves to produce a cough.

Predictive/risk factors
- Smoking history.
- Genetic factors: determine risk of asthma inception and development of allergen sensitization.
- ACE-I.
- Immunosuppression.
- Occupational history.

Section 2: Prevention

> **BOTTOM LINE/CLINICAL PEARLS**
> - Prevention of cough depends upon its etiology.
> - Avoidance of cigarette smoke is most likely the most obtainable method to prevent cough in some subjects.

Screening
Not applicable for this topic.

Primary and secondary prevention
Not applicable for this topic.

Section 3: Diagnosis

> **BOTTOM LINE/CLINICAL PEARLS**
> - Obtain history of recent respiratory tract infections, whether the patient is immunosuppressed, use of ACE-I, smoking, symptoms of allergic rhinitis, GERD.
> - If patient history does not suggest etiology, empiric treatment with a daily intranasal corticosteroid to address UACS is warranted. If there is no improvement after 2–3 weeks, spirometry with pre- and post-bronchodilator response, lung volumes, diffusion capacity should be obtained. If obstruction is not found, methacholine challenge may be indicated.
> - If cough is present >8 weeks, a chest radiograph should be obtained.
> - Esophageal pH monitoring is indicated if therapeutic trials to treat GERD are ineffective.

Differential diagnosis

Differential diagnosis	Features
Upper airway cough syndrome	Frequent nasal discharge, sensation of liquid dripping into back of throat, frequent throat clearing. On examination, cobblestone appearance of nasopharyngeal mucosa and secretions in the nasopharynx
ACE-I induced	Usually begins within 1 week of starting medication and will resolve approximately 1 month after discontinuation
Chronic bronchitis/ obstructive lung disease	Productive cough (clear or white sputum) for most days over a 3-month time period. Frequently associated with smoking history
Lung cancer	Smoking history. Hemoptysis. Pulmonary examination potentially with decreased breath sounds if focal airway obstruction present
Viral infection	Common cause of acute cough
Pertussis	Persistent cough (several weeks to months) with paroxysms
GERD	Cough may be the only symptom of reflux in up to 40% of patients with cough secondary to GERD
Tuberculosis	Chronic cough with sputum production, hemoptysis, fever, weight loss. At-risk populations (e.g. human immunodeficiency virus-seropositive or homeless)
Anatomic abnormalities	e.g. Retrotracheal mass, tracheobronchomalacia
Psychogenic or habitual	Diagnosis of exclusion. Failure to cough during sleep does not exclude this condition
Bronchiectasis	Usually a productive cough that is mucopurulent. High-resolution CT required for diagnosis
Asthma	Airway hyper-responsiveness (AHR), airway inflammation, reversible airway obstruction
Non-asthmatic eosinophilic bronchitis	Elevated sputum eosinophilia. No AHR demonstrated

Typical presentation
- The presentation of cough may be influenced by the underlying etiology.
- Patients with cough secondary to upper airway syndrome frequently have complaints of post-nasal drip or secretions in the back of the throat.

- Cough secondary to asthma should be considered when cough is worse at night and exacerbated by cold air, upper respiratory tract infection, exercise, or pollen exposure.
- Patients with cough secondary to GERD may complain of heartburn or a sour taste in their mouth, but these symptoms may not be present.
- After resolution of an upper respiratory infection, some patients will experience a prolonged cough (post-infectious cough).

Clinical diagnosis

History

- The evaluation of cough includes a thorough history, including smoking status, medication use, history of asthma (past and present), symptoms of allergic rhinitis, occupational exposures, evaluation of immunocompetence, current or recent respiratory tract infections.

Physical examination

- *Nose:* evaluate for pale and swollen turbinates (allergic rhinitis).
- *Throat:* evaluate for cobblestone appearance of oropharyngeal mucosa and mucus in the oropharynx (UACS), tonsillar enlargement.
- *Respiratory:* evaluate for expiratory wheezes and/or wheezing (asthma), bilateral rhonchi or crackles (may suggest bronchiectasis).
- *Extremities:* clubbing and cyanosis.

Laboratory diagnosis

List of diagnostic tests

- *Spirometry:* used to evaluate airway obstruction (asthma or chronic obstructive pulmonary disease, COPD) and if it is reversible after administration of a bronchodilator (asthma).
- *Lung volumes:* determination of air trapping (obstructive lung disease) or airway restriction (interstitial lung disease).
- *Diffusion capacity for carbon monoxide (DLCO):* to distinguish airway obstruction from asthma (DLCO normal or increased) versus COPD (DLCO decreased).
- *Methacholine challenge:* if asthma is suspected, but spirometry does not demonstrate airway obstruction (see Chapter 8).
- *Twenty-four hour esophageal manometry:* determination of GERD.
- *IgE sensitization:* to determine if a patient may have a component of allergic rhinitis (can be done by serum or skin prick testing) (see Procedures section of Chapter 37).
- *Direct laryngoscopic evaluation:* arytenoid erythema and edema suggest laryngeal and pharyngeal reflux.

Lists of imaging techniques

- *Chest X-ray:* persistent cough >8 weeks.
- *High-resolution CT of chest:* persistent cough >8 weeks and if above diagnostic tests and empiric treatments have not identified an etiology.

Potential pitfalls/common errors made regarding diagnosis of disease

- Cough may be the only symptom of asthma in some patients (e.g. cough-variant asthma).
- Symptoms of GERD and post-nasal drip may be absent and cough may be the only symptom.
- Treatment of acute cough secondary to viral infection using antihistamine therapy is not effective.

Section 4: Treatment

Treatment rationale

- Acute cough rarely requires therapy.
- Treatment of subacute and chronic cough involves empiric therapy for the most common causes, treating one potential etiology at a time.
- If cough does not improve with the specific therapy, treatment of the next potential etiology should be pursued.

Table of treatment

Treatment	Comments
Conservative	Most appropriate for acute cough and post-infectious cough Lifestyle modifications for GERD (e.g. weight loss, elevation of head of bed, avoidance of acidic foods, coffee and eating meals 2–3 hours before bed)
Medical • Intranasal corticosteroids (see Chapter 4) • Acid-suppression medications • β-agnostics (see Chapter 10) • Inhaled corticosteroids (and possible addition of long-acting beta-agonists) (see Chapter 10) • Antitussive agents	Patient needs to use on a daily basis; may take 2 weeks to notice improvement Begin proton pump inhibitor (PPI) at moderate dose; may take up to 8 weeks to notice improvement Needed by all patients with asthma for acute rescue For patients with persistent asthma Limited efficacy
Surgical • Nissen fundoplication for GERD	Improvement of symptoms variable

Prevention/management of complications

- *Intranasal corticosteroids:* minimal risk of glaucoma and cataracts (patients should have yearly eye examinations), nasal bleeding (proper teaching of administration may reduce risk).
- *Oral corticosteroids:* risk of adrenal suppression, mood changes, care in diabetics to manage blood glucose level, decreased bone mineral density.
- *Acute cough:* usually associated with the common cold, but occasionally it can be associated with potentially life-threatening conditions (e.g. pulmonary emboli, congestive heart failure). The first step is to evaluate if acute cough is secondary to one of these conditions and treat appropriately. Otherwise, acute cough can be managed conservatively (Algorithm 11.1).
- *Subacute cough:* the initial step in determining treatment for subacute cough is assessing whether the cough follows a respiratory infection. If there is a concern for *Bordetella pertussis* (i.e. whooping cough), a nasopharyngeal swab for culture should be performed and, if positive, treatment with a macrolide antibiotic. In some patients with cough that persists after a respiratory tract infection, treatment with an inhaled corticosteroid for 30 days should be considered. If the cough is not likely post-infectious, management should be the same as for chronic cough (Algorithm 11.2).

Algorithm 11.1 Diagnosis of acute cough for patients ≥15 years of age with cough lasting <3 weeks

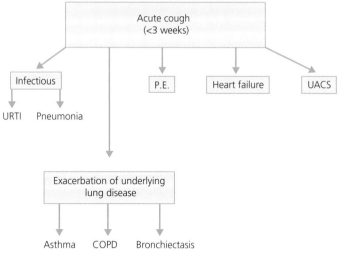

Note: COPD, chronic obstructive pulmonary disease; PE, pulmonary embolism; UACS, upper airway cough syndrome; URTI, upper respiratory tract infection.

Algorithm 11.2 Diagnosis of subacute cough for patients ≥15 years of age with cough lasting 3–8 weeks

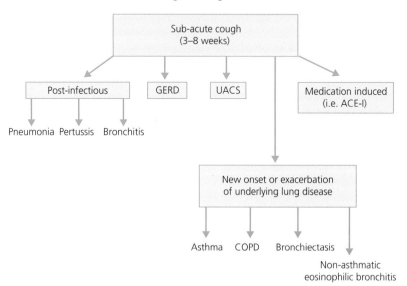

Note: ACE-I, ACE inhibitor; GERD, gastroesophageal reflux disease.

Algorithm 11.3 Diagnosis of chronic cough algorithm for patients ≥15 years of age with cough lasting >8 weeks

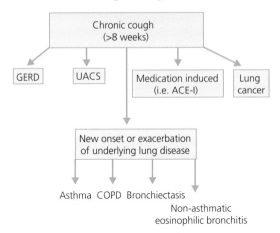

- *Chronic cough:* may be caused by more than one condition. If the etiology is not apparent by history, a sequential and empiric treatment approach is recommended (Algorithm 11.3). In these instances, treatment of the most common etiologies of cough should be addressed as follows:
  - *UACS:* 2-week daily intranasal corticosteroids; patients should be educated that an effect may not be seen before this time (see Chapter 4);
  - *Asthma:* See Chapter 10;
  - *Non-asthmatic eosinophilic bronchitis:* inhaled corticosteroids; and
  - *GERD:* PPI if treatment failure, 24-hour pH monitoring.

If there is partial, but not complete response to therapy, pursuing other etiologies is recommended, which may include the addition of other medications and diagnostic testing.

CLINICAL PEARLS
- The initial step in management of cough is to identify whether patients are immunosuppressed, smokers, or have an emergent condition, which needs to be addressed (e.g. pulmonary emboli, pulmonary edema; more typical of acute cough).
- The most effective approach to treatment of cough is a systematic approach with empiric therapy and, in cases without improvement, objective testing.
- For treatment of suspected UACS, patients should receive a daily intranasal corticosteroid and be instructed that symptoms relief may take 2–3 weeks to begin after initiating daily nasal steroid use.

Section 5: Special populations
Pregnancy
Not applicable for this topic.

Children

- The most common causes of cough in children are asthma, respiratory tract infections, and GERD.
- Foreign body aspiration should be considered as a cause of cough in young children.
- Congenital abnormalities are occasionally a cause of cough in children.

Elderly

Not applicable for this topic.

Others

Not applicable for this topic.

Section 6: Prognosis

> **BOTTOM LINE/CLINICAL PEARLS**
> - Improvement of cough is highly dependent upon the etiology.
> - Complications of cough include headache, dizziness, hoarseness, musculosketal pain, urinary incontinence, and rib fractures in some patients with decreased bone density.

Section 7: Reading list

Birring SS. Controversies in the evaluation and management of chronic cough. Am J Respir Crit Care Med 2011;183:708–15

Chung KF, Pavord ID. Prevalence, pathogenesis, and causes of chronic cough. Lancet 2008;371:1364–74

Haque RA, Usmani OS, Barnes PJ. Chronic idiopathic cough: a discrete clinical entity? Chest 2005;127:1710–3

Irwin RS. Assessing cough severity and efficacy of therapy in clinical research: ACCP evidence-based clinical practice guidelines. Chest 2006;129:232S–7S

Irwin RS. Complications of cough: ACCP evidence-based clinical practice guidelines. Chest 2006;129:54S–8S

Irwin RS, Baumann MH, Bolser DC, Boulet LP, Braman SS, Brightling CE, et al. Diagnosis and management of cough executive summary: ACCP evidence-based clinical practice guidelines. Chest 2006;129:1S–23S

Irwin RS, Madison JM. The diagnosis and treatment of cough. N Engl J Med 2000;343:1715–21

Morice AH, Fontana GA, Sovijarvi AR, Pistolesi M, Chung KF, Widdicombe J, et al. The diagnosis and management of chronic cough. Eur Respir J 2004;24:481–92

Pratter MR. Chronic upper airway cough syndrome secondary to rhinosinus diseases (previously referred to as postnasal drip syndrome): ACCP evidence-based clinical practice guidelines. Chest 2006;129:63S–71S

Woodcock A, Young EC, Smith JA. New insights in cough. Br Med Bull 2010;96:61–73

Woodwell D. National Ambulatory Medical Care Survey: 1998 Summary. Hyattsville, MD: National Center for Health Statistics, 2000

Section 8: Guidelines
National society guidelines

Guideline title	Guideline source	Date
Diagnosis and management of cough executive summary: ACCP evidence-based clinical practice guidelines	American College of Chest Physicians (ACCP)	2006 (http://www.ncbi.nlm.nih.gov/pubmed/16428686)

Section 9: Evidence

See Guideline listed in Section 8.

Section 10: Images

Not applicable for this topic.

Additional material for this chapter can be found online at: www.mountsinaiexpertguides.com
This includes a case study, multiple choice questions, advice for patients, and ICD code

---

CHAPTER 12

Exercise-Induced Asthma

Supinda Bunyavanich

Department of Pediatrics, Department of Genetics and Genomic Sciences, Icahn School of Medicine at Mount Sinai, New York, NY, USA

OVERALL BOTTOM LINE

- Exercise-induced asthma is bronchoconstriction that is induced by exercise.
- Symptoms include wheezing, chest tightness, shortness of breath, and/or coughing 10–15 minutes into prolonged exercise.
- Exercise-induced bronchoconstriction may occur in patients with chronic underlying asthma or may manifest only with exercise in otherwise asymptomatic patients.
- Optimizing cardiovascular fitness, exercising in warm and humid environments, and pre-exercise warm-up can be helpful general measures.
- Symptoms can be prevented with pre-exercise inhaled short-acting beta-2-agonist or cromolyn sodium; inhaled glucocorticosteroids and leukotriene-modifying agents can also be used, but these have longer times to onset.

Section 1: Background

Definition of disease

- Exercise-induced asthma is bronchoconstriction that is triggered by exercise. The preferred term for exercise-induced asthma is exercise-induced bronchoconstriction.

Disease classification

- It is debated whether exercise-induced bronchoconstriction should be grouped as follows:
  - Exercise-induced bronchoconstriction in patients with chronic asthma;
  - Exercise-induced bronchoconstriction in athletes who do not otherwise have asthma.

Incidence/prevalence

- Of the general population, 5–20% are estimated to have exercise-induced bronchoconstriction.
- Of individuals with persistent asthma, 80–90% are thought to have some degree of exercise-induced bronchoconstriction.
- Of elite winter athletes, 30–70% have exercise-induced bronchoconstriction.

Economic impact

Not applicable for this topic.

Mount Sinai Expert Guides: Allergy and Clinical Immunology, First Edition. Edited by Hugh A. Sampson.
© 2015 John Wiley & Sons, Ltd. Published 2015 by John Wiley & Sons, Ltd.
Companion website: www.mountsinaiexpertguides.com

Etiology and pathology/pathogenesis
- Minute ventilation increases with exercise.
- Large volumes of relatively cool and dry air passing through the airways triggers:
  - Changes in airway surface osmolality;
  - Increases in leukotrienes, histamine, and interleukins in the airway;
  - Activation of peripheral Th2 lymphocytes;
  - Eosinophil influx and activation;
  - Release of neurokinins.
- These changes lead to abnormal distribution of alveolar ventilation and perfusion, arterial hypoxemia, and closure or near closure of segmental airways.

Predictive/risk factors
- Chronic asthma.
- Exercise in cold, dry environments.
- History of atopy.

Section 2: Prevention
No interventions have been demonstrated to prevent the development of the disease.

Screening
Not applicable for this topic.

Primary prevention
Not applicable for this topic.

Secondary prevention
- Exercise in warm, humid environment.
- Prophylactic treatment with short-acting beta-2-agonists.
- Prophylactic treatment with inhaled cromolyn sodium.
- Control underlying asthma.

Section 3: Diagnosis

> **BOTTOM LINE/CLINICAL PEARLS**
> - Patient may report wheezing, shortness of breath, chest tightness, and/or coughing during or following exercise.
> - They may not demonstrate any findings on examination at baseline. After 6–8 minutes of vigorous exercise, however, there may be audible wheezing and coughing.
> - An exercise challenge test, which involves monitored exercise with measurement of lung function, may show a $\geq15\%$ decrement in forced expiratory volume (FEV_1).

Differential diagnosis

Differential diagnosis	Features
Central airway obstruction	
Vocal cord dysfunction	Exercise-induced dyspnea and *inspiratory* stridor, with throat tightness during maximal exercise that resolves within 5 minutes of stopping. Common among young adult female patients. Vocal cord adduction may be observed by laryngoscopy when patient is symptomatic. Unresponsive to beta-agonist
Laryngeal dysfunction, laryngeal prolapse, and laryngomalacia	Exercise-induced *inspiratory* stridor, with throat tightness during maximal exercise that resolves within 5 minutes of stopping. Common among young adult female patients. Unresponsive to beta-agonist
Parenchymal pulmonary disease	Dyspnea may be reported during periods of rest as well. Pulmonary findings on examination and imaging. Additional symptoms depending on specific disease
Gastroesophageal reflux	Chronic cough can be an extraesophageal symptom of GERD, which exercise may exacerbate. Arytenoid and interarytenoid edema may be visible on laryngoscopy
Exercise-induced hyperventilation	Not directly from bronchial obstruction, marked by hypocapnia and abnormal ventilator homeostasis during exercise
Coronary artery disease	Patients are typically older and may demonstrate other risk factors such as hyperlipidemia and diabetes
Heart failure	Patients are typically older. Physical findings may include elevated jugular venous pulse and peripheral edema

Typical presentation

- A young adult with asthma describes wheezing, chest tightness, and coughing 10–15 minutes into prolonged exercise, especially when exercising in the cold winter air. Symptoms self-resolve within 30–90 minutes of rest. Symptoms during exercise are worse when the patient forgets to take her maintenance glucocorticosteroid inhaler and her underlying asthma is poorly controlled. Symptoms are attenuated if she takes two puffs of her inhaled short-acting beta-2-agonist inhaler before exercise.

Clinical diagnosis

History

- The clinician should take a detailed history of underlying asthma, including age of onset, past and current treatment, previous emergency department visits and hospitalizations, number of oral steroid courses previously taken, and current symptoms and control (e.g. asthma control test). The clinician should then ask if asthma symptoms are affected by exertion, and, if so, the intensity, duration, and setting of exercise. The patient should also describe if symptoms are modulated by prophylactic use of short-acting beta-2-agonist use before exercise.

Physical examination

- Physical examination should include detailed examination of the ears, nose, throat, chest, heart, and extremities. Heart and extremities may exhibit signs of heart failure and peripheral artery disease that may lend support for alternate etiologies for respiratory symptoms.

Not applicable for this topic.

Not applicable for this topic.

Laboratory diagnosis
- Exercise challenge test. According to the National Heart, Lung, and Blood Institute, this should involve exercise at 5-minute intervals for 20–30 minutes. A post-exercise decrement in FEV_1 of ≥15% compared to baseline is considered a positive result for exercise-induced bronchoconstriction. Different types, durations, and intensities of exercise as well as FEV_1 criteria have been proposed. Ideally, heart rate should reach 80–90% of predicted maximum and pulmonary function should be followed for 30 minutes after exercise.
- Lung function measurements before and after short-acting beta-2-agonist.

Not applicable for this topic.

Potential pitfalls/common errors made regarding diagnosis of disease
- Measurement of peak expiratory flow rates before and after exercise can be inaccurate. Therefore, measurement of FEV_1 before and after exercise is preferred.
- A patient may have no asthma symptoms outside of exercise and still have exercise-induced asthma.

Treatment rationale
- General and pharmacologic measures help with treatment. Good control of any underlying asthma decreases the frequency of exercise-induced bronchoconstriction. Exercising in an environment of warm, humid air also decreases symptoms, and heat exchange mask may help with this. Improving cardiovascular fitness is also helpful, as this reduces the minute ventilation required for a given level of exertion.
- Pharmacologic treatment includes use of inhaled glucocorticosteroids and leukotriene modifiers to control underlying asthma, and prophylactic treatment with inhaled short-acting beta-2-agonists and inhaled cromolyn sodium. Short-acting beta-2-agonist is helpful for symptoms once symptoms are present.

When to hospitalize
- Persistent respiratory distress unresponsive to short-acting beta-2-agonist.

Managing the hospitalized patient
See guidelines for treating acute asthma.

Table of treatment

Treatment	Comment
Conservative	
Improve cardiovascular fitness	Patients with mild symptoms
Exercise in warm and humid environments	Patients who prefer non-pharmacologic
Heat exchange mask (e.g. tie scarf or cloth loosely around nose and mouth during exercise in cold, dry air to provide local humidity and warmth for inspired air)	methods
Pre-exercise warm up for 10–15 minutes to reach 50–60% maximum heart rate	
Breathe through the nose during exercise to allow cool dry air to be humidified and warm	
Medical	
Inhaled short-acting beta-2-agonist (2 puffs 10 minutes before exercise and additionally as needed during exercise)	Peak efficacy 15–60 min, duration of action 3 hours Patients with more severe asthma may require higher doses
Inhaled cromolyn sodium (2–4 puffs 15 minutes before exercise)	Excellent safety profile with few side effects Not as effective as inhaled short-acting beta-2-agonists
Inhaled glucocorticosteroids	Effective for control of underlying asthma that may predispose toward exercise-induced bronchoconstriction Improves airway hyper-responsiveness over weeks to months
Leukotriene modifying agents	Onset within 2 hours and benefit up to 24 hours Also effective for control of underlying asthma Consider in children who exercise intermittently throughout the day

Prevention/management of complications

- Patients should be counseled on appropriate use of maintenance versus fast-acting medications for asthma control, and symptoms and signs of asthma exacerbation that necessitate urgent medical evaluation.
- Daily use of short-acting beta-2-agonists may lead to tachyphylaxis or partial loss of efficacy.

CLINICAL PEARLS
- The main goal of treatment is to allow patients to exercise safely.
- Improving cardiovascular fitness and exercising in warm, humid environments can decrease exercise-induced bronchoconstriction.
- Prophylactic use of short-acting beta-2-agonist and cromolyn sodium inhalers can be helpful.
- Short-acting beta-2-agonist (but not cromolyn sodium) inhaler is effective once exercise-induced bronchoconstriction has occurred.

Section 5: Special populations

Pregnancy

- Shortness of breath during pregnancy may be due to restrictive physiology and not exercise-induced bronchoconstriction.
- It is safer for pregnant women to be treated with asthma medications than to have asthma symptoms and exacerbations.
- Cromolyn sodium inhaler has an excellent safety profile and should be considered for prophylactic treatment before exercise.
- Budesonide is the preferred inhaled glucocorticosteroid during pregnancy.

Children

- Inhaled cromolyn sodium has an excellent safety profile and should be considered.
- Leukotriene modifying agents may be a good choice for children who exert themselves sporadically (thus making frequent prophylactic treatment impractical).

Elderly

- Consider heart failure, coronary artery disease, and parenchymal pulmonary disease in the differential diagnosis of shortness of breath during exercise.

Section 6: Prognosis

BOTTOM LINE/CLINICAL PEARLS

- With good control of underlying asthma (if it exists) and a plan for prophylactic treatment as well as management of breakthrough exercise-induced bronchoconstriction, a patient should be able to continue exercising safely.
- Patients with exercise-induced asthma do not need to avoid exercise. For example, 50% of Olympic cross-country skiers have exercise-induced bronchoconstriction and still exercise strenuously in cold, dry air.

Section 7: Reading list

Hallstrand TS. New insights into pathogenesis of exercise-induced bronchoconstriction. Curr Opin Allergy Clin Immunol 2012;12:42–8

National Heart, Lung, and Blood Institute. National Asthma Education and Prevention Program. Managing asthma long term: special situations. Expert panel report 3: guidelines for the diagnosis and management of asthma. NIH publication no. 07-4051. Bethesda, MD: National Heart, Lung, and Blood Institute; 2007: 363–372. http://www.nhlbi.nih.gov/guidelines/asthma/asthgdln.pdf (accessed October 10, 2014).

O'Byrne PM. Exercise-induced bronchoconstriction. In: UpToDate, Post TW (Ed), UpToDate, Waltham, MA. (Accessed on December 17, 2014.)

Randolph C. Diagnostic exercise challenge testing. Curr Allergy Asthma Rep 2011;11:482–90

Weiller JM, Bonini S, Coifman R, et al. American Academy of Allergy, Asthma and Immunology Work Group Report: Exercise-induced asthma. J. Allergy Clin Immunol 2007;119:1349–58

Suggested websites

American Academic of Allergy, Asthma, and Immunology. http://www.aaaai.org/conditions-and-treatments/library/asthma-library/asthma-and-exercise.aspx

American College of Sports Medicine. http://www.acsm.org/docs/brochures/exercise-induced-asthma.pdf

Section 8: Guidelines
National society guidelines

Guideline title	Guideline source	Date
Guidelines for the Diagnosis and Management of Asthma (EPR-3)	National Heart, Lung, and Blood Institute	2007 (http://www.nhlbi.nih.gov/health-pro/guidelines/current/asthma-guidelines/full-report.htm)

Section 9: Evidence
See Guidelines listed in Section 8.

Section 10: Images
Not applicable for this topic.

Additional material for this chapter can be found online at:
www.mountsinaiexpertguides.com
This includes a case study, multiple choice questions, advice for patients, and ICD codes

CHAPTER 13

Occupational Asthma

Paula J. Busse

Department of Medicine, Division of Clinical Immunology, Icahn School of Medicine at Mount Sinai, New York, NY, USA

OVERALL BOTTOM LINE
- Occupational asthma (OA) is asthma that results from exposure to agents at the workplace.
- OA is classified as either immunologically induced (produced by either high-molecular weight (HMW) or low-molecular weight agents (LMW)) or non-immunologically induced (e.g. irritant or reactive airway dysfunction syndrome, RADS).
- In patients developing late-onset asthma, the possibility of OA should be considered.
- The risk of developing OA depends upon several factors including intensity of exposure, the particular agent, atopy, cigarette smoking, and genetic predisposition.
- Continued exposure to the causative agent in patients with OA leads to a slower rate of recovery.

Section 1: Background

Definition of disease
- OA is defined as new-onset asthma (characterized by variable airway obstruction, airway hyper-responsiveness (AHR) and airway inflammation) which develops secondary to an exposure to a product present at the workplace. It must be distinguished from "work-exacerbated asthma," which is pre-existing asthma that has worsened from workplace exposure.

Disease classification
- OA is typically classified based upon the latency period between exposure and the development of symptoms, and its mechanism of onset as follows:
  - *OA due to immunological sensitizers:* has a latency period; may be IgE or non-IgE mediated;
  - *OA due to non-immunologic provocation:* usually occurs from a single exposure to an inhalation of a high concentration of an irritant gas, aerosol, or smoke (RADS) or from a single or multiple exposures to low doses of irritants. Asthma symptoms develop without a latency period.

Incidence/prevalence
- Between 10% and 25% of adult-onset asthma is attributed to OA.
- OA is one of the most common occupational lung diseases in developed countries.

Economic impact
- The total cost of OA is estimated to be > $1.6 billion per year.

Mount Sinai Expert Guides: Allergy and Clinical Immunology, First Edition. Edited by Hugh A. Sampson.
© 2015 John Wiley & Sons, Ltd. Published 2015 by John Wiley & Sons, Ltd.
Companion website: www.mountsinaiexpertguides.com

Etiology

- Over 350 agents have been identified that may cause OA. Agents that cause immunologic OA are divided into (Table 13.1):
  - High-molecular weight (HMW);
  - Low-molecular weight (LMW).
- Agents that cause non-immunologic OA include irritant gases, fumes, smoke, and aerosols (see Table 13.2).

Pathology/pathogenesis

- *Immunologically mediated:* the underlying lung pathology is similar in this form of OA as in patients with non-occupational asthma in which smooth muscle hyperplasia, subepithelial fibrosis, mucus metaplasia, epithelial desquamation are noted, along with increased eosinophilic and lymphocytic airway inflammation. Many HMW agents act as a complete antigen causing the production of specific IgE molecules; some of the LMW agents act as haptens, binding to proteins

Table 13.1 Principal agents causing immunologic occupational asthma.

Agent		Workers/Occupations at Risk
High-molecular-weight agents		
Cereals (flour)	Wheat, rye, barley, buckwheat	Millers, bakers, pastry makers
Latex	Gloves	Health care workers, laboratory technicians
Animals	Mice, rats, cows, seafood	Laboratory workers, farmers, seafood processors
Enzymes	α-Amylase, maxatase, alcalase, papain, bromelain, pancreatin	Baking products manufacture, bakers, detergent production, pharmaceutical industry, food industry
Low-molecular-weight agents		
Isocyanates	Toluene diisocyanate (TDI), methylene diphenyl-diisocyanate (MDI), hexamethylene diisocyanate (HDI)	Polyurethane production, plastic industry, molding, spray painters, insulation installers
Metals	Chromium, nickel, cobalt, platinum	Metal refinery, metal alloy production, electroplaters, welders
Biocides	Aldehydes, quaternary ammonium compounds	Health care workers, cleaners
Persulfate salts	Hair bleach	Hairdressers
Acid anhydrides	Phthalic, trimellitic, maleic, tetrachlorophthalic acids	Epoxy resin workers
Reactive dyes	Reactive black 5, pyrazolone derivatives, vinyl sulfones, carmine	Textile workers, food industry workers
Acrylates	Cyanoacrylates, methacrylates, di- and triacrylates	Manufacture of adhesives, dental and orthopedic materials, sculptured fingernails, printing inks, paints and coatings
Wood dusts	Red cedar, iroko, obeche, oak	Sawmill workers, carpenters, cabinet and furniture makers

Source: Adkinson et al. (eds). Middleton's Allergy Principles and Practice, 8th edition. Saunders, an imprint of Elsevier Inc. Reproduced with permission of Elsevier.

Table 13.2 Common causes of irritaion in various situations.

Exposure	Agent or process
Acids	Glacial acetic, sulfuric, hydrochloric, hydrofluoric
Alkali	Bleach, calcium oxide, sodium hydroxide, World Trade Center dust, air bag emissions
Gases	Chlorine, sulfur dioxide, ammonia, mustard, ozone, hydrogen sulfide, phosgene, nitrogen dioxide
Sprays	Paints, coatings
Explosion	Irritant gases, vapors, fume releases under pressure
Fire or pyrolysis	Combustion and pyrolysis products of fires, burning paint fumes, pyrolysis products of polyvinylchloride, meat-wrapping film
Confined spaces	Epichlorohydrin, acrolein, floor sealant, metal-coating remover, biocides, fumigating aerosol, cleaning aerosol sprays, mixture of drain-cleaning agents
Workplace	Glass-bottle manufacture, popcorn flavoring manufacture, second-hand tobacco smoke, chlorine gas puffs, pyrite dust explosion, locomotive and diesel exhaust, aerosols of metalworking fluids, aluminum smelting (potroom fumes), metal processing, pulp milling, shoe and leather manufacture (organic solvents), exposure to S02 from apricot sulfurization, aldehydes (formaldehyde, glutaraldehyde), biologic dusts, tunnel construction, coke oven emissions, food industry cleaners and disinfectants, chili pepper picking, cyanoacrylates

Source: Brooks SM, Bernstein IL. Irritant-induced airway disorders. Immunol Allergy Clin North Am 2011;31:747–68. Reproduced with permission of Elsevier.

to form a complete antigen to induce generation of specific IgE molecules. However, most LMW agents act via a non-IgE dependent pathway that has not been clearly established.

- *Non-immunologically mediated:* the underlying airway pathology in this subset of OA is characterized by rapid denudation of the airway mucosa with fibrinohemorrhagic exudates in the submucosa which can develop from loss of epithelial-derived relaxing factors, exposure of the nerve endings with substance P release, non-specific activation of mast cells with release of pro-inflammatory cytokines, and direct beta-2-adrenergic receptor inhibition. Subsequent regeneration of the epithelium with proliferation of the basal and parabasal cells, epithethial edema, and thickening of the airway wall develops.

Predictive/risk factors

Risk factor	Odds ratio
Sex • Male sex • Female sex	Higher in bakers, laundry workers, shoemakers and shoe repair, tanners, metal workers Higher in jewelry engravers, round-timber workers
Geographic location	Low prevalence of OA in Mediterranean and Eastern European countries
Atopy	Risk factor for developing OA due to HMW compounds
Smoking	Risk factor for OA due to some HMW agents (coffee, castor beans, shrimp and snow-crab, but not laboratory animals). Risk factor for OA due to some LMW agents (platinum RR 5, 95% CI 1.7–15.2, phthalic anhydride)

(Continued)

Risk factor	Odds ratio
Type and intensity of workplace exposure: • HMW agents (e.g. laboratory animals, latex, flour)	2–8% person-years of those exposed will develop OA
• LMW agents	5–10% of patients exposed will develop OA
Genetics • HLA antigens DR3, DQ5, DQA1, DQB1, DR1 • Glutathione S-transferase GSTP1 polymorphism	Risk for exposure to diisocyanates, Western red cedar, platinum salts, laboratory animals, anhydrides Diisocyanate-induced asthma

Section 2: Prevention

> **BOTTOM LINE/CLINICAL PEARLS**
> • Control and regulation of the level of exposure to potential agents causing OA is the most important method to prevent the development of disease.
> • Use of respiratory protective equipment reduces the incidence of OA, but may not completely prevent it.

Screening
• Monitoring of workers in the work environment for early detection of antigen sensitization (if possible) and bronchial hyper-responsiveness (see Diagnosis section).
• Patients should not be excluded from employment if they have risk factors for the development of OA.

Primary prevention
• Subjects who are atopic and entering a high-risk workplace with possible exposure to HMW agents should be advised about the potential of developing OA and receive regular medical follow-up.
• Engineering and work practices to control exposure to agents that may cause OA.
• Data on the use of respiratory protection devices to prevent OA are limited.
• Smoking cessation.

Secondary prevention
• Complete avoidance of further exposure to the offending agent.
• Additional study is required to determine if the use of respiratory protection devices (e.g. N95 mask, laminar flow helmets) will allow workers with OA to continue working at the same workplace without causing disease progression.

Section 3: Diagnosis

> **BOTTOM LINE/CLINICAL PEARLS**
> • The clinical history of a patient suspected of having OA must include detailed information about the potential exposures at the workplace, length of time of exposure at work, and history of prior asthma.
> • The initial step in the diagnosis of OA is to demonstrate the patient has asthma (reversible airway obstruction by spirometry and, if necessary, methacholine challenge) (see Chapter 8).
> • A chest radiograph is often required to evaluate new-onset cough and shortness of breath in adults to exclude other etiologies besides OA.
> • Earlier diagnosis of OA and removal of the patient from exposure to the causative agent at work improves chances of clinical improvement.

Differential diagnosis

Differential diagnosis	Features
Work-exacerbated asthma	Asthma onset pre-dates exposure at work
Occupational non-asthmatic eosinophilic bronchitis	New onset non-productive cough without AHR but associated with increased sputum eosinophils (usually exposure to acrylates, latex, lysosyme and mushroom spores)
COPD	Associated with cigarette smoking; DLCO will be decreased
Work-related irritable larynx syndrome (i.e. vocal cord dysfunction)	Hyperkinetic laryngeal symptoms triggered by sensory stimuli in the workplace. Differentiated from asthma by stridor and abnormal inspiratory flow volume loop. No response to bronchodilator. May see paradoxical motion of the vocal cords during symptoms
Hyperventilation syndrome	Hyperventilation without wheezing
Hypersensitivity pneumonitis	Lung volumes with a restrictive pattern

Typical presentation

- *Immunologically mediated OA:* following continued exposure to a causative agent, there is a latency period before the onset of symptoms. The latency is variable in immunologically induced OA and tends to be shorter for LMW agents such as isocyanates (which may occur after 2 years' exposure) and longer for HMW agents (which may take 5 years). Prior to symptom onset many patients experience work-related rhinoconjunctivitis (such as itchy eyes, tearing, sneezing). Symptoms of OA are similar to non-occupational asthma: chest tightness, cough, wheezing, and dyspnea. However, symptoms of OA are typically worse during the work week with exposure and improved on weekends and vacations, especially after initial onset. With progression of OA, symptoms may not improve during these times.
- *Non-immunologically mediated OA:* the clinical symptoms of this type of OA are similar to immunologically induced OA, but the onset of symptoms has no latency period after exposure to the agent. Symptoms are not reproduced by re-exposure of affected patients to lower, non-irritant doses.

Clinical diagnosis

History

- *Immunologic OA:* the history should include exclusion of pre-existing asthma, a detailed current and past work history to determine possible offending agent. The time between starting work and symptom onset, whether there is resolution during weekends and/or vacations needs to be obtained.
- *Non-immunologic OA:* symptoms of RADS and irritant-induced asthma are similar to other forms of asthma. However, the timing of RADS is within 24 hours following exposure to an agent, often leading to an emergency room visit or unscheduled outpatient visit. The time course to onset of symptoms is more gradual in irritant-induced asthma.

Physical examination

- The physical examination may be normal, particularly when away from work. However, as with other patients with asthma, high-pitched wheezing is heard on expirations.
- Some patients with OA who have concomitant occupational rhinitis have pale and swollen nasal mucosa.

Laboratory diagnosis

List of diagnostic tests

- Demonstration of IgE to occupational agents are available for a few HMW antigens (plant and animal) and fewer LMW antigens (platinum salts), and these tests are not standardized. The presence of specific IgE to an agent signifies sensitization, but does not confirm the diagnosis of OA.
- IgE sensitization to common aeroallergens is useful to determine atopic status of the patient.
- *Peak expiratory flow rate* (PEFR)*:* comparison serial measurement of PEFR at work (performed in triplicate done four times per day for 2 weeks) compared to days off (1–2 weeks) to demonstrate if expiratory flow decreases with work exposure.
- *Spirometry:* baseline spirometry is needed to evaluate if airway obstruction is present (FEV_1/FVC below the lower limit of normal). Patients should also have reversibility of obstruction by a significant increase in FEV_1 (12% and >200 mg) after inhalation of a bronchodilator. Reversibility may not be seen in RADS. In some patients, comparison of spirometry should be performed between exposure and non-exposure days (particularly true for immunologically mediated OA).
- *Methacholine challenge* (non-specific bronchoprovocation): performed if spirometry does not demonstrate AHR or obstruction and there is a strong clinical suspicion for OA. It is best to perform methacholine challenges within 24 hours of exposure to the workplace and again when the patient has been away from the workplace for at least 1 week. A decrease of two doublings in the concentration of methacholine that causes a 20% decrease in FEV_1 is considered clinically significant (see Chapter 8).
- *Bronchoprovocation challenge with specific occupational agents:* if spirometry and non-specific bronchoprovocation are normal and there is a high clinical suspension, a specific challenge to the occupational agent may be indicated. This test is performed by exposing the patient to the agent with increasing doses and measuring if lung function changes (e.g. decrease in FEV_1). This is only carried out in specialized centers and for patients with suspected immunologically mediated OA.
- *Sputum cell counts:* the presence of elevated eosinophils or neutrophils suggests asthma, but is not routinely carried out as part of the evaluation of OA.
- *Pulse oximetry:* for patients with RADS.

Lists of imaging techniques

- *Chest X-ray:* typically normal or hyper-inflated. Performed to exclude other etiologies of new-onset cough and shortness of breath.
- *High-resolution CT:* performed only to exclude other etiologies of symptoms.
- *Environmental assessment:* air sampling is not routinely performed as detection of particles may not provide an accurate reflection to what the workers are exposed to. The employer should supply data about possible agents (Box 13.1).

BOX 13.1 DIAGNOSTIC CRITERIA FOR RADS

1. Absence of preexisting respiratory disorder, asthma symptoms, or a history of asthma in remission; and exclusion of conditions that can simulate asthma
2. Onset of asthma after a single exposure or accident
3. Exposure is to irritant vapor, gas, fumes, or smoke in very high concentrations
4. Onset of asthma occurs within minutes to hours and always less than 24 hours after the exposure
5. Finding of a positive methacholine challenge test (<8 mg/ml) following the exposure
6. Possible airflow obstruction on pulmonary function testing
7. Another pulmonary disorder to explain the symptoms and findings is excluded.

Source: Brooks SM, Bernstein IL. Irritant-induced airway disorders. Immunol Allergy Clin North Am 2011;31: 747–68. Reproduced with permission of Elsevier.

Potential pitfalls/common errors made regarding diagnosis of disease
- Compliance obtaining a 2-week record of PEFR often low.
- Methacholine challenge may need to be performed serially – at the end of a work day and >10 days after being away from work.
- Specific inhalation challenge ("gold standard" for diagnosis) is performed only at a few centers.

Section 4: Treatment
Treatment rationale
- A critical step in the treatment of OA is to make the diagnosis and remove the patient from the exposure at the workplace inciting asthma onset.
- The next step is to determine the severity of asthma, following the same guidelines as for non-occupational asthma. This will suggest the appropriate pharmacologic therapy and its dosage (see Chapter 10). Acute presentation of RADS and treatment of exacerbations of other forms of OA is as for the treatment of an acute asthma exacerbation (see Chapter 10).

Table of treatment

Treatment	Comment
Conservative	Prompt removal of worker from exposure to agent. Low levels of exposure, in particular for immunologically mediated OA associated with lower likelihood of improvement and resolution Respiratory protection devices require proper fitting. Not established that use will prevent or attenuate OA
Medical Same as non-occupational asthma Allergen immunotherapy	See Chapter 10 Limited data on effect on the course of OA

CLINICAL PEARLS
- Complete avoidance of the offending agent in OA is the optimal treatment.
- If patients are not able to completely avoid the agent causing OA, the next option (although not ideal) is to reduce the exposure as much as possible and patients should undergo careful medical monitoring to identify worsening of asthma.
- Besides removal from agent exposure, the treatment of asthma should follow standard guidelines of asthma therapy.

Section 5: Special populations
Not applicable for this topic.

Section 6: Prognosis

BOTTOM LINE/CLINICAL PEARLS
- OA is not always reversible after removal from agent exposure.
- Asthma symptoms may persist in approximately 70% of patients several years after removal from environment.
- Better outcome for asthma the shorter the exposure time and sooner the removal of agent.

Natural history of untreated disease

- Most patients with OA due to immunologic mechanisms will have progressive deterioration of lung function with continued exposure to agent.

Prognosis for treated patients

- For patients with immunologically induced OA, a shorter duration of exposure after development of symptoms means they are more likely to undergo remission. Patients with irritant-induced OA, after resolution, should be removed from exposure to the agent, but subsequent exposure at low levels is less likely to induce relapse than immunologically induced OA.

Follow-up tests and monitoring

- For those patients who have milder symptoms and continue at the same workplace, ongoing follow-up (e.g. routine spirometry) is important.

Section 7: Reading list

Brooks SM, Bernstein IL. Irritant-induced airway disorders. Immunol Allergy Clin North Am 2011;31:747–68, vi

Dykewicz MS. Occupational asthma: current concepts in pathogenesis, diagnosis, and management. J Allergy Clin Immunol 2009;123:519–28; quiz 29–30

Fishwick D, Barber CM, Bradshaw LM, Ayres JG, Barraclough R, Burge S, et al. Standards of care for occupational asthma: an update. Thorax 2012;67:278–80

Leigh JP, Romano PS, Schenker MB, Kreiss K. Costs of occupational COPD and asthma. Chest 2002;121:264–72

Maestrelli P, Boschetto P, Fabbri LM, Mapp CE. Mechanisms of occupational asthma. Allergy Clin Immunol 2009;123:531–42; quiz 43–4

Malo JL, Vandenplas O. Definitions and classification of work-related asthma. Immunol Allergy Clin North Am 2011;31:645–62, v

Mapp CE, Boschetto P, Maestrelli P, Fabbri LM. Occupational asthma. Am J Respir Crit Care Med 2005;172:280–305

Tarlo SM, Balmes J, Balkissoon R, Beach J, Beckett W, Bernstein D, et al. Diagnosis and management of work-related asthma: American College of Chest Physicians Consensus Statement. Chest 2008; 134:1S–41S

Venables KM, Dally MB, Nunn AJ, Stevens JF, Stephens R, Farrer N, et al. Smoking and occupational allergy in workers in a platinum refinery. BMJ 1989;299:939–42

Section 8: Guidelines
National society guidelines

Guideline title	Guideline source	Date
An official American Thoracic Society statement: work-exacerbated asthma	American Thoracic Society	2011 (http://www.ncbi.nlm.nih.gov/pubmed/21804122)
Diagnosis and management of work-related asthma	American College of Chest Physicians	2008 (http://www.ncbi.nlm.nih.gov/pubmed/18779187)

Section 9: Evidence

See guidelines listed in Section 8.

Section 10: Images

Not applicable for this topic.

Additional material for this chapter can be found online at:
www.mountsinaiexpertguides.com
This includes a case study, multiple choice questions, advice for
patients, and ICD codes

CHAPTER 14

Status Asthmaticus and Pending Pulmonary Failure

Jacob D. Kattan

Division of Allergy/Immunology, Department of Pediatrics, Icahn School of Medicine at Mount Sinai, New York, NY, USA

OVERALL BOTTOM LINE

- Status asthmaticus is defined as severe asthma unresponsive to repeated courses of beta-agonist therapy.
- Risk factors for a fatal asthma attack include a recent history of poorly controlled asthma or any history of near-fatal asthma (intubation or ICU admission).
- About half of patients with acute severe asthma will have a concomitant respiratory tract infection.
- The goal of therapy is not to restore patients to baseline pulmonary function, but to stabilize them quickly, correct hypoxemia, and improve bronchial obstruction while minimizing and preventing complications such as pneumothorax and respiratory arrest.
- In a patient with status asthmaticus, an arterial blood gas (ABG) demonstrating a normal pH and CO_2 indicates impending respiratory failure.

Section 1: Background

Definition of disease

- Status asthmaticus, or acute severe asthma, is an acute exacerbation of asthma that is unresponsive to repeated treatment with beta-agonists.

Disease classification

- The severity of patients with status asthmaticus may be classified based on the findings of an ABG. ABG in a patient with a less severe exacerbation may demonstrate respiratory alkalosis, a decreased pCO_2, and a normal or slightly decreased pO_2, while a patient with impending respiratory failure or arrest is likely to demonstrate a normal pH or respiratory acidosis, a normal or increased pCO_2, and a decreased pO_2.

Incidence/prevalence

- While the Centers for Disease Control have reported that asthma prevalence in the United States has increased in recent years, the annual death rate from asthma in the United States has declined since 1995.
- In the United States, fatalities from asthma occur more frequently in lower income, non-white, urban populations.
- It is estimated that asthma accounts for about 1 in every 250 deaths worldwide.

Mount Sinai Expert Guides: Allergy and Clinical Immunology, First Edition. Edited by Hugh A. Sampson.
© 2015 John Wiley & Sons, Ltd. Published 2015 by John Wiley & Sons, Ltd.
Companion website: www.mountsinaiexpertguides.com

Economic impact

- There is a considerable cost due to asthma, both from direct costs such as hospital admissions and drug costs as well as indirect costs such as time lost from work or school.

Etiology

- In a patient with asthma, triggers for status asthmaticus include:
  - Respiratory tract infections;
  - Medicinal non-compliance;
  - Lack of inhaled or oral corticosteroid use;
  - Allergen exposure (especially pets);
  - Exercise;
  - Cold temperature;
  - Medications such as beta-blockers or non-steroidal anti-inflammatory drugs; and
  - Irritant inhalation.

Pathology/pathogenesis

- The airway hyper-reactivity and airflow limitation seen in asthma is due to a variety of factors, including airway narrowing, hyperinflation, and plugging of the airways with mucus and inflammatory infiltrates. These infiltrates can vary widely in patients with asthma, but are typically made up of eosinophils, neutrophils, lymphocytes, and plasma cells.

Predictive/risk factors

- A history of near-fatal asthma (intubation or ICU admission).
- Three or more emergency department visits for asthma in the past year.
- Hospitalization for asthma in the past year.
- Recent or current use of oral glucocorticoids.
- Comorbidities such as chronic lung disease.
- A history of poor adherence with asthma medications.
- Use of more than one canister of short-acting beta-agonist per month.

Section 2: Prevention

> **BOTTOM LINE/CLINICAL PEARLS**
> - The prevention of status asthmaticus involves adherence of preventative medications such as inhaled glucocorticoids, smoking cessation, avoidance of known triggers such as aeroallergens or aspirin, and teaching patients to recognize the symptoms of an asthma exacerbation early and to implement an appropriate asthma action plan.

Screening

- While there is no routine screening for status asthmaticus, asthma control may be assessed by clinicians using objective measures such as peak expiratory flow rate, forced expiratory volume in 1 second (FEV_1), and forced vital capacity.

Primary prevention

- Adherence of preventative medications such as inhaled glucocorticoids.
- Smoking cessation.

- Avoidance of known triggers such as aeroallergens or aspirin.
- Teaching patients to recognize the symptoms of an asthma exacerbation early and to implement an appropriate asthma action plan.

Secondary prevention
- Reoccurrence of status asthmaticus or pending pulmonary failure due to asthma may be prevented by the methods discussed in the Primary prevention section.

Section 3: Diagnosis

> **BOTTOM LINE/CLINICAL PEARLS**
> - Patients may report breathlessness, cough, wheezing, or chest tightness.
> - On examination, a patient with a severe asthma exacerbation may have tachypnea, use of accessory muscles of inspiration, inability to speak in full sentences, pulsus paradoxus, diaphoresis, or an inability to lie flat due to breathlessness. Oxygen saturation <90% indicates life-threatening asthma (pending respiratory failure).
> - Decreased expiratory airflow detectable with a peak expiratory flow meter or spirometer may help assess a severe asthma attack. This measurement varies based on patient height, gender, and age, but in general a peak flow rate below 200 L/min indicates severe obstruction in most adults. If the baseline peak flow is known for a patient, a decrease of more than 50% signifies a serious exacerbation.
> - In a patient with status asthmaticus, an ABG demonstrating a normal pH and normal or elevated CO_2 indicates impending respiratory failure.

Differential diagnosis

Differential diagnosis	Features
Anaphylaxis	Frequently associated with cutaneous symptoms including urticaria and angioedema Typical presentation of symptoms is within minutes to 4–6 hours after exposure to a food, drug, insect bite or sting, or other allergen, though signs and symptoms often develop within minutes of exposure May be confirmed by measurement of elevated concentrations of plasma and urinary histamine or serum tryptase levels
Bronchiolitis	Viral upper respiratory prodrome followed by increased respiratory effort and wheezing Difficult to distinguish from asthma during the first episode of wheezing More likely to be asthma with a history of recurrent wheezing episodes or a personal or family history of asthma, eczema, or atopy
Foreign body aspiration	History of choking Radiography may demonstrate a radiopaque object, though most aspirated objects (foods) are radiolucent Bronchoscopy may be necessary for diagnosis and removal of the foreign body
Mediastinal mass	Fever, night sweats, and weight loss can be present in the case of lymphoma Mass is typically diagnosed or suspected based on abnormalities on chest X-ray; a chest CT can confirm the presence of a mediastinal mass

(Continued)

Differential diagnosis	Features
Pneumothorax	Sudden onset dyspnea and pleuritic chest pain Diminished breath sounds, hyper-resonant percussion, decreased chest excursion on the affected side Chest X-ray demonstrates a white visceral pleural line
Vocal cord dysfunction	Stridor that may be inspiratory, expiratory, or both, accompanied by respiratory distress Albuterol typically has little or no beneficial effect In a symptomatic patient, direct observation of the adducted vocal cords by laryngoscopy is diagnostic
Panic disorder	Episodes of intense fear that begin suddenly and last several minutes to an hour Symptoms may include chest pain or shortness of breath Can occur in other anxiety disorders

Typical presentation
- Patients with status asthmaticus will typically present with cough, breathlessness, chest tightness, and wheezing. They may report brief or no response to the use of inhaled beta-agonists. There is often an identifiable trigger such as a respiratory tract infection, allergen exposure, exercise, cold temperature, or inhalation of an irritant.

Clinical diagnosis
History
- Key aspects of the history include a history of asthma, past hospitalizations or emergency department visits, use of inhaled or oral corticosteroids, frequency of inhaled beta-agonist use, current medications, exposure to allergens, and any past admissions to the ICU or intubations for asthma.

Physical examination
- Examination findings with status asthmaticus include tachypnea, use of accessory muscles of inspiration, inability to speak in full sentences, pulsus paradoxus, diaphoresis, or an inability to lie flat due to breathlessness. Oxygen saturation <90% indicates life-threatening asthma (pending respiratory failure).

Disease severity classification
- An asthma exacerbation is moderate when dyspnea interferes with or limits usual activity and the peak expiratory flow is 40–69% of predicted or the patient's personal best. An exacerbation is severe when there is dyspnea at rest or the respiratory status interferes with conversation, with a peak expiratory flow of <40% of predicted or the patient's personal best. Asthma is classified as life-threatening when the patient is too dyspneic to speak or the peak expiratory flow is <25% of predicted or the patient's personal best. When an ABG is obtained, a patient with a less severe exacerbation may demonstrate respiratory alkalosis, a decreased pCO_2, and a normal or slightly decreased pO_2, while a patient with impending respiratory failure or arrest is likely to demonstrate a normal pH or respiratory acidosis, a normal or increased pCO_2, and a decreased pO_2.

Laboratory diagnosis
List of diagnostic tests
- The arterial blood gas is key in the assessment of status asthmaticus and pending respiratory failure.

- A complete blood count may be necessary in patients with fever and a productive cough.
- Electrolytes may be obtained, with a focus on the potassium level, as beta-agonists and steroids may lower serum potassium levels.

Lists of imaging techniques
- Chest X-ray is not required and may be unrevealing in acute asthma exacerbations, although it may help when the diagnosis is uncertain, helping to rule out abnormalities such as a pneumothorax or pneumonia.

Potential pitfalls/common errors made regarding diagnosis of disease
- In a patient presenting with status asthmaticus, a normal pH and CO_2 on an ABG is not a reassuring sign, instead indicating impending respiratory failure.
- Efforts to decrease mortality from asthma focus on educating patients to recognize the symptoms of asthma exacerbations early so that they institute an appropriate action plan and seek prompt medical attention.

Section 4: Treatment (Algorithm 14.1)
Treatment rationale
- Upon first presentation, supplemental oxygen should be administered to relieve hypoxemia with an asthma exacerbation.
- Patients should first be given a short-acting beta-agonist along with inhaled ipratropium bromide to relieve airflow obstruction.
- Systemic corticosteroids should also be administered to decrease airway inflammation in patients who do not respond promptly and completely to a short-acting beta-agonist, although clinical benefits are likely to be delayed.
- Intramuscular epinephrine should be administered if the asthma exacerbation is part of an anaphylactic reaction or if administration of aerosolized albuterol is ineffective or not possible.
- If not responsive to these therapies, other therapies to consider include heliox, as well as intravenous magnesium sulfate.

When to hospitalize
- Admit when a patient has not experienced substantial improvement after 4–6 hours of urgent care management.
- Consider hospital admission when a moderate or severe asthma exacerbation has an incomplete response to therapy, demonstrated by an FEV_1 or peak expiratory flow of 40–69% and mild to moderate symptoms.
- Admit to the hospital if there is a poor response to therapy, including an FEV_1 or peak expiratory flow <40%, a $PCO_2 \geq 42$ mmHg, or severe symptoms.
- When there is impending or actual respiratory arrest the patient should be admitted to the hospital ICU.

Managing the hospitalized patient
- Patients should receive supplemental oxygen as necessary to maintain oxygen saturation ≥92%.
- Inhaled short-acting beta-agonists should be administered from continuously to every 4 hours, depending on the severity of illness.
- Patients should receive systemic glucocorticoids.
- Controller medications should be initiated or adjusted, and asthma education should begin once the patient is admitted and stabilized.

Algorithm 14.1 Management of asthma exacerbations: emergency department and hospital-based care

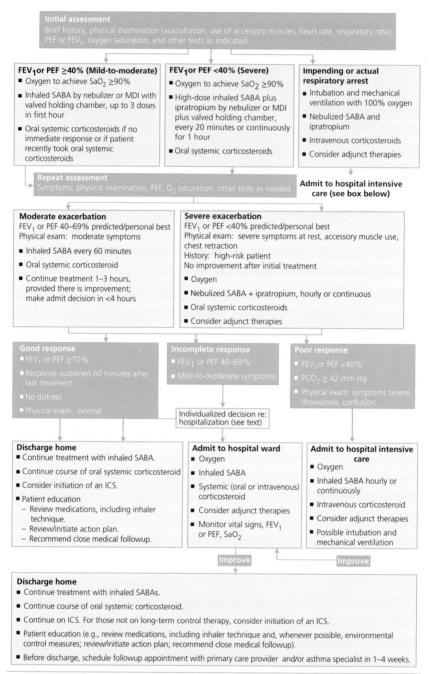

Initial assessment
Brief history, physical examination (auscultation, use of accessory muscles, heart rate, respiratory rate), PEF or FEV₁, oxygen saturation, and other tests as indicated.

FEV₁ or PEF ≥40% (Mild-to-moderate)
- Oxygen to achieve SaO₂ ≥90%
- Inhaled SABA by nebulizer or MDI with valved holding chamber, up to 3 doses in first hour
- Oral systemic corticosteroids if no immediate response or if patient recently took oral systemic corticosteroids

FEV₁ or PEF <40% (Severe)
- Oxygen to achieve SaO₂ ≥90%
- High-dose inhaled SABA plus ipratropium by nebulizer or MDI plus valved holding chamber, every 20 minutes or continuously for 1 hour
- Oral systemic corticosteroids

Impending or actual respiratory arrest
- Intubation and mechanical ventilation with 100% oxygen
- Nebulized SABA and ipratropium
- Intravenous corticosteroids
- Consider adjunct therapies

Repeat assessment
Symptoms, physical examination, PEF, O₂ saturation, other tests as needed

Admit to hospital intensive care (see box below)

Moderate exacerbation
FEV₁ or PEF 40–69% predicted/personal best
Physical exam: moderate symptoms
- Inhaled SABA every 60 minutes
- Oral systemic corticosteroid
- Continue treatment 1–3 hours, provided there is improvement; make admit decision in <4 hours

Severe exacerbation
FEV₁ or PEF <40% predicted/personal best
Physical exam: severe symptoms at rest, accessory muscle use, chest retraction
History: high-risk patient
No improvement after initial treatment
- Oxygen
- Nebulized SABA + ipratropium, hourly or continuous
- Oral systemic corticosteroids
- Consider adjunct therapies

Good response
- FEV₁ or PEF ≥70%
- Response sustained 60 minutes after last treatment
- No distress
- Physical exam: normal

Incomplete response
- FEV₁ or PEF 40–69%
- Mild-to-moderate symptoms

Poor response
- FEV₁ or PEF <40%
- PCO₂ ≥ 42 mm Hg
- Physical exam: symptoms severe, drowsiness, confusion

Individualized decision re: hospitalization (see text)

Discharge home
- Continue treatment with inhaled SABA.
- Continue course of oral systemic corticosteroid
- Consider initiation of an ICS.
- Patient education
  - Review medications, including inhaler technique.
  - Review/initiate action plan.
  - Recommend close medical followup.

Admit to hospital ward
- Oxygen
- Inhaled SABA
- Systemic (oral or intravenous) corticosteroid
- Consider adjunct therapies
- Monitor vital signs, FEV₁ or PEF, SaO₂

Admit to hospital intensive care
- Oxygen
- Inhaled SABA hourly or continuously
- Intravenous corticosteroid
- Consider adjunct therapies
- Possible intubation and mechanical ventilation

Improve   Improve

Discharge home
- Continue treatment with inhaled SABAs.
- Continue course of oral systemic corticosteroid.
- Continue on ICS. For those not on long-term control therapy, consider initiation of an ICS.
- Patient education (e.g., review medications, including inhaler technique and, whenever possible, environmental control measures; review/initiate action plan; recommend close medical followup).
- Before discharge, schedule followup appointment with primary care provider and/or asthma specialist in 1–4 weeks.

Key: FEV₁, forced expiratory volume in 1 second; ICS, inhaled corticosteroid; MDI, metered dose inhaler; PCO2, partial pressure carbon dioxide; PEF, peak expiratory flow; SABA, short-acting beta₂-agonist; SaO₂, oxygen saturation

Source: Management of Asthma Exacerbations: Emergency Department and Hospital-Based Care, p. 388, from: National Heart, Lung, and Blood Institute, National Asthma Education and Prevention Program. Expert panel report 3: guidelines for the diagnosis and management of asthma. NIH publication no. 07-4051. Bethesda, MD: National Heart, Lung, and Blood Institute; 2007. Available here: http://www.nhlbi.nih.gov/guidelines/asthma/asthgdln.pdf. Last accessed November 2014.

Table of treatment

Treatment	Comment
Medical • Oxygen (2–4 L/min) • Short acting beta-2-agonist • Albuterol 0.15 mg/kg (minimum dose 2.5 mg) every 20 minutes for 3 doses then 0.15–0.3 mg/kg up to 10 mg every 1–4 hours as needed, or 0.5 mg/kg/hour by continuous nebulization in children, 2.5–5 mg every 20 minutes for 3 doses, then 2.5–10 mg every 1–4 hours as needed, or 10–15 mg/hour continuously in adults	Only selective beta-2-agonists are recommended in patients with acute severe asthma

• Systemic (injected) beta-2-agonist
  • Epinephrine 0.01 mg/kg up to 0.3 mg IM every 20 minutes for 3 doses in children, 0.3–0.5 mg IM every 20 minutes for 3 doses in adults
  • Terbutaline 0.01 mg/kg subq every 20 minutes for 3 doses then every 2–6 hours as needed in children, 0.25 mg subq every 20 minutes for 3 doses in adults
	Should be administered if the exacerbation is part of an anaphylactic reaction or if administration of aerosolized albuterol is ineffective or not possible
	The systemic therapies have no proven advantage over aerosol

• Ipratropium bromide 0.25–0.5 mg nebulized solution every 20 minutes for 3 doses, then as needed in children, 0.5 mg nebulized solution every 20 minutes for 3 doses then as needed in adults	May be mixed in same nebulizer with albuterol Not recommended for use once patient is admitted

• Systemic glucocorticoids
  • Prednisone 1–2 mg/kg/day PO in divided doses (maximum 60 mg/day) in children, 40–80 mg/day PO in 1 or 2 divided doses in adults
  • Methylprednisolone 1–2 mg/kg/day IV in 2 divided doses up to 60 mg/day in children, 80 mg IV in 1 or 2 divided doses per day in adults
	Glucocorticoid dose should be tailored to patient requirements and can be tapered as patient improves

• Magnesium sulfate 25–75 mg/kg IV up to 2 g in children, 3 g IV in adults • Heliox (mixture of helium and oxygen)	Magnesium sulfate and heliox are for use in life-threatening exacerbations and those unresponsive to 1 hour of intensive conventional therapy

Prevention/management of complications

- Use of continuous nebulized beta-agonist therapy and corticosteroids can lead to decreases in serum potassium, magnesium, and phosphate, and it may be helpful to obtain daily electrolyte levels in these patients.
- Patients should review their asthma action plans with their providers on a regular basis, as adherence to maintenance therapy and appropriate response to exacerbations is vital in the prevention of exacerbations.

> **CLINICAL PEARL**
> - Use of continuous nebulized beta-agonist therapy can lead to transient decreases in serum potassium, magnesium, and phosphate, and it may be helpful to obtain daily electrolyte levels in these patients.

Section 5: Special populations

Pregnancy

- Management of acute asthma exacerbations during pregnancy does not differ greatly from that of non-pregnant patients and includes albuterol, inhaled anticholinergic agents, oral or intravenous glucocorticoids, and, if appropriate, intravenous magnesium sulfate.
- While concerns have been raised that the use of systemic glucocorticoids may lead to a slightly increased risk of congenital malformations, this potential risk is considered small compared to the substantial risk to the mother and fetus resulting from severe, uncontrolled asthma.

Children

- Infants require special attention, as they are at greater risk for respiratory failure than other populations. Assessment depends on the physical examination rather than objective measurements. Signs of serious distress include inspiratory and expiratory wheezing, use of accessory muscles, cyanosis, paradoxical breathing, and a respiratory rate >60 breaths per minute.

Elderly

Not applicable for this topic.

Others

Not applicable for this topic.

Section 6: Prognosis

> **BOTTOM LINE/CLINICAL PEARLS**
> - In general, status asthmaticus has a good prognosis when appropriate therapy is administered.
> - While the mortality rate from asthma had been increasing in the 1990s, it has decreased in recent years. In 2008 and 2009, there were about 11 deaths from asthma per million people in the United States population.

Natural history of untreated disease

- When left untreated, status asthmaticus can be fatal.

Prognosis for treated patients

- Good in the vast majority of cases.

Follow-up tests and monitoring

- Patients should follow- up with their primary care provider or an asthma specialist 3–5 days following hospital discharge.

Section 7: Reading list

Akinbami L. Asthma prevalence, health care use and mortality: United States, 2003–2005. National Center for Health Statistics, Centers for Disease Control and Prevention. http://www.cdc.gov/nchs/data/hestat/asthma03-05/asthma03-05.htm (accessed October 10, 2014)

British Guideline on the Management of Asthma. British Thoracic Society and Scottish Intercollegiate Guidelines Network. 2012. Available from: https://www.brit-thoracic.org.uk/document-library/clinical-information/asthma/btssign-guideline-on-the-management-of-asthma/ (accessed October 30, 2014)

Camargo CA Jr, Spooner CH, Rowe BH. Continuous versus intermittent beta-agonists in the treatment of acute asthma. Cochrane Database Syst Rev 2003;4:CD0011115

Griffiths B, Ducharme FM. Combined inhaled anticholinergics and short-acting beta2-agonists for initial treatment of acute asthma in children. Cochrane Database Syst Rev 2013;8:CD000060

Kim IK, Phrampus E, Venkataraman S, Pitetti R, Saville A, Corcoran T, et al. Helium/oxygen-driven albuterol nebulization in the treatment of children with moderate to severe asthma exacerbations: a randomized, controlled trial. Pediatrics 2005;116:1127–33

Krishnan V, Diette GB, Rand CS, Bilderback AL, Merriman B, Hansel NN, et al. Mortality in patients hospitalized for asthma exacerbations in the United States. Am J Respir Crit Care Med 2006;174:633–8

Manser R, Reid D, Abramson M. Corticosteroids for acute severe asthma in hospitalised patients. Cochrane Database Syst Rev 2001;1:CD001740

National Heart, Lung, and Blood Institute, National Asthma Education and Prevention Program. Expert panel report 3: Guidelines for the diagnosis and management of asthma. NIH publication no. 07-4051. Bethesda, MD: National Heart, Lung, and Blood Institute; 2007. Available from: http://www.nhlbi.nih.gov/guidelines/asthma/asthgdln.pdf (accessed October 10, 2014)

Paasche-Orlow MK, Riekert KA, Bilderback A, Chanmugam A, Hill P, Rand CS, et al. Tailored education may reduce health literacy disparities in asthma self-management. Am J Respir Crit Care Med 2005;172:980–6

Suggested websites

Centers for Disease Control and Prevention FastStats. http://www.cdc.gov/nchs/fastats/asthma.htm

National Heart, Lung and Blood Institute. http://www.nhlbi.nih.gov/health/prof/lung/asthma/naci/asthma-info/asthma-guidelines.htm

Section 8: Guidelines
National society guidelines

Guideline title	Guideline source	Date
Expert Panel Report 3: Guidelines for the Diagnosis and Management of Asthma	National Heart, Lung, and Blood Institute (NHLBI), National Asthma Education and Prevention Program (NAEPP)	2007 (http://www.nhlbi.nih.gov/files/docs/guidelines/asthgdln.pdf)
British Guideline on the Management of Asthma	British Thoracic Society and Scottish Intercollegiate Guidelines	2012 (http://www.sign.ac.uk/pdf/SIGN141.pdf)

Section 9: Evidence
See Guidelines listed in Section 8.

Section 10: Images
Not applicable for this topic.

Additional material for this chapter can be found online at:
www.mountsinaiexpertguides.com
This includes a case study, multiple choice questions, advice for patients, and ICD codes

CHAPTER 15

Evaluation of Food Allergy

Scott H. Sicherer

Department of Pediatrics, Division of Allergy/Immunology, Mount Sinai Hospital, New York, NY, USA

OVERALL BOTTOM LINE

- Food allergy is distinct from other adverse food reactions to foods because it is caused by an adverse immune response.
- Diagnosis relies upon a careful history and is confirmed by tests including skin prick tests, serum tests for food-specific IgE, elimination diets, and oral food challenges.
- Treatment relies upon allergen avoidance and preparation to treat severe reactions promptly with epinephrine.
- Prognosis is excellent for resolution of many childhood food allergies, although allergies to peanut, tree nuts, fish, and shellfish are likely to persist.

Section 1: Background

Definition of disease

- A food allergy is an adverse health effect arising from a specific immune response that occurs reproducibly on exposure to a given food. A food allergy is distinct from other adverse health consequences from food such as intolerance (non-immunologic, e.g. lactose intolerance) or other non-immune-mediated reactions (e.g. toxic, pharmacologic).

Disease classification

- Immune responses may primarily be IgE antibody mediated, typically with acute onset of symptoms, or cell-mediated (non-IgE) in which symptoms may be subacute or chronic. Disease classification is also related to the organ systems affected, such as the skin, gastrointestinal or respiratory tract, cardiovascular system, or combinations of these (see chapters on individual diseases).

Incidence/prevalence

- Food allergy is estimated to affect more than 1–2% and less than 10% of the population.
- Significant food allergies appear to be more common in children than adults.
- Although over 170 foods have been noted to cause allergic reactions, peanut, tree nuts, milk, egg, fish, shellfish, soy, and wheat account for the majority of significant allergies.
- Immune responses to chemical, in contrast to protein, food additives/preservatives appears uncommon.

Mount Sinai Expert Guides: Allergy and Clinical Immunology, First Edition. Edited by Hugh A. Sampson.
© 2015 John Wiley & Sons, Ltd. Published 2015 by John Wiley & Sons, Ltd.
Companion website: www.mountsinaiexpertguides.com

Economic impact
- Treatment of allergic reactions to foods is estimated to cost $25 billion annually in the United States.

Etiology
- Food allergy is a failure of normal oral tolerance induction.
- The etiology is not completely understood, but appears to be related to a Th2 immune bias.
- IgE-mediated allergy requires sensitization (perhaps oral, cutaneous, or respiratory exposure) where antigen-presenting cells and T cells orchestrate production of allergen-specific IgE antibodies by plasma cells.
- Cell-mediated allergy is not completely understood but may involve homing of effector cells, such as eosinophils, to affected organs.

Pathology/pathogenesis
- Food protein-specific IgE antibodies populate the high affinity IgE receptors on mast cells and basophils where, upon re-exposure, protein binding to IgE and cross-linking of antibodies results in mediator release (e.g. histamine) thereby inducing symptoms.
- Disorders with chronic symptoms may involve homing of effector cells to sites of inflammation (e.g. eosinophilic esophagitis and atopic dermatitis).

Predictive/risk factors
- Children with moderate to severe atopic dermatitis appear to be at increased risk of having food allergies (e.g. 35% risk versus 8% population risk).
- The risk of peanut allergy for a sibling of a child with peanut allergy is approximately 7% (compared with a population risk of approximately 1.4%).
- Having a pollen allergy increases the risk of having mild allergic responses to raw fruits and vegetables (pollen-related food allergy).
- Based on case series, those at highest risk of fatal, food-induced anaphylaxis are teenagers/young adults, those with asthma, a known food allergy, and, most importantly, a delay in treatment with epinephrine.

Section 2: Prevention

> **BOTTOM LINE/CLINICAL PEARLS**
> - There are limited data supporting any intervention to prevent food allergy, although breastfeeding is encouraged and, if not possible, the use of a protein hydrolysate formula may reduce the risk of atopic dermatitis and perhaps milk allergy compared to using a cow's milk or soy infant formula. Secondary prevention (treatment) is based on allergen avoidance.

Screening
- General screening tests in healthy individuals are not recommended.
- Screening for peanut allergy in a younger sibling of a child with peanut allergy might be considered.
- For patients with food allergies who have not already tolerated potential allergens (based on individual circumstances), screening may be considered (i.e. testing for cashew allergy in a person with walnut, pecan, and macadamia allergies who has not yet ingested cashew).

Primary prevention

- Exclusive breastfeeding is recommended for the first 4–6 months but evidence for the prevention of food allergy is uncertain.
- For at-risk infants (parent or sibling with an allergic disorder) who are not breast fed, a hydrolyzed infant formula, as opposed to cow's milk or soy formula, may be considered to prevent cow's milk allergy or atopic dermatitis.
- The introduction of solid foods should not be delayed beyond 4–6 months, including potentially allergenic foods.
- Maternal avoidance diets during pregnancy or lactation are not proven to prevent food allergy.
- Studies of probiotics, prebiotics, and synbiotics suggest a potential to reduce atopic disease, but studies remain inconclusive.

Secondary prevention

- Avoidance of foods proven to be allergens for the individual is the primary means of prevention of food-allergic reactions.

Section 3: Diagnosis (Algorithm 15.1)

BOTTOM LINE/CLINICAL PEARLS
- The history is necessary to determine if symptoms are likely caused by food allergy, and, if so, what the underlying pathophysiology may be (IgE-mediated or not) and which foods are triggers.
- Skin and serum tests to determine food-specific IgE antibodies are recommended to diagnose IgE-mediated food allergy but are not in and of themselves diagnostic.
- Elimination diets and other modalities may be needed to diagnose non-IgE-mediated food allergies.
- The oral food challenge is recommended to diagnose food allergies, and the double-blind, placebo-controlled oral food challenge is considered the "gold standard."
- Pitfalls in diagnosis include clinically irrelevant cross-reactivity, sensitization without clinical reactivity, tests that are positive because of binding to proteins that are unlikely to trigger allergic reactions, misidentification of triggers, having negative tests despite clinical reactions due to cell-mediated allergy, or IgE-mediated reactions to proteins not represented on the test.

Differential diagnosis

Differential diagnosis	Features or examples
Anaphylaxis or allergic reactions from another cause	History of another exposure (e.g. insect sting, drug) or lack of food ingestion or lack of consistent responses
Food intolerance	Symptoms typically affect the gut without signs or symptoms of typical allergic responses
Toxic reactions to spoiled food	Bacterial food poisoning. Scombroid fish poisoning may mimic anaphylaxis
Pharmacologic reactions to foods	Caffeine may induce tachycardia, sweating

Typical presentation

- The most common presentation is an acute reaction in childhood. For example, an 18-month-old child who has had moderate atopic dermatitis ingests peanut butter for the first time and

Algorithm 15.1 General approach to diagnosis of food allergy

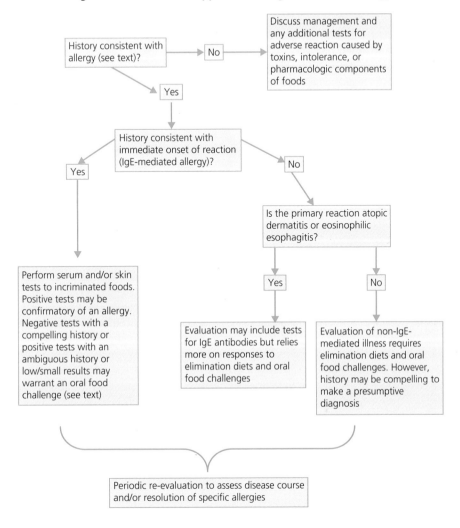

within minutes his lips swell, urticaria develops on the face and becomes generalized, and he coughs repetitively and vomits.

Clinical diagnosis

History

- A detailed history should focus upon the symptoms, timing in relation to ingestion, the possible causal food(s), consistency of reactions upon exposure, how the food was prepared, whether additional factors were occurring at the time (exercise, illness, use of aspirin), whether symptoms also occur without a relationship to ingestion, what treatments were given, and the time course of symptoms.
- A diet diary may be helpful.
- The nature of the reaction is important in determining if food allergy is a likely cause, what food may be a trigger, and whether the pathophysiology may be IgE-mediated or cell-mediated.

Physical examination

- The physical examination alone cannot diagnose a food allergy but may reveal ongoing symptoms or signs of atopic disease.

Laboratory diagnosis

List of diagnostic tests

- Skin prick tests are recommended to assist in identifying foods that may be provoking an IgE-mediated allergic reaction. The test cannot be used as the sole means to diagnose food allergy (see Potential pitfalls section). Some studies suggest that increasingly larger positive tests correlate with a higher chance of clinical allergy.
- Allergen-specific serum IgE is recommended to assist in identifying foods that may be provoking an IgE-mediated allergic reaction. The test cannot be used as the sole means to diagnose food allergy (see Potential pitfalls section). Some studies suggest that increasingly higher antibody concentrations correlate with a higher chance of clinical allergy. Particularly high "diagnostic points" may confirm an allergy. Testing to specific proteins within a food, component testing, is available for select foods and may assist in confirming an allergy when binding is observed to proteins that are stable to digestion and are associated with clinical reactions.
- Food elimination diets may be used to investigate if a select number of suspected allergens are triggering chronic symptoms, especially in non-IgE-mediated disorders or mixed IgE/non-IgE-mediated disorders. However, confirmatory diagnostic studies should be considered.
- Oral food challenges (medically supervised) are recommended for diagnosing food allergy. They are typically performed when the medical history and ancillary tests do not confirm an allergy, or to test for resolution. The may be the only means to identify non-IgE-mediated allergic reactions. The double-blind, placebo-controlled oral food challenge is a "gold standard" for diagnosis (see Chapter 25).
- A variety of tests are not routinely recommended (total serum IgE, the atopy patch test), not recommended (intradermal skin testing), or not recommended because they are non-standardized or unproven (provocation-neutralization, basophil histamine activation, applied kinesiology, IgG/IgG4, cytotoxicity assays, electrodermal testing, hair analysis, facial thermography, gastric juice analysis, and mediator release assays, among others).
- Serum tryptase levels may not be elevated during food-induced anaphylaxis, and are not a reliable means of diagnosis.

Lists of imaging techniques

Not applicable for this topic.

Potential pitfalls/common errors made regarding diagnosis of disease

- A positive prick skin test or food-specific IgE antibody test indicates "sensitization" but does *not* indicate clinical allergy. For example, approximately 8% of the US population is sensitized to peanut but only about 1% are clinically allergic. Also, about 50% of those with peanut allergy test positive to other legumes, but 95% tolerate ingestion of these related foods. Persons with pollen allergy may test positive to many foods with homologous proteins but may tolerate the food or have only mild reactions to raw forms. The history is essential in interpretation of the test results. Screening a battery of foods without a specific suspicion can be misleading.
- Patients may be clinically allergic to a food despite negative tests either because the disorder is not IgE-mediated, the test does not display a protein to which they react, or there is a laboratory error. If there is a high suspicion of an allergy, retesting, possibly with a different modality such as prick testing with a fresh food extract or using an alternative test whether serum or skin test. If these are negative, an oral food challenge should be considered.

Section 4: Treatment
Treatment rationale
- There are no medications currently recommended to prevent food-allergic reactions.
- Allergen avoidance is required to prevent allergic reactions. Disorder-specific treatment advice is provided in separate chapters (see chapters on individual diseases). Physicians should instruct patients on allergen avoidance including careful reading of product ingredient labels, discussing the allergy when obtaining food at restaurants, and avoiding cross contact, whereby a safe food is tainted by an allergen during preparation (e.g. chopping nuts and lettuce on the same cutting board).
- Young children require close supervision to prevent unintended ingestion of avoided foods.
- Approximately 70% of persons allergic to egg or milk may tolerate these allergens in bakery goods (extensive heating), but caution is needed in identifying individuals who may tolerate such foods because anaphylaxis to these foods is possible.
- Treatment of food allergy using immunotherapy and other measures is under study.
- Patients with life-threatening IgE-mediated food allergies should carry epinephrine, wear medical identification jewelry, and have emergency plans in place to treat anaphylaxis promptly. They should be instructed on emergency management including recognizing and treating anaphylaxis and seeking emergency care.
- The management of food-induced anaphylaxis is similar to anaphylaxis from other causes.

When to hospitalize
- Hospitalization may be required for severe or prolonged anaphylaxis.

Table of treatment

Treatment	Comment
Allergen avoidance	Allergen avoidance is the basis of prevention of allergic reactions
Epinephrine autoinjector, 0.15 or 0.3 mg	Patients with potentially life-threatening food allergies should have immediate access to autoinjectors. Delay in treatment with epinephrine is associated with fatal outcomes
Antihistamines	Provides additional relief of minor symptoms

Prevention/management of complications
- Complications of allergen avoidance include nutritional deficiencies.
- Height and weight should be followed in children and nutritional counseling provided.
- Clinical evaluations should address whether the diet can be expanded.
- Food allergy can affect quality of life, induce anxiety, and affect social activities.
- Responsibilities of management should be age-appropriate. Counseling about addressing these issues is warranted.

CLINICAL PEARLS
- Education about avoidance and emergency management is key to successful management.
- Exposure by ingestion, rather than skin contact or inhalation, is the main concern in preventing anaphylaxis.
- Patients should be reminded not to "test" their allergens by home trials.
- Anaphylaxis can occur without urticaria.

Section 5: Special populations

Pregnancy

Not applicable for this topic.

Children

Not applicable for this topic.

Elderly

Not applicable for this topic.

Others

- Teenagers and young adults are at highest risk of fatal anaphylaxis, presumably as a result of risk-taking and delay in treatment. Additional focus on avoidance and emergency management, and possibly psychosocial issues that could affect treatment, should be considered.

Section 6: Prognosis

BOTTOM LINE/CLINICAL PEARLS
- Allergies to milk, egg, wheat, and soy typically resolve in childhood.
- Allergies to peanuts, tree nuts, fish, and shellfish are likely to persist.
- Fatalities are rare, but vigilance is needed to prevent and treat severe reactions.
- Non-IgE-mediated gastrointestinal food allergies (enterocolitis, proctocolitis) typically resolve in childhood, but eosinophilic esophagitis is more likely to persist.

Natural history of untreated disease

- Peanut allergy diagnosed in young children remits for approximately 20% of patients.
- Milk, egg, wheat, and soy allergies typically remit by adulthood.
- Allergies to tree nuts, fish, and shellfish are persistent, with generally under 10% remitting.
- Non-IgE-mediated gastrointestinal food allergies (enterocolitis, proctocolitis) typically resolve in childhood, but food-induced eosinophilic esophagitis appears to be more likely to persist.

Follow-up tests and monitoring

- Periodic retesting is recommended, but the timing depends upon the age of the patient and food involved. Annual testing for children with allergies to milk, egg, wheat, and soy is generally undertaken. Testing may be less frequent for other foods or in older individuals. However, there is no specified schedule of retesting. Physician re-evaluations, for example annually, may be warranted to provide updates and education on management even if testing is not indicated.

Section 7: Reading list

Bernstein IL, Li JT, Bernstein DI, Hamilton R, Spector SL, Tan R, et al. Allergy diagnostic testing: an updated practice parameter. Ann Allergy Asthma Immunol 2008;100(Suppl 3):S1–148

Boyce JA, Assa'ad A, Burks AW, Jones SM, Sampson HA, Wood RA, et al. Guidelines for the diagnosis and management of food allergy in the United States: report of the NIAID-sponsored expert panel. J Allergy Clin Immunol 2010;126(Suppl):S1–58

Burks AW, Jones SM, Boyce JA, Sicherer SH, Wood RA, Assa'ad A, et al. NIAID-sponsored 2010 guidelines for managing food allergy: applications in the pediatric population. Pediatrics 2011;128:955–65

Greer FR, Sicherer SH, Burks AW. Effects of early nutritional interventions on the development of atopic disease in infants and children: the role of maternal dietary restriction, breastfeeding, timing of introduction of complementary foods, and hydrolyzed formulas. Pediatrics 2008;121:183–91

Nowak-Wegrzyn A, Assa'ad AH, Bahna SL, Bock SA, Sicherer SH, Teuber SS. Work Group report: oral food challenge testing. J Allergy Clin Immunol 2009;123(Suppl):S365–83

Sampson HA, Gerth vW, Bindslev-Jensen C, Sicherer S, Teuber SS, Burks AW, et al. Standardizing double-blind, placebo-controlled oral food challenges: American Academy of Allergy, Asthma and Immunology-European Academy of Allergy and Clinical Immunology PRACTALL consensus report. J Allergy Clin Immunol 2012;130:1260–74

Sampson, HA, Aceves S, Bock SA, James J, Jones S, Lang D, et al. Food allergy: a practice parameter update–2014. J Allergy Clin Immunol 2014; pii:S0091-6749(14)00672-1. Available from: http://www.ncbi.nlm.nih.gov/pubmed/25174862 (accessed October 13, 2014)

Sicherer SH, Sampson HA. Food allergy. J Allergy Clin Immunol 2010;125(Suppl 2):S116–25

Sicherer SH, Vargas PA, Groetch ME, Christie L, Carlisle SK, Noone S, et al. Development and validation of educational materials for food allergy. J Pediatr 2012;160:651–6

Sicherer SH, Wood RA. Allergy testing in childhood: using allergen-specific IgE tests. Pediatrics 2012;129:193–7

Suggested websites

www.aaaai.org

www.acaai.org

www.cofargroup.org

www.foodallergy.org

Section 8: Guidelines
National society guidelines

Guideline title	Guideline source	Date
Food allergy: a practice parameter update	Joint Council of Allergy and Immunology	2014 (http://www.ncbi.nlm.nih.gov/pubmed/25174862)
Guidelines for the diagnosis and management of food allergy in the United States: report of the NIAID-sponsored expert panel	National Institutes of Allergy and Infectious Diseases	2010 (http://www.ncbi.nlm.nih.gov/pubmed/21134576)

Section 9: Evidence
See Guidelines listed in Section 8.

Section 10: Images
Not applicable for this topic.

Additional material for this chapter can be found online at:
www.mountsinaiexpertguides.com
This includes a case study, multiple choice questions
(provided by Hugh Sampson), advice for patients,
and ICD codes

CHAPTER 16

Oral Allergy Syndrome

Julie Wang

Department of Pediatrics, Division of Allergy/Immunology, Icahn School of Medicine at Mount Sinai, New York, NY, USA

OVERALL BOTTOM LINE

- Oral allergy syndrome (OAS) is a contact allergy that affects patients with allergic rhinitis and is a result of homologous proteins in pollens and fresh fruits and vegetables.
- Symptoms are primarily mild and limited to the oropharyngeal area.
- Anaphylaxis can occur in 2% of cases.
- Patients with OAS should avoid the fresh foods that trigger symptoms, but may continue to include heated forms of those foods in the diet as well as other related foods that do not trigger symptoms.

Section 1: Background

Definition of disease

- OAS describes localized symptoms with ingestion of fresh fruits and vegetables in patients with allergic rhinitis.

Disease classification

Not applicable for this topic.

Incidence/prevalence

- OAS is the most common food allergy in adults.
- The prevalence of OAS is variable by region and affects 30–70% of patients with allergic rhinitis.
- OAS is more common in women.

Economic impact

- While OAS can significantly impact quality of life, the economic burden of this disorder has not been investigated.

Etiology

- OAS is an IgE-mediated allergy that is due to cross-reacting homologous proteins between pollens and food proteins.
- These proteins are sensitive to heat, acid, and digestion, thus symptoms are often limited to the oropharynx, and cooked forms of the foods are well tolerated.
- Birch pollen allergy is most commonly associated with symptoms with Rosacea fruits (i.e. apple, pear, cherry, peach), Apicaceae vegetables (i.e. carrot, celery), and some tree nuts (e.g. hazelnuts, and occasionally peanuts).

Mount Sinai Expert Guides: Allergy and Clinical Immunology, First Edition. Edited by Hugh A. Sampson.
© 2015 John Wiley & Sons, Ltd. Published 2015 by John Wiley & Sons, Ltd.
Companion website: www.mountsinaiexpertguides.com

- Lipid transfer proteins (LTPs), the major allergens involved in non-pollen allergy plant food allergies, are primarily seen in the Mediterranean area and are associated with higher rates of systemic reactions, including anaphylaxis.
- Other associations have been described, including celery-birch-mugwort-spice syndrome, ragweed-melon-banana association, and latex-fruit syndrome.

Pathology/pathogenesis
- The primary event is sensitization to inhaled pollen allergens (or latex allergen) via the respiratory tract, leading to production of pollen-specific IgE. When exposure to homologous proteins in plant-derived foods occurs, cross-linking of IgE on mast cells and basophils in the oropharyngeal mucosa leads to mediator release (i.e. histamine) which results in symptoms of OAS. These food allergens are generally heat labile and susceptible to gastric digestion, therefore these proteins are denatured in the stomach.

Predictive/risk factors
- Sensitization to tree pollens (particularly birch pollen).
- Sensitization to multiple pollens.
- More severe symptomatic allergic disease.
- Higher pollen-specific IgE levels.
- High-risk areas where pollens are prevalent (e.g. birch, LTP).
- Sensitization to LTPs.

Section 2: Prevention

> **BOTTOM LINE/CLINICAL PEARLS**
> - No interventions have been demonstrated to prevent the development of this disease.

Screening
Not applicable for this topic.

Primary prevention
Not applicable for this topic.

Secondary prevention
Not applicable for this topic.

Section 3: Diagnosis (Algorithm 16.1)

> **BOTTOM LINE/CLINICAL PEARLS**
> - History is the most important diagnostic tool for OAS.
> - Physical findings include signs and symptoms of allergic rhinitis.
> - Skin prick tests and measurement of serum-specific IgE levels are not very reliable for the diagnosis of OAS.
> - Oral food challenges are diagnostic for food allergy; however, difficulties in standardizing the procedure include variations in allergen levels in different parts of the fruits, in different cultivars, or due to different ripeness or storage conditions, which may lead to different food challenge outcomes.

Differential diagnosis

Differential diagnosis	Features
Class I food allergy	Symptoms are triggered by fresh and cooked forms of the foods Systemic reactions are more common
Contact urticaria	Tomato, citrus, garlic, berries can cause local urticaria This is suggested by lack of pollen sensitization
Contact dermatitis	Delayed-type hypersensitivity reaction Symptoms may be triggered by contact allergens (particularly metals) and drugs
Gastroesophageal reflux	Symptoms are not specific to raw fruits and vegetables There is no association with atopy
Eosinophilic esophagitis	Throat symptoms due to dysphagia may be mistaken for OAS Symptoms are not limited to raw fruits and vegetables Other gastrointestinal symptoms including vomiting and failure to thrive may be seen
Burning mouth syndrome	Characterized by recurrent or chronic burning symptoms of the mouth Not triggered by food ingestion

Typical presentation
- A patient with allergic rhinitis typically complains of oropharyngeal symptoms such as lip and/or mouth itching and swelling after eating fresh fruits or vegetables. The onset of symptoms is often within 5 minutes of exposure. Heated fruits or vegetables are generally well tolerated. Symptoms can extend outside of the oropharynx, with 14% having gastrointestinal symptoms, 14% reporting laryngeal edema, and 2% having anaphylaxis. For some, seasonal variations are seen, with symptoms being more pronounced during the associated pollen season.

Clinical diagnosis
History
- History is important for the diagnosis of OAS. Patients should be asked about rhinitis symptoms, foods triggering symptoms, type of symptoms, medications used to treat symptoms, whether symptoms occur with only the fresh fruit or vegetables or whether heated foods trigger symptoms as well.

Physical examination
- Physical examination may reveal signs and symptoms of allergic rhinitis (e.g. ocular redness, nasal congestion or rhinorrhea, allergic shiners, nasal crease).

Useful clinical decision rules and calculators
Not applicable for this topic.

Disease severity classification
Not applicable for this topic.

Laboratory diagnosis
List of diagnostic tests
- Skin prick tests and measurement of serum-specific IgE levels can identify the pollens that are triggering allergic rhinitis.
- Skin prick tests and serum-specific IgE are less reliable for identifying the triggering foods for OAS.
- While skin prick tests with fresh fruits and vegetables correlate better with clinical symptoms when compared with commercial extracts, this is not standardized. Variations in test results

Algorithm 16.1 Diagnosis of oral allergy syndrome (OAS)

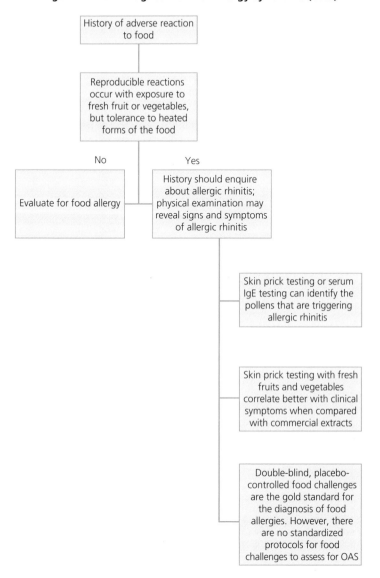

from testing with fresh fruits and vegetables can be due to differences in part of the fruit used for testing, cultivars, ripeness, and storage conditions.

- Double-blind, placebo-controlled food challenges are the gold standard for the diagnosis of food allergies; however, there are no standardized protocols for food challenges to assess for OAS. Furthermore, difficulties blinding fresh foods and variations in allergen level as a result of different parts of the fruit, different cultivars, ripeness, or storage conditions complicate the standardization of the food challenge procedure.

Lists of imaging techniques
No imaging studies are indicated for OAS.

Potential pitfalls/common errors made regarding diagnosis of disease

- OAS should be distinguished from class I food allergy in which food allergens are the sensitizers and elicitors of symptoms. The risk for anaphylaxis is greater for class I food allergy.
- Skin testing and serum IgE testing are not reliable predictors of OAS because standard reagents may not contain the relevant proteins.

Section 4: Treatment (Algorithm 16.2)

Treatment rationale

- There are currently no consensus guidelines for the management of OAS. As symptoms with one food do not necessarily predict symptoms with all members within a botanical family, patients are advised to avoid only the fruits and/or vegetables that trigger symptoms. For related foods that patients have not yet been exposed to, oral challenges may be performed to determine whether it is safe to include these new foods in the diet. Heating the food allergens that trigger OAS denatures the relevant protein, therefore cooked forms of the foods are well tolerated.
- In addition to education on allergen avoidance, patients should understand that OAS can lead to systemic reactions and anaphylaxis in some cases. Thus, it is important to be knowledgeable

Algorithm 16.2 Management of oral allergy syndrome

Food allergen avoidance

Avoid the fresh fruits and vegetables that cause symptoms

Heated forms of the fruits and vegetables causing symptoms should be well tolerated

Foods that are tolerated may continue to be included in the diet

Oral food challenges may be performed for related foods that have not yet been introduced

Management of acute reactions

Oral antihistamines can relieve mild symptoms of OAS

In ~2% of cases, OAS symptoms can result in anaphylaxis. Intramuscular epinephrine is the treatment of choice for anaphylaxis

about the identification and treatment of systemic reactions, including indications for self-injectable epinephrine.
- There are currently no effective therapies to prevent or cure OAS. While subcutaneous immunotherapy is effective to treat symptoms of allergic rhinitis, it remains an unproven therapeutic approach for OAS.

When to hospitalize
- OAS is managed in the outpatient setting.

Managing the hospitalized patient
Not applicable for this topic.

Table of treatment

Treatment	Comment
Conservative • Avoid the fresh fruits and vegetables that cause symptoms. However, foods that are tolerated may continue to be included in the diet • Heated forms of the fruits and vegetables causing symptoms should be well tolerated • Oral food challenges may be performed for related foods that have not yet been introduced • Patients should be educated on the potential risk for severe reactions and be prepared to identify and treat allergic reactions, including having self-injectable epinephrine available	This is applicable to all patients with OAS
Medical • Oral antihistamines can relieve symptoms of OAS	Chronic use of antihistamines may mask mild symptoms of OAS, prompting increased consumption of the triggering food and increasing the risk of systemic reactions

Prevention/management of complications
- In approximately 2% of cases, OAS symptoms can result in anaphylaxis. Intramuscular epinephrine is the treatment of choice for anaphylaxis (see Chapter 29).

CLINICAL PEARLS
- Only the fresh fruits and vegetables that cause symptoms should be avoided.
- Heated forms of these foods are generally well tolerated.
- Systemic reactions can occur in some cases so patients need to be educated regarding the identification and treatment of acute allergic reactions, including the use of self-injectable epinephrine.

Section 5: Special populations
Not applicable for this topic.

Section 6: Prognosis

> **BOTTOM LINE/CLINICAL PEARLS**
> - OAS is a mild disorder for most.
> - Risk factors for systemic reactions include prior history of systemic reaction to the food, reactions to the cooked forms of the food, positive skin prick tests with the food extract, lack of pollen sensitization, and sensitization to lipid transfer protein.

Natural history of untreated disease
- There is no treatment available to alter the natural history of OAS.
- Immunotherapy with pollen or food allergens have been investigated; however, results have been inconsistent so this remains an unproven therapeutic approach for OAS.

Prognosis for treated patients
Not applicable for this topic.

Follow-up tests and monitoring
Not applicable for this topic.

Section 7: Reading list

Geroldinger-Simic M, Zelniker T, Aberer W, Ebner C, Egger C, Greiderer A, et al. Birch pollen-related food allergy: clinical aspects and the role of allergen-specific IgE and IgG$_4$ antibodies. J Allergy Clin Immunol 2011;127:616–22

Ma S, Sicherer SH, Nowak-Wegrzyn A. A survey on the management of pollen-food allergy syndrome in allergy practices. J Allergy Clin Immunol 2003;112:784–8

Ortolani C, Ispano M, Pastorello EA, Ansaloni R, Magri GC. Comparison of results of skin prick tests (with fresh foods and commercial food extracts) and RAST in 100 patients with oral allergy syndrome. J Allergy Clin Immunol 1989;83:683–90

Valenta R, Kraft D. Type 1 allergic reactions to plant-derived food: a consequence of primary sensitization to pollen allergens. J Allergy Clin Immunol 1996;97:893–5

Suggested websites
American Academy of Allergy, Asthma and Immunology (AAAAI). www.aaaai.org

American College of Allergy, Asthma and Immunology (ACAAI). www.acaai.org

Section 8: Guidelines
National society guidelines

Guideline title	Guideline source	Date
Food allergy: A practice parameter update—2014	American Academy of Allergy, Asthma and Immunology (AAAAI); American College of Allergy, Asthma and Immunology (ACAAI)	2014 (http://www.allergyparameters. org/published-practice-parameters/ alphabetical-listing/food-allergy-download/)

Section 9: Evidence

Not applicable for this topic.

Section 10: Images

Not applicable for this topic.

Additional material for this chapter can be found online at:
www.mountsinaiexpertguides.com
This includes a case study, multiple choice questions, advice for
patients, and ICD codes

CHAPTER 17

Food Allergy and Atopic Dermatitis

Kate Welch and Hugh A. Sampson

Jaffe Food Allergy Institute, Icahn School of Medicine at Mount Sinai, New York, NY, USA

OVERALL BOTTOM LINE
- Atopic dermatitis (AD) is a chronic inflammatory skin disorder characterized by intense pruritus and a variable course of exacerbations and remissions (see Chapters 1 and 2).
- While there is some controversy with regard to the role of food allergy in atopic dermatitis, these two conditions are often seen in the same patient.
- Food allergy is considered to be a provoking cause of AD in a subset of patients, particularly in about one-third of infants and young children with moderate to severe AD.
- Patients with AD often have elevations of serum food-specific IgE antibodies.
- Food elimination diets followed by oral food challenges are the best way to determine whether food allergy or sensitivity is an exacerbating factor of a patient's AD.

Section 1: Background

Definition of disease

- Patients with AD have a higher rate of allergic disease, including allergic rhinitis and food allergy, than the general population. There is clearly an increased rate of sensitization to food allergens in patients with AD, but the degree to which food triggers or exacerbates AD varies between patients.

Disease classification

- Food-induced AD affects a subset of patients with AD. Food allergies are more likely to have a role in exacerbating symptoms in patients who have more severe forms of AD as measured by the SCORAD index.

Incidence/prevalence

- AD affects roughly 10% of children and 1–3% of adults worldwide.
- Food allergens are considered to provoke AD in approximately 35% of pediatric patients.
- They have a role in exacerbating AD in up to 33% of patients with moderate to severe AD, 10–20% of patients with mild to moderate AD, and 6% of patients with mild AD.
- Milk, egg, wheat, soy, and peanut account for nearly 75% of the cases of food-induced AD.

Mount Sinai Expert Guides: Allergy and Clinical Immunology, First Edition. Edited by Hugh A. Sampson.
© 2015 John Wiley & Sons, Ltd. Published 2015 by John Wiley & Sons, Ltd.
Companion website: www.mountsinaiexpertguides.com

Economic impact

Not applicable for this topic.

Etiology

- AD is thought to occur as a result of a genetic predisposition coupled with environmental triggers.
- Atopic conditions, including eczema, allergic rhinitis, food allergy, and asthma, are often seen in the same patient.
- Patients with AD generally have increased serum IgE levels as well as food allergen-specific IgE levels initially and environmental aeroallergens later.
- In the subset of patients with food-induced AD, ingestion of certain allergens leads to an immediate or delayed exacerbation of eczematous skin eruptions.

Pathology/pathogenesis

- AD, which typically begins in early infancy, has numerous trigger factors, including foods, inhalant allergens, bacterial colonization of the skin (especially with *Staphylococcus aureus*), irritating substances, temperature change, psychologic stress, systemic infections, and hormones, among others. T cells have an important role in mediating hypersensitivity reactions in AD. Once ingested, food proteins enter the circulation and are distributed throughout the body, including to skin. Food antigens can directly interact with food-specific IgE bound to mast cells, basophils, and skin-infiltrating T lymphocytes, thus setting off the inflammatory response.

Predictive/risk factors

Not applicable for this topic.

Section 2: Prevention

BOTTOM LINE/CLINICAL PEARLS

- Management of food-induced AD ultimately involves the identification and elimination of culprit foods from the diet.
- Not all foods to which a patient has evidence of IgE sensitivity will cause an exacerbation of eczema symptoms, so a systematic approach must be undertaken.

Screening

- Given that there are a wide range of triggers for AD, from allergens to environmental factors such as heat, humidity, irritants, and stress, the question of whom to screen for food hypersensitivity arises. In general, any patient who responds poorly to the usual AD treatment regimen of hydrating baths, topical steroids, lubricating ointments, and antihistamines should be screened for evidence of food hypersensitivity. Furthermore, if an obvious pattern is noted between ingestion of a food and exacerbation of skin conditions, an evaluation should be pursued.

Primary prevention

- There is no consensus on methods of primary prevention for food-induced AD.

Secondary prevention

- Once a specific food has been identified to exacerbate a patient's AD, that food should be eliminated from the patient's diet. Because certain food allergies are frequently outgrown, particularly milk and egg in the pediatric population, routine monitoring for clinically relevant allergy is essential.

Section 3: Diagnosis (Algorithm 17.1)

> **BOTTOM LINE/CLINICAL PEARLS**
> - AD is a clinical diagnosis based on identification of the classic pruritic skin eruption that occurs by the age of 5 years in nearly 85% of cases.
> - For patients who have additional atopic conditions, or for patients who do not seem to improve on the classic regimen of skincare treatment, an investigation into food hypersensitivity should be undertaken.
> - The diagnosis involves identification of food sensitization (via skin testing or serum IgE evaluation) and confirmation of clinical allergy with oral food challenges.
> - Ingestion of a causal food can provoke a flare of eczema within minutes to hours if the reaction is IgE-mediated, or infrequently can take hours to days if the reaction is non-IgE-mediated. Consequently, history of food-induced symptoms is often not evident in patients with AD and food allergy.
> - A patient may have persistent lesions if the food is eaten chronically.
> - Food elimination with subsequent monitoring for skin clearing is the key to diagnosis.

Differential diagnosis

Differential diagnosis	Features
Allergic contact dermatitis	Suspicion of reaction to a medication or skincare product
Exposure to irritants	Environmental history
Severe AD unrelated to food	No improvement on elimination diet and/or spontaneous relapses without dietary intervention

Typical presentation

- Food-induced AD is more commonly seen in the pediatric population. Typically, an infant will present who has severe eczema and is starting to eat solid foods. The parents note that when a certain food, such as egg, is fed to the child, he/she will have a flare of eczema within 24 hours. The same scenario may be seen at a younger age with introduction of milk- or soy-based formulas. There is often a family history of atopy in such cases. Allergy testing for milk, egg, peanut, wheat, and soy can be undertaken, and sensitivity to one or more food allergens likely noted (egg allergy is the most frequent cause of food-induced AD exacerbations). Once the sensitized food is completely eliminated from the child's diet, the eczema should improve.

Clinical diagnosis

History

- The clinician should enquire about periods of exacerbation and remission. Patients are unlikely to have food-induced AD if they have extended periods of clear skin with little need for topical corticosteroids while on a regular diet. Food allergy is more likely a trigger if the onset or worsening of skin symptoms correlates with exposure to the food, but this is often not evident, especially in children with moderate to severe disease.

Algorithm 17.1 Diagnosis of atopic dermatitis

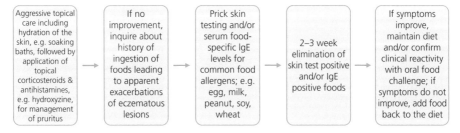

Physical examination
- A complete skin examination to evaluate the extent and severity of eczematous involvement is key to diagnosis. Clinicians should look for other signs of atopic conditions such as asthma or allergic rhinitis. This includes a lung examination to evaluate potential wheezing as well as an ENT examination to evaluate for signs of rhinitis or ocular allergy.

Useful clinical decision rules and calculators
- Food-induced AD is more common in infants and young children.
- In general, the more severe the AD, the more likely that food allergy is present.

Disease severity classification
- Food-induced AD is clinically indistinguishable from classic food allergy with risk for severe systemic reaction, including anaphylaxis. An evaluation for the latter condition may be needed based on the patient's history. While patients with AD may appear to tolerate certain food allergens with no evidence of acute allergic symptoms, elimination of these foods from their diet for a 2–3 week period may result in the development of acute allergic symptoms (e.g. dyspnea and wheezing, vomiting) with reintroduction of the food.

Laboratory diagnosis
List of diagnostic tests
- Prick skin testing to common food allergens as well as suspected foods.
- Serum food-specific IgE evaluation.

Lists of imaging techniques
Not applicable for this topic.

Potential pitfalls/common errors made regarding diagnosis of disease
- Not all foods to which a patient is sensitized will result in a challenge-confirmed food allergy or lead to eczema flares.
- Clinicians must be careful not to overly restrict a patient's diet, particularly in the pediatric population, and thereby place the patient at risk of nutritional deficiency.
- Foods should not be eliminated from the diet without firm clinical suspicion.

Section 4: Treatment
Treatment rationale
- A hydrating skincare regimen with use of topical steroids or antibiotics as needed is necessary in the initial management of all forms of eczema.
- For patients with food-induced symptoms, elimination of the food from the patient's diet should lead to improvement.
- Patients should be evaluated at regular intervals to determine if the food allergy is resolved, especially to milk and egg. However, children with serum IgE levels greater than 25 kU$_A$/L to major food allergen are unlikely to "outgrow" the food allergy in the short term.

When to hospitalize
- Patients with food-exacerbated AD rarely need to be hospitalized. Reasons for hospitalization might include a severe anaphylactic reaction to food or a severe skin infection resulting from excoriations of eczematous skin lesions.

Managing the hospitalized patient
Not applicable for this topic.

Table of treatment

Treatment	Comment
Conservative	Elimination of foods to which a patient has hypersensitivity and which exacerbate skin symptoms
Medical	Lubricating emollients, topical steroids, and antibiotics may be needed for management of skin lesions and super-infections

Prevention/management of complications
- It is important to note that once a food allergen is identified as a trigger of AD and removed from a patient's diet, there is a risk for severe allergic reaction upon reintroduction of that food, particularly if hypersensitivity persists. Routine monitoring of sensitivity via skin and serum testing as well as introduction of a food in a monitored setting is generally necessary.

> **CLINICAL PEARLS**
> - Not all foods to which an atopic patient has evidence of IgE sensitivity will result in clinically significant food allergy or eczema exacerbations.
> - Do not overly restrict a patient's diet without firm clinical evidence of hypersensitivity.
> - There is a risk for anaphylaxis upon reintroduction of a food that was eliminated from the diet for reasons of food-exacerbated AD.

Section 5: Special populations
Pregnancy
No change in management.

Children

No change in management. Attention to nutritional status upon food elimination.

Elderly

No change in management. Overall, less common issue in this population.

Others

Not applicable for this topic.

Section 6: Prognosis

> **BOTTOM LINE/CLINICAL PEARLS**
> * AD is characterized by relapses and exacerbations of disease.
> * Removal of an inciting food can improve overall skin condition in food-exacerbated eczema.
> * Pediatric patients will often outgrow their food hypersensitivities that are associated with AD.

Natural history of untreated disease

* Continued feeding of food allergens may lead to more severe AD lesions and secondary infection due to severe pruritus.

Prognosis for treated patients

Not applicable for this topic.

Follow-up tests and monitoring

* Serum food-specific IgE levels.

Section 7: Reading list

Caubet JC, Eigenmann PA. Allergic triggers in atopic dermatitis. Immunol Allergy Clin North Am 2010;30:289–307

Eigenman PA, Sicherer SH, Borkowski TA, Cohen BA, Sampson HA. Prevalence of IgE-mediated food allergy among children with atopic dermatitis. Pediatrics 1998;101:E8

Hill DJ, Hosking CS, de Benedictis FM, Oranje AP, Diepgen TL, Bauchau V; EPAAC Study Group. Confirmation of the association between high levels of immunoglobulin E food sensitization and eczema in infancy: an international study. Clin Exp Allergy 2008;38:161–8

NIAID-Sponsored Expert Panel, Boyce JA, Assa'ad A, Burks AW, Jones SM, Sampson HA, Wood RA, et al. Guidelines for the diagnosis and management of food allergy in the United States: report of the NIAID-sponsored expert panel. J Allergy Clin Immunol 2010;126(Suppl):S1–58

Sicherer SH, Sampson HA. Food hypersensitivity and atopic dermatitis: pathophysiology, epidemiology, diagnosis, and management. J Allergy Clin Immunol 1999;104:S114–22

Tollefson MM, Bruckner AL. Atopic dermatitis: Skin-directed management. Pediatrics 2014;134(6):e1735–44

Werfel T, Breuer K. Role of food allergy in atopic dermatitis. Curr Opin Allergy Clin Immunol 2004;379–85

Suggested websites

www.acaai.org
www.aaaai.org
www.aad.org

Section 8: Guidelines
National society guidelines

Guideline title	Source	Date
Atopic dermatitis: A practice parameter update.	American Academy of Allergy, Asthma & Immunology	2012 (http://www.allergyparameters. org/published-practice- parameters/alphabetical-listing/ dermatitis-download/)
Guidelines for the Diagnosis and Management of Food Allergy in the United States: Report of the NIAID-Sponsored Expert Panel	NIH, National Institute of Allergy and Infectious Disease	2010 (http://www.ncbi.nlm.nih.gov/ pubmed/21134576)

Section 9: Evidence
Not applicable for this topic.

Section 10: Images
Not applicable for this topic.

Additional material for this chapter can be found online at:
www.mountsinaiexpertguides.com
This includes a case study, multiple choice questions, advice for patients, and ICD codes

CHAPTER 18

Food Protein-Induced Enterocolitis Syndrome

Elizabeth J. Feuille and Anna Nowak-Węgrzyn
Jaffe Food Allergy Institute, Icahn School of Medicine at Mount Sinai, New York, NY, USA

OVERALL BOTTOM LINE

- Food protein-induced enterocolitis syndrome (FPIES) is a non-IgE-mediated food hypersensitivity. Patients typically present with profuse vomiting, diarrhea, and dehydration in the acute setting, or with weight loss and failure to thrive in the chronic form.
- The most common inciting foods are cow's milk (CM) and soy formulas, and rice in young infants.
- FPIES is diagnosed based on history and typical symptoms, which improve with food avoidance, and exclusion of other etiologies.
- Management of FPIES includes rehydration in the acute setting and food avoidance and provision of an emergency treatment plan for reactions after accidental ingestion.
- The majority of patients with FPIES caused by CM and soy resolve within the first 3–5 years of life; solid food FPIES or FPIES associated with positive food-specific IgE may have a more protracted course.

Section 1: Background
Definition of disease

- FPIES is a non-IgE-mediated food hypersensitivity in which patients present in infancy with profuse vomiting, sometimes accompanied by diarrhea, resulting in dehydration, lethargy, weight loss, and failure to thrive.

Incidence/prevalence

- Non-IgE-mediated or mixed gastrointestinal immune hypersensitivities to CM account for 40% of all CM protein allergy in children.
- The incidence of CM FPIES in a large Israeli birth cohort was found to 0.34% (44/33 019); by comparison, the incidence of IgE-mediated CM allergy in this population was 0.5%.
- The prevalence of FPIES in the United States is not known.

Etiology

- The mechanisms through which FPIES develops are as yet unclear.
- The most common triggering foods causing FPIES are CM and soy, although FPIES may also occur upon ingestion of solid foods, including grains (rice, oats, barley, corn), meat and poultry

---

Mount Sinai Expert Guides: Allergy and Clinical Immunology, First Edition. Edited by Hugh A. Sampson.
© 2015 John Wiley & Sons, Ltd. Published 2015 by John Wiley & Sons, Ltd.
Companion website: www.mountsinaiexpertguides.com

(beef, chicken, turkey), egg white, vegetables (white potato, sweet potato, squash, string bean), fruit (tomato, banana), legumes (peanut, green pea, lentil), seafood (fish, crustaceans, mollusks), and the probiotic *Saccharomyces boulardii*.

Pathology/pathogenesis

- The mechanisms underlying FPIES are not known.
- It is hypothesized that T-cell activation by food allergens may mediate local intestinal inflammation through release of pro-inflammatory cytokines, causing increased intestinal permeability and fluid shifts. This local inflammation may be mediated by activated peripheral mononuclear cells, increased TNF-β, and decreased expression of TGF-β receptors in the intestinal mucosa.
- Patients with FPIES have decreased food-specific IgG_4 and increased serum food-specific IgA levels. Though systemic food-specific IgE is typically absent in FPIES, intestinal mucosal IgE antibodies may facilitate antigen uptake and intestinal inflammation.
- Increased eosinophils present in intestinal biopsies, blood and stool samples from patients with FPIES point to possible overlap of the immunopathogenic mechanisms underlying food protein-induced syndromes and eosinophilic gastroenteropathies.

Predictive/risk factors

- There is only one study using a large unselected birth cohort in Israel with sufficient data to calculate odds ratios.

Risk factor	Odds ratio
Cesarean delivery	2.57
Jewish race	10
Male gender	52–60% of infants with FPIES are male*
FPIES to other food protein	30–50% of patients with FPIES to one food develop FPIES to another*
Personal history of atopic disease	Present in 30% of FPIES patients*
Family history of atopic disease	Present in 40–80% of FPIES patients*
Family history of food allergy	Present in 20% of FPIES patients*

*Sufficient data are not available to calculate odds ratio.

Section 2: Prevention

> **BOTTOM LINE/CLINICAL PEARLS**
> - Prevention of FPIES has not been studied; however, breastfeeding appears to be protective as FPIES is very rare in exclusively breastfed infants.

Screening

There are no screening methods for FPIES.

Primary prevention

- Primary prevention in FPIES has not been well studied.
- Breastfeeding appears to have a role in preventing FPIES. CM FPIES in exclusively breastfed infants is rare, with only four case reports in the literature.

Section 3: Diagnosis (Algorithm 18.1)

Algorithm 18.1 Diagnosis of food protein-induced enterocolitis syndrome (FPIES)

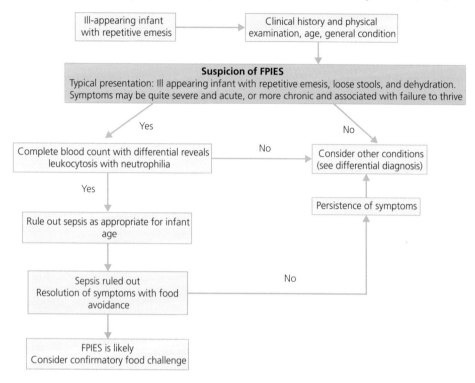

- FPIES is diagnosed based on history of typical presenting symptoms, which improve with removal of the offending food from the diet, and exclusion of other etiologies.
- On examination, infants with FPIES often appear dehydrated and lethargic; infants with chronic FPIES may additionally have failure to thrive.
- Though there are no laboratory or radiographic findings specific to FPIES, findings of an elevated white blood count with neutrophilia and methemoglobinemia following food ingestion and vomiting are consistent with FPIES.
- Oral food challenge (OFC) is the gold standard for diagnosis, but may not be necessary for the initial diagnosis if the child presents with recurrent symptoms consistent with typical FPIES.

Differential diagnosis

Differential diagnosis	Features
Food protein-induced proctitis/ proctocolitis	Blood-streaked stools, otherwise well
Food protein-induced enteropathy	Malabsorption, failure to thrive, intermittent emesis, and blood-streaked diarrhea

(Continued)

Differential diagnosis	Features
Eosinophilic gastrointestinal disorders	Nausea, emesis, abdominal pain and distension, early satiety, diarrhea, weight loss, difficulty swallowing, and food impaction; insidious and chronic in onset
Anaphylaxis	Emesis, lethargy, rash (urticaria), oropharyngeal swelling, and bronchoconstriction; within minutes to hours after ingestion of offending food
Sepsis	Lethargy, emesis, diarrhea, hypothermia, and hypotension; associated fever and respiratory symptoms when present are distinguishing features
Infectious gastroenteritis or enteritis (viral, bacterial, or parasitic)	Emesis, lethargy, diarrhea, and dehydration; reported sick contacts and presence of other manifestations of infection are distinguishing features
Intestinal obstruction due to volvulus or other	Acute onset of bilious emesis and feeding intolerance
Gastroesophageal reflux disease (GERD)	Emesis and discomfort after feeding, persisting despite formula changes
Necrotizing enterocolitis	Variable presentation that includes emesis, feeding intolerance, diarrhea, abdominal distension, and lethargy; when present, temperature instability, abdominal distension, and gastric retention are distinguishing features
Metabolic disease	May manifest acutely with emesis, dehydration, and lethargy, and chronically with failure to thrive; findings of hypoglycemia, anion gap metabolic acidosis, or hyperammonemia should raise suspicion for a metabolic disorder
Congenital methemoglobinemia	Typically mild symptoms, including headache and easy fatigability

Typical presentation
- FPIES occurs in chronic and acute forms.
  - Chronic FPIES occurs with frequent ingestion of the inciting food. It typically occurs in a formula-fed infant in the first weeks of life, with symptoms of intermittent emesis, watery or mucus-containing diarrhea, poor weight gain, and dehydration.
  - Acute FPIES occurs with intermittent ingestion of the inciting food, with the onset of symptoms 1–3 hours after ingestion, typically with somewhat more severe presentation than chronic FPIES. In addition to profuse emesis (which may be projectile and occur up to 10–20 times) and dehydration, infants may develop lethargy, pallor, and hypotension.

Clinical diagnosis
History
- Detailed history regarding the timing and number of vomiting episodes, diarrhea, and association with feeding changes; the infant's growth since birth; any associated symptoms including choking, breathing difficulty, cyanosis, abdominal distension; and office or emergency department visits for symptoms.

Physical examination
- The clinician should pay particular attention to the following, which indicate the need for resuscitation: lethargy, depressed fontanelle, sunken eyes, dry mucous membranes, poor skin turgor, prolonged capillary refill, pallor, and cyanosis.

Laboratory diagnosis

List of diagnostic tests

- A complete blood count (CBC) with differential may reveal leukocytosis with neutrophilia, anemia, eosinophilia, and thrombocytosis.
- Blood chemistries in significantly dehydrated infants may reveal electrolyte abnormalities.
- A blood gas assessment should be ordered for infants who are ill-appearing or lethargic, and may reveal non-anion gap metabolic acidosis (with a mean pH of 7.03 in one series).
- Co-oximetry to assess for methemoglobinemia is important when an infant appears ashen, gray, or cyanotic on physical examination.
- Food-specific IgE and/or skin prick testing may be ordered non-emergently to provide complete evaluation for food sensitization, particularly when considering a food challenge. Though more than 90% of patients with FPIES have undetectable serum IgE at the time of diagnosis, 18–30% of patients with FPIES develop IgE-mediated food sensitivity to the same food at some point during their course.
- Endoscopy with biopsy may be indicated to rule out other gastrointestinal disorder when symptoms do not resolve with bowel rest or amino acid based formula.
- Stool studies may reveal elevated leukocytes, frank or occult blood, and/or eosinophils.
- OFC is the gold standard for diagnosis, but may not be necessary for initial diagnosis if the child presents with recurrent symptoms typical of FPIES. OFC in patients with FPIES is considered a high-risk procedure, and is best performed under physician supervision in a facility capable of administering intravenous fluids. OFC involves administering 0.06–0.6 g of food protein divided in three equal portions, eaten over 30 minutes, and followed by observation for 4–6 hours prior to discharge. OFC is positive if typical symptoms and laboratory findings occur. Symptoms include emesis (onset 1–3 hours), lethargy (onset 1–3 hours), and, less often, diarrhea (onset 2–10 hours, mean 5 hours). CBC with differential should be sent prior to and about 6 hours after challenge if there are symptoms. If diarrhea is present, stool guaiac tests and other stool investigations may be required.
- In research studies, gastric juice analysis showing >10 leukocytes/high-powered field (hpf) 3 hours after a food challenge and atopy patch testing have been evaluated in patients with FPIES, but the utility of these tests has not yet been confirmed.

Lists of imaging techniques

- Radiologic studies are not part of the routine diagnostic investigation for FPIES but may be obtained when the diagnosis is not clear in order to rule out other etiologies. Abdominal X-ray may reveal distension of small bowel loops, air–fluid levels, non-specific narrowing, and thumb-printing of the rectum and sigmoid, intramural gas, thickening of the plicae circulares in the duodenum and jejunum with excess luminal fluid.

Potential pitfalls/common errors made regarding diagnosis of disease

- Infants with FPIES often present with multiple reactions and extensive evaluations before the diagnosis of FPIES is considered.
- Factors contributing to delays in diagnosis of FPIES include the non-specific nature of symptoms and lack of classic allergic skin and respiratory symptoms, broad differential diagnosis, relative lack of knowledge among physicians, and, in the case of FPIES to solid foods, the perception that grains and vegetables are hypoallergenic (Table 18.1).

Table 18.1 Empirical recommendations for dietary management of food protein-induced enterocolitis (FPIES). No controlled trials have been performed to determine optimal timing of introduction in infants and toddlers with FPIES.

	Milk/soy FPIES	Solid food FPIES	Milk/soy and solid food FPIES
0–12 months			
Avoid cow's milk and soy	X		X
Exclusive breastfeeding[a] or extensively hydrolyzed casein formula[b] or consider soy OFC in case of milk FPIES	X		X
Introduce yellow vegetables	X	X	X
Avoid grains[c], legumes, poultry		X[d]	X[d]
>12 months			
Avoid trigger foods, OFC with reactive food every 18 months	X	X	X
Exclusive breastfeeding[a] or extensively hydrolyzed casein formula[b] or consider soy OFC in case of milk FPIES	X		X
Consider OFC with milk or soy if not tried	X	X	X
Consider OFC with grains, legumes, poultry if not tried		X[d]	X[d]

[a]No maternal elimination diet recommended unless reactions to food through breast milk.
[b]If not tolerated, an amino acid based formula should be initiated.
[c]Including oat, rice, wheat, barley, rye.
[d]Oral food challenges may be necessary to introduce new solid foods to children with multiple food FPIES.
Source: Järvinen KM, Nowak-Wegrzyn A. Food protein induced enterocolitis syndrome: current management strategies. J Allergy Clin Immunol 2013;1:317. Reproduced with permission from Elsevier.

Section 4: Treatment (Algorithm 18.2)

Treatment rationale

- Treatment of acute and chronic FPIES consists of dietary food elimination, supportive therapies for acute and chronic FPIES on presentation, and providing an emergency treatment plan for episodes resulting from accidental exposures.
- *Acute episode:* the first line in management of an acute episode of FPIES is vigorous intravenous hydration, usually 10–20 mL/kg bolus of normal saline, repeated as needed. The second line includes a single dose of intravenous methylprednisolone (dosed at 1 mg/kg, with a maximum of 60–80 mg), in order to decrease presumed cell-mediated inflammation. Patients may need other supportive therapies as necessary including supplemental oxygen, vasopressors, bicarbonate, and methylene blue. A recent case report described the use of ondansetron for the management of severe emesis during the food challenge in FPIES.
- *Elimination diet:* infants with suspected FPIES to cow's or soy milk protein should strictly avoid all forms of the inciting food, including baked and processed foods. They may be either exclusively breastfed or start a casein hydrolysate-based formula. Ten to 20% may require an amino acid-based formula. For the rare cases of FPIES in breastfed infants, breastfeeding mothers should eliminate the suspected trigger food(s) from her diet.

Algorithm 18.2 Management of FPIES

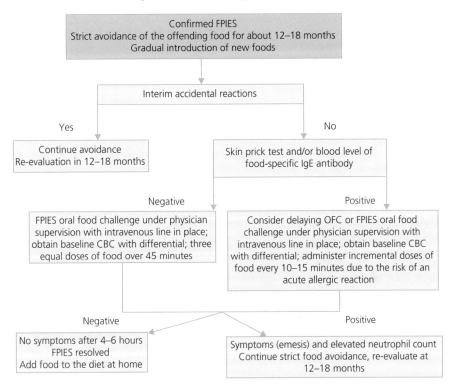

- *Food introduction:* for infants with FPIES to one food, experts recommended delaying the introduction of grain, legumes, poultry, as well as cow's and soy milk until the first year because of the high rate of FPIES to multiple foods.
- *Emergency treatment plan:* emergency treatment plans outlining clinical features and management of acute reactions should be provided to patients with FPIES (a template can be accessed on the International Association for Food Protein Enterocolitis, http://iaffpe.org/docs/Emergency_Plan.pdf). Mild reactions may be managed with careful oral rehydration at home. Infants with more severe reactions require resuscitation in the emergency department or inpatient unit (see Treatment rationale for acute episode).

When to hospitalize
- Significant dehydration, with inability to continue rehydration or keep up with ongoing losses with fluid intake by mouth.
- Persistent tachycardia, acidosis, hypotension, or lethargy despite administration of intravenous fluids in the emergency department.
- Methemoglobinemia requiring intravenous methylene blue.

Prevention/management of complications
- Treatment complications are minimal as the mainstay of treatment consists of dietary food elimination and provision of an emergency plan for accidental ingestions. Nutritional consultation may be necessary.

> **CLINICAL PEARLS**
> - Infants with moderate to severe reactions should be resuscitated in the emergency department or inpatient unit with intravenous fluids and other supportive therapies. Intravenous methylprednisolone may be used for more severe reactions, although its therapeutic benefit has not been proven in controlled clinical trials.
> - The mainstay of treatment is dietary elimination of the inciting food and provision of an emergency plan.
> - Currently, experts recommend avoiding the inciting food until 1 year of life, after which OFC should be considered every 18–24 months.

Section 5: Special populations

Not applicable for this topic.

Section 6: Prognosis

> **BOTTOM LINE/CLINICAL PEARLS**
> - Infants with acute FPIES reactions generally recover rapidly with rehydration alone.
> - Infants with chronic FPIES usually return to usual state of health within 3–10 days of switching to a hypoallergenic formula.
> - FPIES to one food increases likelihood of developing FPIES to other foods.
> - Age of FPIES resolution varies widely depending on the inciting foods, the country, and the population being studied.

Natural history of untreated disease

- For CM FPIES, resolution rates by age 3 years ranges from about 50% in a US referral population to 90% in an Israeli birth cohort. For soy FPIES, resolution rates range from 25% by age 3 years in a US referral population to 90% by age 10 months in a Korean cohort. For solid food FPIES, a retrospective study in Italy reported a resolution rate of 48%. In US referral populations, resolution rates are approximately 40% for rice, 66% for oat, and 67% for vegetables.
- Though the majority of patients with FPIES have negative specific IgE antibodies and skin prick tests at diagnosis, those with positive testing tend to have a more protracted course and are at risk for developing IgE-mediated food allergy.

Follow-up tests and monitoring

- After 1 year of life, consider OFC to inciting foods every 18–24 months, along with testing to evaluate for development of food-specific IgE.

Section 7: Reading list

Järvinen KM, Nowak-Wegrzyn A. Food protein induced enterocolitis syndrome: current management strategies. J Allergy Clin Immunol 2013;1:317

Katz Y, Goldberg MR, Rajuan N, Cohen A, Leshno M. The prevalence and natural course of food protein-induced enterocolitis syndrome to cow's milk: a large-scale, prospective population-based study. J Allergy Clin Immunol 2011;127:647–53

Leonard SA, Nowak-Wegrzyn A. Manifestations, diagnosis, and management of food protein-induced entero-colitis syndrome. Pediatr Ann 2013;42:135–40

Mehr S, Kakakios A, Frith K, Kemp AS. Food protein induced enterocolitis: 16-year experience. Pediatrics 2009;123:e459

Sicherer SH. Food protein-induced enterocolitis syndrome: case presentations and management lessons. J Allergy Clin Immunol 2005;115:149–56

Suggested websites

www.fpies.org

http://www.niaid.nih.gov/topics/foodallergy/clinical/Pages/default.aspx

Section 8: Guidelines
National society guidelines

Guideline title	Guideline source, comment	Date
Guidelines for the Diagnosis and Management of Food Allergy in the United States	National Institute of Allergy and Infectious Disease (NIAID) **Comment:** These guidelines were developed by a panel of experts in the field, through review and evaluation of recent publications about food allergy	2011 (http://www.niaid.nih.gov/topics/foodallergy/clinical/Pages/default.aspx)

Section 9: Evidence

Type of evidence	Title, comment	Date
Prospective, cohort study	The prevalence and natural course of food protein-induced enterocolitis syndrome to cow's milk: a large-scale, prospective population-based study **Comment:** This is the only study assessing the prevalence of FPIES; it describes the natural course of FPIES in a large birth cohort	2011 (Katz Y et al. J Allergy Clin Immunol 2011;127;647–53)
Cohort study	Indexes of suspicion of typical cow's milk protein-induced enterocolitis **Comment:** In this analysis of 142 consecutive infants admitted with vomiting and diarrhea, authors identify independent predictors of FPIES to cow's milk (versus infants with infection), which included failure to thrive and hypoalbuminemia	2007 (Hwang JB et al. J Korean Med Sci 2007;94:425)
Retrospective study	A multicenter retrospective study of 66 Italian children with food protein-induced enterocolitis syndrome: different management for different phenotypes **Comment:** This study demonstrated an increase in FPIES diagnosis over the 7 years of the study. It documented presentations and natural course of FPIES in 66 children	2012 (Sopo SM et al. Clin Exp Allergy 2012;42:326)

(Continued)

Type of evidence	Title, comment	Date
Restrospective study	Food protein-induced enterocolitis: a 16-year experience **Comment:** In reviewing the cases of 35 children with FPIES, the authors highlight the frequent misdiagnosis and delays in diagnosis of FPIES; they identify hypothermia and thrombocytosis as features of FPIES	2009 (Mehr S et al. Pediatrics 2009;123:e459)
Cohort study	Prospective follow-up oral food challenge in food protein-induced enterocolitis syndrome **Comment:** The authors determined resolution rates for 23 infants with FPIES in a Korean cohort	2009 (Hwang JB et al. Arch Dis Child 2009;94:425)
Retrospective study	Clinical features of food protein-induced enterocolitis syndrome **Comment:** Thorough discussion of 16 patients with FPIES in a referral population, this article clarifies the diagnostic features, laboratory evaluation, food challenge results, and clinical course of FPIES	1998 (Sicherer SH et al. J Pediatr 1998;133:214)
Retrospective study	Food protein-induced enterocolitis syndrome caused by solid food proteins **Comment:** The clinical characteristics and natural course of 14 infants with solid food FPIES are described and compared with 30 infants with cow's milk or soy FPIES	2003 (Nowak-Wegrzyn et al. Pediatrics 2003;111:829)

Section 10: Images

Not applicable for this topic.

Additional material for this chapter can be found online at:
www.mountsinaiexpertguides.com
This includes a case study, multiple choice questions, advice for patients, and ICD codes

CHAPTER 19

Food Protein-Induced Proctocolitis Syndrome

Jean-Christoph Caubet[1] and Anna Nowak-Węgrzyn[2]

[1] Division of Allergy, Department of Pediatrics, University Hospitals of Geneva, Geneva, Switzerland
[2] Jaffe Food Allergy Institute, Icahn School of Medicine at Mount Sinai, New York, NY, USA

OVERALL BOTTOM LINE

- Food protein-induced proctocolitis (FPIP) should be suspected in well-appearing infants presenting with isolated bloody stools.
- No specific diagnostic test is available and the diagnosis is based mainly on the clinical response to a strict elimination diet and exclusion of other etiologies.
- FPIP is characterized by an eosinophil-dominated inflammation limited to the rectum and distal sigmoid colon.

Section 1: Background

Definition of disease

- Food protein-induced proctocolitis or proctitis is a benign and transient non-IgE-mediated food allergy, characterized by an inflammatory response limited to the rectum and distal sigmoid colon induced by ingested food proteins. From a clinical point of view, the typical presentation is blood-streaked stools appearing in the first few weeks of life in otherwise healthy breastfed infants or infants receiving infantile formulas (i.e. milk or soy formulas).

Disease classification

- According to the current nomenclature of allergy, FPIP is classified as a non-IgE-mediated allergic disorder.

Incidence/prevalence

- The overall prevalence of rectal bleeding and of FPIP is not well established.
- In one study, rectal bleeding was the chief complaint in 0.3% of more than 40 000 patients presenting to a referral hospital emergency department.
- FPIP appears to be a common cause of rectal bleeding in otherwise healthy infants, with a prevalence in the range of 18–64%; one study estimated the prevalence of isolated rectal bleeding attributed to cow's milk consumption to be 0.16%.

Economic impact

Not applicable for this topic.

Mount Sinai Expert Guides: Allergy and Clinical Immunology, First Edition. Edited by Hugh A. Sampson.
© 2015 John Wiley & Sons, Ltd. Published 2015 by John Wiley & Sons, Ltd.
Companion website: www.mountsinaiexpertguides.com

Etiology

- FPIP typically occurs in breastfed infants, with cow's milk and soy proteins from the mother's diet being the most common causes.
- FPIP is also common in infants fed with cow's milk or soy-based formulas.

Pathology/pathogenesis

- The exact pathogenic mechanism of FPIP is not well defined.
- This disorder most commonly affects the distal colon and the rectum. The reason why specific food proteins induce an inflammatory response limited to this part of the digestive tract is not known.
- Endoscopy typically reveals focal erythema with lymphoid nodular hyperplasia. Biopsy shows an eosinophil-dominated inflammation. These cells are often degranulated and localized next to the lymphoid nodules. Eosinophil mediators may be responsible for mast cells' degranulation, smooth muscle constriction, gastric dismotility, and stimulation of chloride secretion from colonic epithelium. Of note, these pathologic features are similar to other forms of eosinophilic gastrointestinal disorders, suggesting that they could correspond to different forms and grades of the same fundamental process.

Predictive/risk factors

Risk factors have not been determined.

Section 2: Prevention

No interventions have been demonstrated to prevent the development of the disease.

Screening

No screening tests have been shown to be useful in this disease

Primary prevention

Not applicable for this topic.

Secondary prevention

- Secondary prevention relies on the avoidance of the offending food in the diet.

Section 3: Diagnosis (Algorithm 19.1)

> **BOTTOM LINE/CLINICAL PEARLS**
> - The diagnosis is based on a positive clinical history (mild rectal bleeding in an otherwise healthy infant) and resolution of symptoms following elimination of the causative food protein, usually within 48–96 hours.
> - Skin prick tests and specific IgE are usually negative in FPIP.
> - Exclusion of other causes of rectal bleeding, particularly infection, anal fissure, necrotizing enterocolitis, and intussusception, is of major importance.

Differential diagnosis

Differential diagnosis	Features
Anal fissure	Most common cause of rectal bleeding in children younger than 1 year; clinical examination lead to correct diagnosis
Infection	Fever, abdominal pain, diarrhea, vomiting, tenesmus
Food protein-induced enterocolitis syndrome (FPIES)	Severe, repetitive emesis in 1–3 hours, diarrhea in 2–10 hours after food intake; tends to persist longer; chronic form may cause failure to thrive

Differential diagnosis	Features
Swallowed maternal blood	Transient, self-resolving, blood in the stool not associated with any other symptoms
Meckel's diverticulum	Painless rectal bleeding in an otherwise healthy individual
Necrotizing enterocolitis	Typically occurs in infants born prematurely, associated with fever or hypothermia, septic appearance, abdominal distension and presence of intramural gas on abdominal X-ray
Intussusception	Sudden-onset, severe, crampy, progressive abdominal pain, crying, lethargy associated with bloody mucus in the stool (currant jelly stool). Uncommon prior to 3 months of age

Algorithm 19.1 Diagnosis of food protein-induced proctocolitis

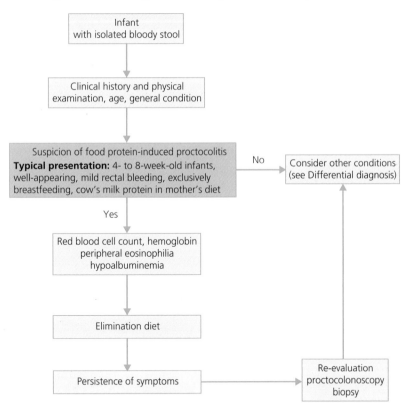

Typical presentation

- The patient typically presents at 2–8 weeks of age with gradual onset of intermittent blood-streaked stools having a normal or soft consistency.
- Infants with FPIP are otherwise healthy and thriving. Most of them are either breastfed or fed with standard infant cow's milk or soy-based formulas.
- The symptoms increase in frequency if the incriminated food is continuously ingested and resolves only after complete elimination of the offending food, usually within 3 days.

Clinical diagnosis
History
- The diagnosis is mainly based on a typical clinical history and resolution of symptoms following withdrawal of the presumed food antigen.
- Although FPIP typically occurs before the age of 4 months, the age of onset ranges from 1 week of life to 14 years of age. Breastfed infants are often older at the time of initial presentation and have less severe disease.
- In addition to the bloody stools, associated digestive symptoms have been described in up to one-third of the patients (i.e. increased gas, intermittent emesis, pain on defecation, or abdominal pain).
- A careful dietary history is essential to diagnose FPIP. In formula-fed infants, cow's milk and/or soy proteins are typically incriminated; in breastfed infants, it is usually caused by cow's milk and soy proteins.
- Although there is often a prolonged latent interval between the introduction of food proteins and the initial presentation, the onset of symptoms may occur within 12 hours after the first feeding of the offending food.
- Elimination of the offending food leads to complete resolution of the symptoms, typically within 48–96 hours, but it may take longer for some patients (i.e. up to 2 weeks).

Physical examination
- The physical examination should particularly focus on the digestive system and evaluation for anal fissures, as well as on the evaluation of the growth. No specific sign is characteristic of this disorder.

Useful clinical decision rules and calculators
Not applicable for this topic.

Disease severity classification
Not applicable for this topic.

Laboratory diagnosis
List of diagnostic tests
- A complete blood count (CBC) is recommended in children with persistent symptoms, particularly as some rare patients may develop mild anemia. Approximately one-third of the older children have peripheral eosinophilia, which does not correlate with the level of eosinophils in the biopsy.
- Although rare, an associated hypoalbuminemia can be found in some patients with more severe symptoms.
- Approximately one-quarter of patients have a history of atopy and elevated serum IgE levels, which correspond to the prevalence in the general population. Thus, skin prick tests and specific IgE are not recommended for an initial diagnosis, except for patients presenting with symptoms suggestive of a concomitant IgE-mediated food allergy.
- Smears of the fecal mucus usually reveal increased polymorphonuclear neutrophils.
- Colonoscopy should be reserved for patients with persistent bleeding despite implementation of an elimination diet, mainly to exclude another cause. The colonoscopy usually shows a mild colitis with focal erythema, rectal ulcerations, and lymphoid nodular hyperplasia.
- Biopsy reveals a high number of eosinophils (6 to >20 per 40× high power field) in the lamina propria and muscularis mucosa, features of eosinophils degranulation, and, occasionally, crypt abscesses.

Not applicable for this topic.

Potential pitfalls/common errors made regarding diagnosis of disease

- Some patients falsely diagnosed with anal fissures can present with symptoms lasting for several weeks.
- Distinction with food protein-induced enterocolitis syndrome (FPIES) could be difficult as the initial symptoms (bloody stools) may be similar to those of FPIP. Some authors have suggested that these disorders may represent a continuum of the same disease with similar underlying immunopathogenic mechanisms.

Section 4: Treatment (Algorithm 19.2)

Treatment rationale

- Treatment is based on dietary restriction.
- Mothers should be encouraged to continue breastfeeding, but will have to strictly avoid the offending food proteins in their diet.
- Initially, milk products are avoided. In the absence of clinical response, soy followed by egg should be eliminated. Usually, the symptoms resolve gradually within 72 hours, although it may take up to 2 weeks for complete resolution.
- In formula-fed children, casein hydrolysates are the first line of treatment; only a few infants (i.e. approximately 5–10%) will need amino acid-based formulas.
- Gradual reintroduction of the offending food is proposed usually at 8–12 months of age, usually at home. Recurrence of bleeding will appear within 6–72 hours if the infant is still allergic to the food.
- In infants with significant atopic dermatitis and/or IgE-mediated allergy to other foods, skin prick tests or serum measurement of food-specific IgE can be performed at that time. If food-specific IgE to the offending food is negative, food reintroduction can be carried out at home. If food-specific IgE to the offending food is positive, a supervised oral food challenge in the physician's office may be necessary.

When to hospitalize

Patients with FPIP do not usually require hospitalization.

Managing the hospitalized patient

Not applicable for this topic.

Table of treatment

Treatment	Comment
Dietary restriction	In breastfed infants, elimination of cow's milk from the maternal diet is recommended in the first place. If there is no improvement, elimination of soy followed by egg should be carried out. Rarely, weaning the baby from breast milk may be required In infants fed with artificial formula, formulas based on casein hydrolysate, or, in rare instances, an amino acid-based formula may be required
Iron supplementation	May be required in infants with an associated anemia
Psychological	The psychological impact of strict dietary restriction as well as the onset of the symptoms during the first few weeks of life may have important psychological consequences, which need to be managed appropriately

Algorithm 19.2 Management of food protein-induced proctocolitis

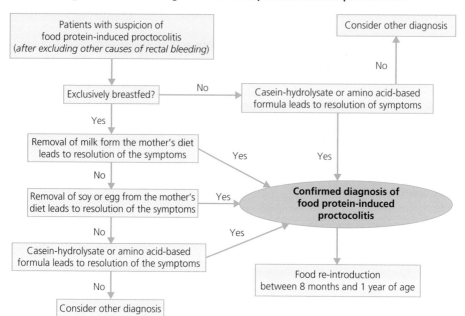

Prevention/management of complications
- Dietary restrictions may be responsible for nutrient deficiencies and may require additional supplementations, especially with calcium.
- Large dietary restrictions should be avoided and only limited to selected foods known to cause this disorder (i.e. milk, soy, egg, corn).
- The decision to start a diet should always be discussed with the pediatrician and/or the allergist. A nutritional consultation may be considered.

CLINICAL PEARLS
- In breastfed infants, it is recommended to eliminate milk products from the mother's diet first, followed by soy and egg in the absence of clinical response. Resolution of visible blood usually occurs within 48–96 hours.
- In infants fed by soy or milk formulas, an extensively hydrolyzed formula is recommended.
- Amino acid-based formula is rarely needed to control patients with FPIP.
- Food reintroduction is usually attempted at 8–12 months of age. If allergy tests to the offending food are negative, reintroduction can be carried out at home. If allergy food tests are positive, reintroduction may require an oral food challenge under physician supervision.

Section 5: Special populations
Not applicable for this topic.

Section 6: Prognosis

> **BOTTOM LINE/CLINICAL PEARLS**
> - The prognosis is excellent, the majority of patients achieve tolerance by 1 year of age and usually before 2 years of age.
> - Up to 20% of breastfed infants have spontaneous resolution of bleeding without changes in the maternal diet.
> - The long-term prognosis is excellent, and there are no report of inflammatory bowel disease in infants with FPIP followed for more than 10 years.

Natural history of untreated disease
- Some patients with a satisfying growth rate may have persistent bleeding despite maternal avoidance of food(s). These patients may develop anemia even though receiving iron supplementation, so regular laboratory monitoring is important for the follow-up.
- Persistence of bleeding may be a result of a partial elimination diet or because the allergen has not been correctly identified. Reaction to the human breast milk protein is another possible explanation.

Prognosis for treated patients
Not applicable for this topic.

Follow-up tests and monitoring
Not applicable for this topic.

Section 7: Reading list

Arvola T, Ruuska T, Keranen J, Hyoty H, Salminen S, Isolauri E. Rectal bleeding in infancy: clinical, allergological, and microbiological examination. Pediatrics 2006;117:e760–8

Elizur A, Cohen M, Goldberg MR, Rajuan N, Cohen A, Leshno M, et al. Cow's milk associated rectal bleeding: a population based prospective study. Pediatr Allergy Immunol 2012;23:766–70

Lake AM. Food-induced eosinophilic proctocolitis. J Pediatr Gastroenterol Nutr 2000;30(Suppl):S58–60

Maloney J, Nowak-Wegrzyn A. Educational clinical case series for pediatric allergy and immunology: allergic proctocolitis, food protein-induced enterocolitis syndrome and allergic eosinophilic gastroenteritis with protein-losing gastroenteropathy as manifestations of non-IgE-mediated cow's milk allergy. Pediatr Allergy Immunol 2007;18:360–7

Xanthakos SA, Schwimmer JB, Melin-Aldana H, Rothenberg ME, Witte DP, Cohen MB. Prevalence and outcome of allergic colitis in healthy infants with rectal bleeding: a prospective cohort study. J Pediatr Gastroenterol Nutr 2005;41:16–22

Suggested websites
Not applicable for this topic.

Section 8: Guidelines
National society guidelines

Guideline title	Guideline source	Date
Guidelines for the diagnosis and management of food allergy in the United States: Summary of the NIAID-Sponsored Expert Panel Report	J Allergy Clin Immunol	2010 (http://www.ncbi.nlm.nih.gov/pubmed/21134576)
Summary and recommendations: Classification of gastrointestinal manifestations due to immunologic reactions to foods in infants and young children	J Pediatr Gastroenterol Nutr	2000 (http://www.ncbi.nlm.nih.gov/pubmed/10634304)

Section 9: Evidence

Type of evidence	Title, comment	Date
Birth cohort study	Cow's milk associated rectal bleeding: a population based prospective study **Comment:** This is one of the largest studies evaluating the prevalence of rectal bleeding induced by cow's milk	2012 (http://www.ncbi.nlm.nih.gov/pubmed/23050491)
Prospective	Allergic proctocolitis in infants: a prospective clinicopathologic biopsy study Comment: This is a large prospective clinicopathologic biopsy study demonstrating the focal eosinophil-dominant inflammation in patients with FPIP	1993 (http://www.ncbi.nlm.nih.gov/pubmed/8505043)
Retrospective	Allergic proctitis and gastroenteritis in children. Clinical and mucosal biopsy features in 53 cases **Comment:** This is important large study on the clinical characteristics of patients with FPIP	1986 (http://www.ncbi.nlm.nih.gov/pubmed/3953938)

Section 10: Images
Not applicable for this topic.

Additional material for this chapter can be found online at:
www.mountsinaiexpertguides.com
This includes a case study, multiple choice questions, advice for patients, and ICD codes

CHAPTER 20

Eosinophilic Esophagitis

Mirna Chehade

Division of Allergy/Immunology, Department of Pediatrics, Icahn School of Medicine at Mount Sinai, New York, NY, USA

OVERALL BOTTOM LINE

- Eosinophilic esophagitis (EoE) is a chronic, immune/antigen-mediated esophageal disease characterized clinically by symptoms related to esophageal dysfunction and histologically by eosinophil-predominant inflammation.
- Although it is a relatively newly recognized disease, EoE has been reported worldwide, and its prevalence has been increasing over time.
- EoE seems to be triggered by multiple foods, and possibly aeroallergens.
- The pathogenesis of EoE is poorly understood; histopathology points towards an allergic phenomenon.
- Age-related differences in presenting symptoms are noticed in EoE. Children typically present with abdominal pain, gastroesophageal reflux symptoms, vomiting, feeding difficulties, and, at times, failure to thrive. Older children and adults present with dysphagia and esophageal food impactions.
- There are no FDA-approved therapies for EoE. If left untreated, EoE may lead to complications such as esophageal narrowing and strictures. Treatment has so far consisted of various forms of dietary restrictions and/or topical corticosteroids to the esophagus with variable success.

Section 1: Background
Definition of disease

- EoE is a chronic, immune/antigen-mediated esophageal disease characterized clinically by symptoms related to esophageal dysfunction and histologically by eosinophil-predominant inflammation.

Disease classification

Not applicable for this topic.

Incidence/prevalence

- EoE has been reported to occur worldwide. It seems to be reported more frequently in westernized, developed countries. The reason for this is unclear.
- The incidence and prevalence have been increasing over time. This is because of a true increase in the incidence in addition to improving awareness of the disease by health care providers.

Mount Sinai Expert Guides: Allergy and Clinical Immunology, First Edition. Edited by Hugh A. Sampson.
Companion website: www.mountsinaiexpertguides.com

- Using the International Classification of Diseases, 9th revision, code 530.13 for EoE, its prevalence is calculated to be 56.7/100 000 in the United States. This is deemed to be an underestimate, given that knowledge of the code and recognition of EoE have been suboptimal but improving over time.
- Approximately 1% of children and adults with gastroesophageal reflux symptoms prove to have EoE.
- Approximately 12–15% of adults referred to endoscopy for dysphagia are eventually diagnosed with EoE.
- Approximately 50% of adults with esophageal food impactions have EoE.

Etiology
- Multiple food allergens and possibly aeroallergens can act as triggers for EoE.

Pathology/pathogenesis
- The pathogenesis of EoE is poorly understood.
- Histopathologically similar to other allergic diseases, EoE is characterized by an inflammatory infiltrate in the epithelial layers of the esophagus, consisting of an increased number of T lymphocytes (both T-helper (CD4) and T-suppressor (CD8) cells), mast cells, and eosinophils. Finding 15 or more intraepithelial eosinophils per high power field (HPF) on microscopic examination of esophageal mucosal biopsy sections is considered diagnostic for EoE in the proper clinical setting.
- Mast cells and eosinophils residing in the esophagus seem to be activated in a large number of patients, as evidenced by degranulation on histopathologic examination.
- Increased number of mast cells and IgE-positive cells in the esophagus, and a tissue cytokine profile consistent with a T-helper type 2 phenotype, suggest an allergic etiology for EoE. Whether T-lymphocytes largely contribute to the T-helper type 2 allergic cytokine profile is still unknown.

Predictive/risk factors
- *Family history:* sibling recurrence risk ratio for EoE is estimated at approximately 80.
- *IgE-mediated food hypersensitivity:* rate of IgE-mediated food allergy in patients with EoE is reported to be 15–43%.
- *Allergic rhinitis:* rate of allergic rhinitis in patients with EoE is reported to be 40–75%.
- *Asthma:* rate of asthma in patients with EoE is reported to be 14–70%.
- *Atopic dermatitis:* rate of atopic dermatitis in patients with EoE is reported to be 40–75%.

Section 2: Prevention
No interventions have been demonstrated to prevent the development of the disease.

Screening
Not applicable for this topic.

Primary prevention
Not applicable for this topic.

Secondary prevention
- If the disease is food-responsive (i.e. disease remission is achieved by avoidance of certain food triggers), then continued avoidance of those food triggers may prevent recurrence of EoE.

Section 3: Diagnosis (Algorithm 20.1)

Algorithm 20.1 Diagnosis of eosinophilic esophagitis (EoE)

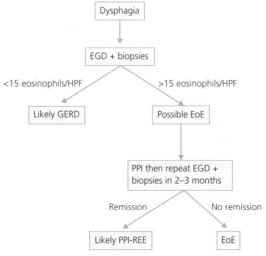

Note: EGD, esophagogastroduodenoscopy; GERD, gastroesophageal reflux disease; HPF, high power field; PPI-REE, proton pump inhibitor-responsive esophageal eosinophilia. Note that whenever remission is mentioned, it refers to clinical and histologic remission.

BOTTOM LINE/CLINICAL PEARLS
- Age-related differences in presenting symptoms are noticed with EoE. Children typically present with abdominal pain, gastroesophageal reflux symptoms including nausea and vomiting, and, at times, failure to thrive. Discerning EoE from acid-induced gastroesophageal reflux disease (GERD) by symptoms alone can be difficult, although dysphagia and early satiety/anorexia are more commonly seen in EoE than GERD. In infants and younger children, symptoms are harder to delineate, as EoE may simply manifest as feeding difficulties, such as food refusal and gagging with foods. In adults, symptoms are better defined, with dysphagia, food impactions, and heartburn and/or chest pain being the most common presenting symptoms.
- Physical examination is useful in children to identify any abnormal growth pattern, and in both children and adults to identify any comorbid allergic diseases. However, no features on physical examination are specific in making the diagnosis of EoE.
- The diagnosis of EoE is confirmed by esophagogastroduodenoscopy (EGD) with biopsies, demonstrating esophageal eosinophilia (15 or more eosinophils per HPF in the maximally infiltrated area of the esophageal epithelium) in the absence of increased eosinophils in other parts of the gastrointestinal tract, and after ruling out acid-induced GERD by negative pH probe or by empiric trial with proton pump inhibitor therapy for 8 weeks. Multiple esophageal biopsies need to be obtained, because the disease is patchy in nature.
- Radiologic tests are not routinely recommended for the diagnosis of EoE. They can be helpful in selected cases to characterize esophageal abnormalities that are difficult to identify by endoscopy, and can provide information on the length and diameter of complicated esophageal strictures in EoE.

- No specific blood test has shown utility in serving as a surrogate peripheral marker of esophageal eosinophilia in patients with EoE. Peripheral eosinophilia (absolute eosinophil count >300–350/mm³) was reported in 40–50% of patients with EoE. Total serum IgE levels are increased in 50–60% of patients with EoE. These tests can be influenced by the presence of comorbid allergic diseases in some patients with EoE.
- Sensitization to foods (positive skin prick tests to foods, positive serum food-specific IgE) is common in children with EoE, but the significance of these positive test results remains unclear.

Differential diagnosis

Differential diagnosis	Features
Gastroesophageal reflux disease (GERD)	The vast majority of patients with GERD respond to antacids Failure to thrive is very rare in children with GERD Erosive features may be seen on endoscopy Intraepithelial esophageal eosinophils are rare or very low in number
Infectious esophagitis (*Candida*, herpes, cytomegalovirus)	Intraepithelial esophageal eosinophils are low in number Neutrophils are often present in the esophageal epithelium The organisms can be seen in the esophageal epithelium with special staining
Connective tissue disease	Intraepithelial esophageal eosinophils are rare or very low in number Esophageal mucosal abnormalities are rarely seen

Typical presentation

- A typical presentation in adults is that of a Caucasian male in his second or third decade of life, who presents with dysphagia and food impaction. This is because the disease seems to have a male predominance of 2:1 to 3:1, and is more common in the non-elderly. Racial disparity is also described, with most patients being white, non-Hispanic. The reasons for this observation are still not clear. Often the patient also gives a history of IgE-mediated food allergy, allergic rhinitis, asthma, and/or atopic dermatitis, and at times family history of atopy or esophageal food impactions.
- Children typically present differently, often with abdominal pain, intermittent emesis, and feeding difficulties. The child is typically described as the picky eater by his/her family. Some children also suffer from growth failure.

Clinical diagnosis

History

- In addition to enquiring about the symptoms described, as well as any medical history of food allergies and atopic diathesis, it is helpful to enquire about family history of esophageal food impactions or esophageal dilatations, because EoE is a relatively newly recognized disease, therefore it may have been under-diagnosed in the past. Furthermore, dysphagia can be a difficult symptom to elicit in some patients because of the development of feeding adaptational behaviors to cope with symptoms and prevent food impactions, such as eating slowly, prolonged chewing, drinking liquids with every bite of food, cutting foods into very small pieces, and at times avoiding foods with harder/lumpier textures altogether. Therefore, enquiring about feeding patterns is important.

Physical examination
- Physical examination should include a neck examination to exclude any masses or an enlarged thyroid gland interfering with swallowing. Evaluation for growth failure should be carried out in children. At times, epigastric tenderness may be elicited on physical examination, especially in children.

Useful clinical decision rules and calculators
Not applicable for this topic.

Disease severity classification
Not applicable for this topic.

Laboratory diagnosis
List of diagnostic tests
- Endoscopy may reveal one or more of the following features:
  - Longitudinal furrows;
  - White plaques or exudates;
  - Rings (appearance referred to as trachealization of the esophagus);
  - Shearing (crepe paper esophagus);
  - Stricture; and
  - At times, the esophagus appears normal, highlighting the importance of obtaining biopsies for accurate diagnosis.
- Esophageal biopsies reveal some of the following features on hematoxylin and eosin (H&E) staining of biopsy sections:
  - *Esophageal eosinophilia:* eosinophilic infiltration of the epithelial layer (at least 15 eosinophils per HPF in the maximally involved area), at times with eosinophilic degranulation, surface layering of the eosinophils, and/or formation of eosinophilic microabscesses.
  - *Infiltration of the epithelium by other cells:* lymphocytes (commonly referred to as squiggle cells on H&E sections) and other immune cells that can only be seen by special staining, including mast cells, dendritic cells, and basophils.
  - *Epithelial alterations:* epithelial basal zone hyperplasia, along with papillary elongation and dilated intercellular spaces in the epithelium.
  - *Lamina propria changes:* subepithelial lamina propria fibrosis is seen in some patients, with occasional infiltration of the lamina propria by eosinophils and plasma cells.

Lists of imaging techniques
- Radiologic tests are not routinely recommended for the diagnosis of EoE. They can be helpful in patients with EoE and esophageal stricture or narrowing, to evaluate the length and diameter of the stricture.

Potential pitfalls/common errors made regarding diagnosis of disease
- To under-diagnose EoE in children with non-specific abdominal symptoms such as abdominal pain and vomiting.
- To under-diagnose EoE in adults who do not report dysphagia because of behavioral feeding modifications to prevent symptoms, such as eating slowly, prolonged chewing, drinking liquids with every bite of food, cutting foods into very small pieces, and at times avoiding foods with harder or lumpier textures altogether.

- To misdiagnose EoE as chronic GERD because of similar symptoms in some patients, and the fact that patients with EoE can feel better with the use of proton pump inhibitor therapy despite persistent esophageal eosinophilia.

Section 4: Treatment (Algorithm 20.2)
Treatment rationale

- Goals of therapy are to relieve symptoms and prevent disease progression from inflammatory to fibrostenosis, as delay in diagnosis and increasing patient age seem to correlate with fibrostenotic disease.
- No FDA-approved therapies for EoE yet exist. Therefore, therapy consists mostly of dietary restriction or topical corticosteroids to the esophagus. Dietary therapy can consist of an elemental diet (amino acid-based formula, at times with continued ingestion of only 1–2 foods), an allergy test-directed elimination diet (removing foods that test positive on skin prick tests and atopy patch tests), or an empiric elimination diet (removing foods known to be typical food allergens in the general population, such as milk, wheat, egg, soy, nuts, and seafood). Success rate of these dietary elimination therapies, defined as clinical and histologic disease remission, range from 50% to 95%.
- Topical corticosteroid therapies to the esophagus have also been used. These consist of off-label use of various doses of inhaled medications to swallow, such as fluticasone sprayed and swallowed, or oral viscous budesonide (liquid budesonide that is thickened with a sugar substitute so that it coats the esophagus when swallowed), with very variable success rates.

Algorithm 20.2 Treatment of EoE

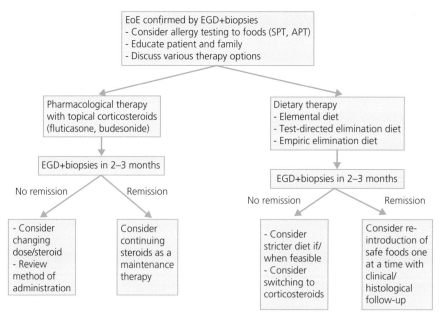

Note: APT, atopy patch tests; EGD, esophagogastroduodenoscopy; SPT, skin prick tests. Note that whenever remission is mentioned, it refers to clinical and histologic remission.

When to hospitalize

- Hospitalization is rare for patients with EoE. It may occur for a few reasons:
  - Observation following a complicated emergency removal of a food impacted in the esophagus;
  - Esophageal perforation (occurring spontaneously with a severe food impaction, or following a complicated esophageal dilatation for a stricture); or
  - Hydration in a patient who develops severe anxiety and refusal to eat or drink following a severe esophageal food impaction.

Table of treatment

Treatment	Comment
Conservative Observation only	Being debated for truly asymptomatic patients with EoE, due to the risk of esophageal narrowing and stricture formation over time
Medical Off-label use of fluticasone inhalation spray to swallow	Monitor for risk of oropharyngeal and/or esophageal candidal infection; unknown long-term risks
Off-label use of budesonide to swallow (thickened with a sugar substitute to render it viscous)	Monitor for risk of oropharyngeal and/or esophageal candidal infection; unknown long-term risks
Oral corticosteroids	Not advisable as a chronic therapy option, because of the plethora of potential systemic side effects
Psychological Counseling	Recommended for reduced quality of life; maladaptive coping with the disease or its therapy
Dietary Elemental diet (amino acid-based formula ±1–2 foods)	Difficult to implement in older children and adults because of its very restrictive nature; food introductions under close monitoring are advised as soon as disease remission is achieved
Test-directed elimination diet (based on positive skin prick tests and atopy patch tests to foods)	Consultation with a dietitian is recommended to ensure adequate restriction and proper caloric intake and balance
Empiric elimination diet (avoiding milk, wheat, egg, soy, nuts, seafood)	Consultation with a dietitian is recommended to ensure adequate restriction and proper caloric intake and balance

Prevention/management of complications

- Esophageal stricture or narrowing may be present with prolonged disease, requiring esophageal dilatation at times.
- Risk of osteoporosis, cataract formation, or other systemic side effects with long-term use of topical corticosteroids to the esophagus is unknown.
- Dietary therapies can be associated with decreased quality of life or malnutrition if not properly monitored and difficulties addressed.

CLINICAL PEARLS
- Monitor patients on dietary elimination therapy to ensure adequate caloric intake and balance. A dietitian with expertise in food allergy is important for this.
- Reintroduce foods as soon as disease remission is achieved, with clinical and histologic follow-up, to ensure that foods that are not EoE triggers for the patient are being consumed again.
- Verify for any risk of immediate allergic reactivity to the newly introduced food following a long period of avoidance of that food, prior to offering it to the patient. An allergist with expertise in food allergy is important for this.
- Monitor patients for any decreased quality of life or coping difficulties and provide counseling when needed. A mental health professional may be needed for this.

Section 5: Special populations

Not applicable for this topic.

Section 6: Prognosis

BOTTOM LINE/CLINICAL PEARLS
- Untreated EoE seems to progress from an inflammatory to a fibrostenotic disease over time.
- Esophageal cancer has not been described in EoE. However, the disease is relatively new in terms of its recognition and follow-up.

Natural history of untreated disease
- If left untreated, EoE may lead to complications such as esophageal narrowing and strictures.

Prognosis for treated patients
Not applicable for this topic.

Follow-up tests and monitoring
Not applicable for this topic.

Section 7: Reading list

Chehade M, Lucendo AJ, Achem SR, Souza RF. Causes, evaluation, and consequences of eosinophilic esophagitis. Ann N Y Acad Sci 2013:1300:110–8

Liacouras CA, Furuta GT, Hirano I, Atkins D, Attwood SE, Bonis PA, et al. Eosinophilic esophagitis: updated consensus and recommendations for children and adults. J Allergy Clin Immunol 2011;128:3–20

Lieberman JA, Chehade M. Eosinophilic esophagitis: diagnosis and management. Immunol Allergy Clin N Am 2012;32:67–81

Schoepfer AM, Safroneeva E, Bussmann C, Kuchen T, Portmann S, Simon HU, et al. Delay in diagnosis of eosinophilic esophagitis increases risk for stricture formation in a time-dependent manner. Gastroenterology 2013;145:1230–6

Straumann A, Aceves SS, Blanchard C, Collins MH, Furuta GT, Hirano I, et al. Pediatric and adult eosinophilic esophagitis: similarities and differences. Allergy 2012;67:477–90

Suggested websites
American Partnership for Eosinophilic Disorders. www.apfed.org

Section 8: Guidelines
National society guidelines

Guideline title	Guideline source	Date
ACG clinical guideline: Evidenced based approach to the diagnosis and management of esophageal eosinophilia and eosinophilic esophagitis	American College of Gastroenterology (ACG)	2013 (http://gi.org/guideline/evidenced-based-approach-to-the-diagnosis-and-management-of-esophageal-eosinophilia-and-eosinophilic-esophagitis-eoe/)

International society guidelines

Guideline title	Guideline source	Date
Management guidelines of eosinophilic esophagitis in childhood	European Society for Pediatric Gastroenterology, Hepatology, and Nutrition (ESPGHAN)	2014 (http://www.ncbi.nlm.nih.gov/pubmed/24378521)

Section 9: Evidence

Type of evidence	Title, comment	Date
Systematic review	Eosinophilic esophagitis: Updated consensus and recommendations for children and adults **Comment:** Summary of what is known and what still needs to be investigated in EoE, with consensus recommendations for diagnosis and management	2011 (http://www.ncbi.nlm.nih.gov/pubmed/21477849)

Section 10: Images

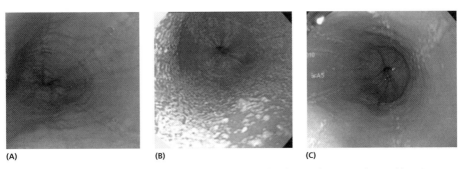

(A)   (B)   (C)

Figure 20.1 Inflammatory features of eosinophilic esophagitis (EoE) on endoscopy. Patients with EoE can present with furrows (A), white plaques (B), or white plaques aligning along the furrows (C) on endoscopy. See color plate 20.1.

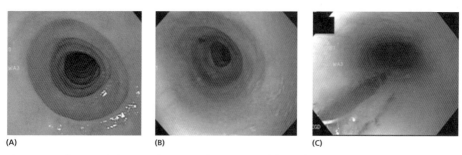

(A)   (B)   (C)

Figure 20.2 Fibrostenotic features of EoE on endoscopy. Rings (A), esophageal stricture (B), or esophageal shearing (C) can be present in patients with advanced EoE on endoscopy. See color plate 20.2.

Additional material for this chapter can be found online at:
www.mountsinaiexpertguides.com
This includes a case study, multiple choice questions, advice for
patients, and ICD codes

CHAPTER 21

Eosinophilic Gastroenteritis

Mirna Chehade

Division of Allergy/Immunology, Department of Pediatrics, Icahn School of Medicine at Mount Sinai, New York, NY, USA

OVERALL BOTTOM LINE

- Eosinophilic gastroenteritis (EG) is a disease characterized by eosinophilic infiltration of the gastric and/or duodenal mucosae with related symptoms, in the absence of other causes of tissue eosinophilia.
- EG is rare, but seems to affect all age groups.
- The pathogenesis of EG is poorly understood.
- Symptoms relate to the depth of tissue that the eosinophils infiltrate. Mucosal disease manifests with abdominal pain, emesis, and diarrhea; muscular disease leads to obstructive symptoms; and serosal disease is associated with ascites. The mucosal type is the most common. Children with EG can also present with growth failure. Gastrointestinal bleeding can rarely occur in children and adults with EG, likely secondary to ulcer formation. A subset of patients with EG can also have anemia and edema thought to be secondary to an associated protein-losing enteropathy (PLE), where occult blood and protein losses occur.
- There are no FDA-approved therapies for EG. Systemic corticosteroids have been shown to be effective but disease relapse may occur following discontinuation. Elemental diets have shown effectiveness in some children with EG.

Section 1: Background

Definition of disease

- EG is a disease characterized by eosinophilic infiltration of the gastric and/or duodenal mucosae with related symptoms, in the absence of other causes of tissue eosinophilia.

Disease classification

Not applicable for this topic.

Incidence/prevalence

- No data exist as to the incidence or prevalence of EG. EG seems to be much less prevalent than eosinophilic esophagitis (EoE).
- EG can affect adults, children, and infants.

Etiology

- Multiple food allergens can act as triggers for EG, especially in children.

Pathology/pathogenesis

- The pathogenesis of EG is poorly understood.

Mount Sinai Expert Guides: Allergy and Clinical Immunology, First Edition. Edited by Hugh A. Sampson.
© 2015 John Wiley & Sons, Ltd. Published 2015 by John Wiley & Sons, Ltd.
Companion website: www.mountsinaiexpertguides.com

- Histopathologically, while eosinophils are normally present in the gastric and duodenal mucosae, they are significantly increased in number in EG.
- Eosinophils can infiltrate various depths of the gastric and duodenal mucosae, resulting in mucosal, muscular, and/or serosal disease, with varying clinical manifestations as a result.

Predictive/risk factors
- *Allergic rhinitis:* allergic rhinitis is common in patients with EG, especially the mucosal type.
- *Asthma:* asthma is common in patients with EG, especially the mucosal type.
- *Atopic dermatitis:* atopic dermatitis is common in patients with EG, especially the mucosal type.

Section 2: Prevention
No interventions have been demonstrated to prevent the development of the disease.

Screening
Not applicable for this topic.

Primary prevention
Not applicable for this topic.

Secondary prevention
- If the disease is food-responsive (i.e. remission is achieved by avoidance of certain food triggers), then continued avoidance of these food triggers may prevent recurrence of EG. This is particularly true in children.

Section 3: Diagnosis (Algorithm 21.1)

BOTTOM LINE/CLINICAL PEARLS
- Symptoms relate to the depth of tissue that the eosinophils infiltrate. Mucosal disease manifests with abdominal pain, emesis, and diarrhea; muscular disease leads to obstructive symptoms; and serosal disease is associated with ascites. The mucosal type is the most common. Children with EG can also present with growth failure. Gastrointestinal bleeding can rarely occur in children and adults with EG, likely secondary to ulcer formation. A subset of patients with EG can also have anemia and edema thought to be secondary to an associated PLE, where occult blood and protein losses occur.
- Physical examination may reveal abdominal tenderness, pallor in those with anemia, and edema in those with PLE. Abdominal distension may be seen in EG patients with muscular involvement resulting from obstruction. Ascites may be detected in patients with serosal disease.
- The diagnosis of mucosal EG (the most common type) is confirmed by esophagogastroduodenoscopy (EGD) with biopsies, demonstrating gastric and/or duodenal eosinophilia that is not accompanied by other inflammatory cells such as neutrophils. Deeper involvement with eosinophilia may require a laparotomy for diagnosis.
- Blood tests may reveal anemia in those with a bleeding ulcer or those with PLE, and hypoproteinemia and hypoalbuminemia in those with PLE. Peripheral eosinophilia is variable in patients with EG.
- Radiological tests are helpful in EG patients with symptoms of obstruction (e.g. abdominal X-ray, upper gastrointestinal series) and those with suspected ascites (e.g. abdominal sonogram).

Algorithm 21.1 Diagnosis of eosinophilic gastroenteritis (EG)

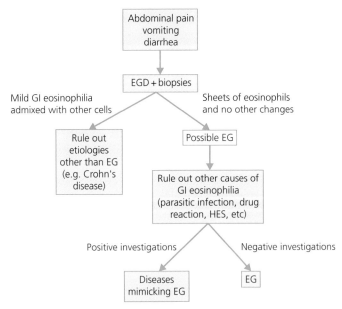

Note: EGD, esophagogastroduodenoscopy; GI, gastrointestinal; HES, hypereosinophilic syndrome; IBS, irritable bowel syndrome.

Differential diagnosis

Differential diagnosis	Features
Irritable bowel syndrome	No inflammation and no increase in eosinophil numbers are seen on gastric and duodenal biopsies
Inflammatory bowel disease	Gastrointestinal eosinophilia not as severe as in EG, and is admixed with other inflammatory infiltrates
Hypereosinophilic syndrome	Other organs are involved with eosinophilia
Parasitic infection	History of travel to areas or settings with high rates of parasitic infections Recovery of ova or parasites upon stool testing
Drug reaction	History of taking medications or supplements associated with eosinophilia
Collagen vascular disease	Suggestive history is present

Typical presentation

- A typical presentation is that of a patient with abdominal pain, and at times bloating. Vomiting and/or diarrhea can often be present as well. Children also often suffer from growth failure. Often, the patient also gives history of atopy, including allergic rhinitis, asthma, and/or atopic dermatitis.

Clinical diagnosis

History

- In addition to enquiring about the symptoms described, as well as any medical history of food allergies and atopic diathesis, it is helpful to enquire about symptoms suggestive of Crohn's disease, medication history, joint symptoms, and history of travel or swimming in stagnant water ponds, to rule out other diseases mimicking EG.

Physical examination

- Abdominal examination is important, noting for any tenderness. Severe epigastric tenderness may suggest an ulcer or severe eosinophilic inflammation. In addition, examine for abdominal distension and for ascites. Presence of pallor, and periorbital or peripheral pitting edema should be noted.

Useful clinical decision rules and calculators

Not applicable for this topic.

Disease severity classification

Not applicable for this topic.

Laboratory diagnosis

List of diagnostic tests

- The diagnosis of EG requires performing an EGD with biopsies of the gastric and duodenal mucosae. Grossly, the mucosa may appear normal, or may reveal erosions or even ulcers. Ulcers can be deep enough in some patients to result in occult bleeding and anemia, and can result in the appearance of pseudopolyps in the stomach.
- Histologically, dense gastric and/or duodenal mucosal eosinophilic infiltration, not accompanied by other inflammatory cells such as neutrophils, is present. Eosinophils may infiltrate the glands or the surface epithelium in some patients.
- Peripheral eosinophilia and elevated serum total IgE are seen in half of the patients with EG.
- In patients with associated PLE, anemia, hypoproteinemia, and hypoalbuminemia are present. Confirmation of PLE can be done by checking for stool alpha-1-antitrypsin, which will be elevated, and by checking stools for occult blood, which will be positive. As only small protein molecules leak through the gut in PLE, serum IgG levels can sometimes be low while IgM and IgA levels remain normal.

Lists of imaging techniques

- Radiologic tests are not routinely recommended for the diagnosis of EG. They may be helpful in assisting with the diagnosis of obstruction or ascites in those patients with the muscular or serosal type of EG, respectively.

Potential pitfalls/common errors made regarding diagnosis of disease

- To misdiagnose EG as irritable bowel syndrome in adults with chronic non-specific abdominal pain and intermittent or mild diarrhea.
- To confuse Crohn's disease with EG, since early Crohn's disease can present with gastrointestinal tissue eosinophilia.
- To confuse hypereosinophilic syndrome (HES) as EG in patients with gastrointestinal eosinophilia, the latter being one possible feature of HES.

Section 4: Treatment (Algorithm 21.2)

Treatment rationale

- Goals of therapy are to relieve symptoms and prevent disease complications such as bleeding ulcers. No FDA-approved therapies for EG yet exist.
- Dietary restriction therapies may be effective in some patients, mostly in the pediatric population. An elemental diet consisting of an amino acid-based formula is highly effective in children. Food allergy test-directed dietary elimination therapy has not been successful because the food allergic mechanism in EG seems to be non-IgE mediated.
- Oral corticosteroids are effective in treating EG. However, long-term use may be needed in some patients to prevent disease relapse, therefore risking potential systemic side effects of corticosteroids. Topical corticosteroids to the stomach were attempted in a case series of patients with EG with symptomatic relief, although histologic verification for disease remission was not available in those patients. Cromolyn and montelukast have been reported to be successful in some patients with EG. However, data on these two drugs are limited to case reports. As for biologic therapies, the monoclonal humanized anti-IgE antibody omalizumab was given to adults with EG at one center, with a resultant decrease in gastric and duodenal eosinophilia, but not to a significant degree. Symptoms, however, significantly improved in the EG patients, suggesting that anti-IgE therapy may be a potential candidate for future therapeutic trials in EG patients, alone or in combination with other therapies.

When to hospitalize

- Hospitalization is rare for patients with EG. It may occur for a severely bleeding ulcer, complications from obstruction in EG with muscular involvement, or peritonitis in the case of EG with serosal disease.

Algorithm 21.2 Treatment of EGD

Note: APT, atopy patch tests; EGD, esophagogastroduodenoscopy; SPT, skin prick tests. Note that whenever remission is mentioned, it refers to clinical and histologic remission.

Managing the hospitalized patient

Not applicable for this topic.

Table of treatment

Treatment	Comment
Conservative Observation only	Being debated for truly asymptomatic patients with EG, due to the risk of ulcers and bleeding
Medical Off-label use of budesonide (crushed beads in water) to take at bedtime Oral corticosteroids	Efficacy uncertain, unknown short-term and long-term risks Not advisable as a chronic therapy option, due to plethora of systemic side effects
Psychological Counseling	Recommended for reduced quality of life; maladaptive coping with the disease or its therapy
Dietary Elemental diet (amino acid-based formula ±1–2 foods)	Difficult to implement in older children and adults because of its very restrictive nature; may be less effective in adults; food introductions under close monitoring needed as soon as disease remission is achieved

Prevention/management of complications

- Risk of osteoporosis or cataract formation with repeated or chronic use of oral corticosteroids.
- Dietary therapies can be associated with decreased quality of life or malnutrition if not properly monitored and difficulties addressed.

CLINICAL PEARLS
- Monitor patients on dietary elimination therapy to ensure adequate caloric intake and balance. A dietitian with expertise in food allergy is important for management.
- Reintroduce foods as soon as disease remission is achieved, with clinical and histologic follow-up, to ensure that foods that are not EG triggers for the patient are being consumed again.
- Wean off corticosteroid therapy whenever possible to prevent systemic complications of the medication.
- Monitor patients for any decreased quality of life or coping difficulties and provide counseling when needed. A mental health professional may be needed for this.

Section 5: Special populations

Not applicable for this topic.

Section 6: Prognosis

BOTTOM LINE/CLINICAL PEARL
- Treatment is needed to alleviate symptoms and prevent serious complications such as bleeding ulcers during flare-ups of EG.

Natural history of untreated disease

- Untreated EG may have three possible courses over time: no relapse following therapy, remitting/relapsing, or chronic.

Prognosis for treated patients

Not applicable for this topic.

Follow-up tests and monitoring

Not applicable for this topic.

Section 7: Reading list

Chang JY, Choung RS, Lee RM, Locke GR 3rd, Schleck CD, Zinsmeister AR, et al. A shift in the clinical spectrum of eosinophilic gastroenteritis toward the mucosal disease type. Clin Gastroenterol Hepatol 2010;8:669–75

Chehade M, Magid MS, Mofidi S, Nowak-Wegrzyn A, Sampson HA, Sicherer SH. Allergic eosinophilic gastroenteritis with protein-losing enteropathy: intestinal pathology, clinical course, and long-term follow-up. J Pediatr Gastroenterol Nutr 2006;42:516–21

Chehade M, Sicherer SH, Magid MS, Rosenberg HK, Morotti RA. Multiple exudative ulcers and pseudopolyps in allergic eosinophilic gastroenteritis that responded to dietary therapy. J Pediatr Gastroenterol Nutr 2007;45:354–7

Foroughi S, Foster B, Kim N, Bernardino LB, Scott LM, Hamilton RG, et al. Anti-IgE treatment of eosinophil-associated gastrointestinal disorders. J Allergy Clin Immunol 2007;120:594–601

Goldman H, Proujansky R. Allergic proctitis and gastroenteritis in children: clinical and mucosal biopsy features in 53 cases. Am J Surg Pathol 1986;10:75–86

Klein NC, Hargrove RL, Sleisenger MH, Jeffries GH. Eosinophilic gastroenteritis. Medicine 1970;49:299–319

Pineton de Chambrun G, Gonzalez F, Canva JY, Gonzalez S, Houssin L, Desreumaux P, et al. Natural history of eosinophilic gastroenteritis. Clin Gastroenterol Hepatol 2011;9:950–6

Prussin C, Lee J, Foster B. Eosinophilic gastrointestinal disease and peanut allergy are alternatively associated with IL-5+ and IL-5(–) T(H)2 responses. J Allergy Clin Immunol 2009;124:1326–32

Talley NJ, Shorter RG, Phillips SF, Zinsmeister AR. Eosinophilic gastroenteritis: a clinicopathological study of patients with disease of the mucosa, muscle layer, and subserosal tissues. Gut 1990;31:54–8.

Suggested website

American Partnership for Eosinophilic Disorders. www.apfed.org

Section 8: Guidelines
National society guidelines

Not applicable for this topic.

International society guidelines

Not applicable for this topic.

Section 9: Evidence

Type of evidence	Title, comment	Date
Systematic review	Summary and recommendations: Classification of gastrointestinal manifestations due to immunologic reactions to foods in infants and young children **Comment:** Comprehensive summary of the IgE-mediated and non-IgE-mediated food allergies in children, including EG	2000 (http://journals.lww.com/jpgn/ Fulltext/2000/01001/Summary_ and_Recommendations__ Classification_of.13.aspx#)

Section 10: Images

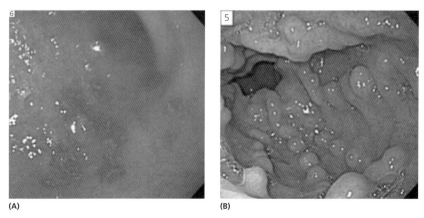

(A)   (B)

Figure 21.1 Possible features of eosinophilic gastroenteritis (EG) on endoscopy include multiple erosions of the gastric mucosa (A) or multiple gastric pseudopolyps in advanced cases (B). See color plate 21.1.

Additional material for this chapter can be found online at:
www.mountsinaiexpertguides.com
This includes a case study, multiple choice questions, advice for patients, and ICD codes

CHAPTER 22

Food Allergy-Induced Anaphylaxis

Kate Welch and Hugh A. Sampson

Jaffe Food Allergy Institute, Icahn School of Medicine at Mount Sinai, New York, NY, USA

OVERALL BOTTOM LINE
- Anaphylaxis is a severe and life-threatening allergic reaction that can be caused by the ingestion of a food to which a patient is allergic.
- It is caused by the release of inflammatory mediators from mast cells and basophils after cross linkage of food allergen with allergen-specific IgE antibodies bound to these cells.
- Symptoms often involve the skin and mucosal tissue in conjunction with respiratory or cardiovascular compromise and occur within minutes to hours after ingestion of the allergen.
- Treatment includes the intramuscular injection of epinephrine and immediate medical attention for supportive care.
- Without treatment, food-induced anaphylaxis can result in death.

Section 1: Background
Definition of disease
- Food-induced anaphylaxis is a severe allergic reaction resulting from the ingestion of a food allergen. It most commonly involves the rapid onset of skin or mucosal tissue symptoms (e.g. hives, flushing, or oral mucosal swelling) *in addition to* respiratory compromise (dyspnea, shortness of breath, wheezing) and/or cardiovascular symptoms (light-headedness, dizziness, hypotension).
- Alternatively, it can be defined as the involvement of two or more of the following areas after the ingestion of a known food allergen: skin/mucosal tissue symptoms, respiratory compromise, hypotension/syncope, and persistent gastrointestinal symptoms, such as abdominal pain and vomiting.

Disease classification
- Food-induced anaphylaxis is, by definition, a severe reaction, but may be classified as mild, moderate, or severe. It is most commonly caused by ingestion of a food to which a patient has an IgE-mediated allergy.
- A less common form of the disease, known as food-dependent, exercised-induced anaphylaxis (FDEIA) occurs only after exercise is undertaken within several hours after a known allergen is ingested. In rare cases, this can occur with exercise after the ingestion of any food, not simply foods to which a patient has a known allergy.

Incidence/prevalence
- Food allergy is the leading cause of anaphylaxis outside of the hospital setting.

Mount Sinai Expert Guides: Allergy and Clinical Immunology, First Edition. Edited by Hugh A. Sampson.
© 2015 John Wiley & Sons, Ltd. Published 2015 by John Wiley & Sons, Ltd.
Companion website: www.mountsinaiexpertguides.com

- Food allergic reactions account for more than 200 000 emergency room visits each year, and the CDC estimates that food allergies among children increased approximately 50% between 1997 and 2011.
- Episodes of anaphylaxis from all causes are estimated at a lifetime prevalence of 0.05–2%.
- Less than 1% of all-cause cases of anaphylaxis prove fatal.

Economic impact

- The economic cost of food-related anaphylaxis is difficult to measure, but the estimated cost of food allergies in the pediatric population alone is nearly $25 billion per year.

Etiology

- Food-related anaphylaxis occurs after a patient ingests a food to which he or she has an IgE-mediated food allergy.
- The most common allergens to trigger an anaphylactic reaction include peanuts, tree nuts, and shellfish, although in children, milk, egg, and sesame are also common culprits.
- Anaphylaxis caused by mere contact with a food rather than actual ingestion has not been reliably validated, although inhalation of cooking vapors (steam), particularly involving seafood, has been implicated in rare reactions.

Pathology/pathogenesis

- Once a food allergen is ingested and crosses the oral or gastrointestinal lining, it enters the circulation, where it can bind to allergen-specific IgE antibodies. These antibodies are attached to receptors on basophils and mast cells, which when cross-linked by allergen, degranulate and release their pro-inflammatory cytokines. Such inflammatory mediators lead to the classic symptoms of flushing, swelling, urticaria, respiratory distress, and potentially intravascular collapse.

Predictive/risk factors (H2)

- Any person with a food allergy, whether diagnosed or undiagnosed, is potentially at risk of anaphylaxis following the ingestion of a food allergen. Several risk factors put patients at slightly higher risk: large quantity of ingested food allergen, presence of asthma (especially poorly controlled asthma), extreme sensitivity (i.e. prior reaction to only a small amount of ingested food), and a prior history of anaphylaxis.

Section 2: Prevention

BOTTOM LINE/CLINICAL PEARLS

- The key to prevention involves avoiding the ingestion of known allergens. If the ingestion of a food allergen is suspected, prompt treatment with a liquid antihistamine is warranted. If symptoms of anaphylaxis begin to develop, epinephrine should be injected intramuscularly and medical attention sought immediately. In individuals who experienced a previous severe anaphylactic reaction following ingestion of a food allergen, administration of epinephrine even prior to the development of obvious symptoms is warranted. Unfortunately, there is no way to predict the severity of an allergic reaction.

Screening
- While there is no way to screen for risk of anaphylaxis, food allergy testing, in the form of a detailed history as well as skin prick testing and serum IgE evaluation, helps to identify food allergies and guide avoidance patterns.

Primary prevention
- Education on how to recognize hidden sources of food allergens and avoidance of those known allergens.
- Education on how to recognize early signs of a pending anaphylactic reaction.
- Adherence to a patient-specific "emergency action plan" which guides dosing of antihistamines and need for epinephrine injections based on severity of symptoms.

Secondary prevention
- Education and avoidance are the best ways to prevent recurrent severe allergic reactions.

Section 3: Diagnosis

BOTTOM LINE/CLINICAL PEARLS
- Food-induced anaphylaxis is a clinical diagnosis based upon a detailed history of ingestion and evaluation of characteristic signs and symptoms (see Table: Diagnosis of anaphylaxis).
- A panel of experts has agreed upon the clinical criteria needed for diagnosis as any one of the following three scenarios:
  - Acute onset of an illness (minutes to several hours) with involvement of the skin, mucosal tissue, or both (i.e. generalized hives, pruritus or flushing, swollen lips-tongue-uvula) *and* at least one of the following:
    - respiratory compromise (i.e. dyspnea, wheeze-bronchospasm, stridor, hypoxemia);
    - reduced BP or associated symptoms of end-organ dysfunction (i.e. hypotonia, collapse, syncope, incontinence).
  - Two or more of the following that occur rapidly after exposure to a likely allergen for that patient (minutes to several hours):
    - involvement of the skin-mucosal tissue (i.e. generalized hives, pruritus or flushing, swollen lips–tongue–uvula);
    - respiratory compromise (i.e. dyspnea, wheeze–bronchospasm, stridor, hypoxemia);
    - reduced BP or associated symptoms of end-organ dysfunction (i.e. hypotonia, collapse, syncope, incontinence);
    - persistent gastrointestinal symptoms (i.e. crampy abdominal pain, vomiting).
  - Reduced blood pressure (BP) after exposure to a known allergen for that patient (minutes to several hours):
    - infants and children: low systolic BP or greater than 30% decrease in systolic BP;
    - adults: systolic BP of less than 90 mmHg or greater than 30% decrease from the person's baseline.
- Biphasic anaphylactic reactions occur in up to 20% of anaphylactic reactions and are defined as a recurrence of symptoms after the apparent resolution of the initial event. It typically occurs within 1–4 hours following the initial event and should be diagnosed and managed similarly.

Differential diagnosis

Differential diagnosis	Features
Asthma exacerbation	Wheezing is predominant symptom
Aspiration	Airway symptoms predominate; no ingestion of allergen
Acute urticaria	No mucosal or airway involvement
Panic attack	No evidence of mucosal or gastrointestinal involvement; able to be calmed or "talked down"
Vasovagal reactions	Clinical history of precipitant
Reactions caused by excess endogenous production of histamine	Laboratory tests confirm such disorders as mastocytosis, urticarial pigmentosa
Other forms of shock	History of bleeding, infection, hypoglycemia, cardiac disease, etc.
"Restaurant syndromes"	Ingestions of MSG, sulfites, fish (scombroidosis)

Typical presentation

- Food-induced anaphylaxis is typically seen in the emergency room, as it is a severe reaction necessitating urgent care. Upon ingestion of a previously unknown food allergen or accidental ingestion of a known culprit, a patient will develop the acute onset of symptoms varying from mucosal, skin, gastrointestinal, or respiratory involvement. There is slight variability in presentation between children and adults. In the pediatric population, gastrointestinal and cutaneous symptoms tend to predominate; shock is less common than in adults. Ideally, symptoms are recognized as those of anaphylaxis, and an epinephrine auto-injector is used prior to presentation to the hospital.

Clinical diagnosis

History

- The clinician should enquire about the timing of previously ingested foods, as most anaphylactic reactions to foods will occur within minutes to several hours of ingestion. Concomitant use of NSAIDs or alcohol may exacerbate symptoms, and this should be discussed as well. A history of asthma is important to note, as these patients may have more severe symptoms. Also, a history of beta-blocker use may render anaphylactic symptoms more difficult to treat.

Physical examination

- A rapid assessment of vital signs is critical as well as evaluation of the airway. Any hypoxia or hypotension should be treated immediately with supplemental oxygen and intravenous fluids.
- ENT examination should look for signs of oropharyngeal swelling that may obstruct the airway and necessitate intubation.
- Lung examination should focus on signs of wheezing.
- An assessment of the skin for rash or hives and an abdominal examination complete the initial evaluation.

Useful clinical decision rules and calculators (Table 22.1)

- Some cases of food-induced anaphylaxis require multiple injections of epinephrine. If a patient is still symptomatic after the initial injection, subsequent doses can be given at 10-minute intervals. Ideally, the patient is in an emergent setting at this point, where attention can also be given to other means of supportive care.

Table 22.1 Diagnosis of anaphylaxis

Anaphylaxis is highly likely when any one of the following 3 criteria are fulfilled

1. Acute onset of an illness (minutes to several hours) with involvement of the skin, mucosal tissue, or both (eg, generalized hives, pruritus or flushing, swollen lips-tongue-uvula)
   AND AT LEAST ONE OF THE FOLLOWING
   a. Respiratory compromise (eg, Dyspnea, wheezed-bronchospasm, stridor, reduced PEF, hypoxemia)
   b. Reduced BP or associated symptoms of end-organ dysfunction (eg, hypotonia [collapse], syncope, incontinence)
2. Two or more of the following that occur rapidly after exposure *to a likely allergen for that patient* (minutes to several hours):
   a. Involvement of the skin-mucosal tissue (eg, generalized hives, itch-flush, swollen lips-tongue-uvula)
   b. Respiratory compromise (eg, dyspnea, wheeze-bronchospasm, stridor, reduced PEF, hypoxemia)
   c. Reduced BP or associated symptoms (eg, hypotonia [collapse], syncope, incontinence)
   d. Persistent gastrointestinal symptoms (eg, crampy abdominal pain, vomiting)
3. Reduced BP after exposure to *known allergen for that patient* (minutes to several hours):
   a. Infants and children: low systolic BP (age specific) or greater than 30% decrease in systolic BP*
   b. Adults: systolic BP of less than 90mmHg or greater than 30% decrease from that person's baseline

PEF, Peak expiratory flow; *BP*, blood pressure.
*Low systolic blood pressure for children is defined as less than 70mmHg from 1 month to 1 year, less than (70mm Hg + [2 × age]) from 1 to 10 years, and less than 90mmHg from 11 to 17 years.
Source: Sampson HA, et al. Second symposium on the definition and management of anaphylaxis: summary report—Second National Institute of Allergy and Infectious Disease/Food Allergy and Anaphylaxis Network symposium. Journal of Allergy and Clinical Immunology 2006;117:391–7. Reproduced with permission of Elsevier.

Disease severity classification

- Anaphylaxis is by definition a severe reaction.
- Biphasic symptoms, which occur in up to 20% of reactions, typically occur within 1–4 hours after initial symptom resolution. However, some cases have been reported up to 78 hours later.

Laboratory diagnosis

List of diagnostic tests

- There is no reliable laboratory test to define food-induced anaphylaxis.
- Elevated serum tryptase, which may be present in other forms of anaphylaxis, are often not found in food-induced cases.
- Elevated urine or serum, typically histamine, occurs during anaphylactic reactions, but requires special handling procedures because of the lability of histamine and therefore is not available in emergency room settings.

Lists of imaging techniques

- There are no imaging techniques routinely used in the diagnosis of food-induced anaphylaxis.

Potential pitfalls/common errors made regarding diagnosis of disease

- Delay of self-treatment because of fear of epinephrine use or under-estimation of symptom severity are the major pitfalls seen outside of the professional setting.

Section 4: Treatment (Algorithm 22.1)

Treatment rationale

- When food-induced anaphylaxis is suspected or recognized, self-injection of epinephrine is the mainstay of treatment. Other methods of supportive care, such as supplemental oxygen or intravenous fluids, can be provided as needed in a hospital setting. Bronchodilators and intravenous steroids or antihistamines may be added as secondary management.

Algorithm 22.1 Management of anaphylaxis

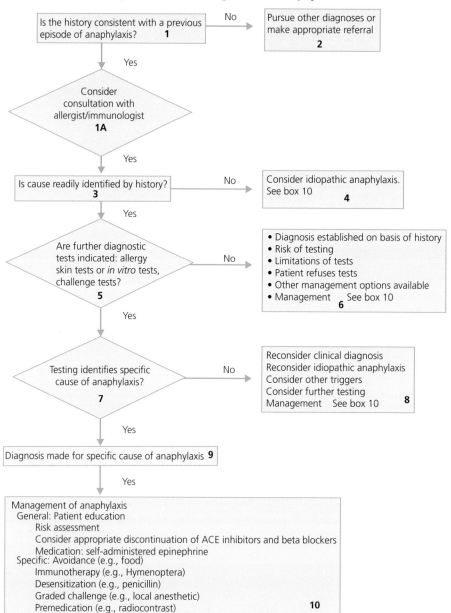

Source: Lieberman P, et al. The diagnosis and management of anaphylaxis practice parameter: 2010 update. J Allergy Clin Immunol 2010;126:477–80. Reproduced with permission of Elsevier.

When to hospitalize

- Any patient suspected of having a severe allergic reaction should seek medical care in an emergency room setting immediately, and all patients are advised to call 911 or go to the nearest emergency room after administering injectable epinephrine.
- Cases of severe food allergy can often be managed in the emergency room with close attention to vital signs and patency of the airway. Further doses of epinephrine or treatment with IV antihistamines, steroids, and fluids may be warranted.

- Patients with severe symptoms or those needing intensive treatment should be admitted for further observation until resolution of symptoms.

Managing the hospitalized patient

- If a patient is hospitalized, attention must be paid to serial evaluation of vital signs, O_2 saturation, physical examination, and symptoms such as shortness of breath, abdominal pain, and mucocutaneous irritation. This will guide the need for further treatment or supportive care.

Table of treatment

Treatment	Comment
Conservative	Oral antihistamines are used in the management of minor food allergic reactions but are second line treatment for anaphylaxis
Medical	Injectable epinephrine is the mainstay of treatment Intravenous steroids and antihistamines can also be used for symptom control
Radiological	Chest X-ray should be considered in cases where foreign body aspiration is high on the differential diagnosis
Psychological	Some patients, particularly in the pediatric population, can suffer anxiety and fear after an episode of anaphylaxis. Behavioral therapy is recommended in this population of patients

Prevention/management of complications

- Injectable epinephrine will likely cause a sensation or rapid heartbeat or sometimes palpitations, and patients should be educated on this when the injector is prescribed.

CLINICAL PEARLS
- Injectable epinephrine should be used at the first suspicion of a serious food allergic reaction or for any signs of anaphylaxis.
- Particularly in the pediatric population, err on the cautious side and treat a possible anaphylactic event, rather than delay treatment as symptoms develop.
- Patients should call 911 or go to the nearest emergency room once epinephrine is used.

Section 5: Special populations

Pregnancy

- Management of food-induced anaphylaxis in a pregnant patient is no different, because emergency epinephrine use is equally important for survival of mother and fetus.

Children

- Food-induced anaphylaxis is more prevalent in the pediatric population. Injectable epinephrine is available in a pediatric dose. Education and avoidance of allergens in this population is key, as children may not be able to distinguish allergens, and there is a propensity for food sharing among young children. Allergy to foods such as milk, egg and soy is more prevalent in children but often outgrown by school age.

Elderly

- There is no change in management for elderly patients.

Others

- Certain medications, such as beta-blockers, may blunt the effect of epinephrine and render anaphylaxis more difficult to treat. Glucagon may be needed as a beta-blocker antagonist in this population.

Section 6: Prognosis

> **BOTTOM LINE/CLINICAL PEARLS**
> - If managed appropriately, food-induced anaphylaxis is completely treatable.
> - Patients who have one episode of anaphylaxis are at increased risk of experiencing a second episode.
> - Anxiety and fear of certain foods is a common side effect, particularly in the pediatric patient, for patients who have experienced anaphylaxis.

Natural history of untreated disease

- Untreated, anaphylaxis can lead to death through respiratory or cardiovascular collapse.

Prognosis for treated patients

- Treated patients experience a full recovery.

Follow-up tests and monitoring

- In patients who experience a first-time episode of anaphylaxis, thorough allergy testing should be undertaken to identify potential triggers. This includes a detailed history as well as skin prick testing and serum IgE analysis.

Section 7: Reading list

Lieberman P. Biphasic anaphylactic reactions. Ann Allergy Asthma Immunol 2005;95:217

Lieberman P, Nicklas RA, Oppenheimer J, Kemp SF, Lang DM, Bernstein DI, et al. The diagnosis and management of anaphylaxis practice parameter: 2010 Update. Joint Task Force on Practice Parameters, representing the AAAAI, ACAAI, and the Joint Council of Allergy, Asthma and Immunology. J Allergy Clin Immunol 2010;126:477–80

Sampson HA, Munoz-Furlong A, Campbell RL, Adkinson NF Jr, Bock SA, Branum A, et al. Second symposium on the definition and management of anaphylaxis: Second National Institute of Allergy and Infectious Disease/Food Allergy and Anaphylaxis Network Symposium. J Allergy Clin Immunol 2006;117:391–7

Sampson, HA. Anaphylaxis and emergency treatment. Pediatrics 2003;111:1601–8

Sicherer SH, Sampson HA. Food allergy. J Allergy Clin Immunol 2010;125(Suppl 2):S116–25

Wang J, Sampson HA. Food anaphylaxis. Clin Exp Allergy 2007;37:651–60

Suggested websites

www.foodallergy.org

www.aaaai.org

www.acaai.org

www.niaid.nih.gov

Section 8: Guidelines
National society guidelines

Guideline title	Source	Date
Guidelines for the Diagnosis and Management of Food Allergy in the United States: Report of the NIAID-Sponsored Expert Panel	NIH, National Institute of Allergy and Infectious Disease	2010 (http://www.ncbi.nlm.nih.gov/pubmed/21134576)

International society guidelines

Guideline title	Source	Date
The diagnosis and management of anaphylaxis practice parameter	American Academy of Allergy, Asthma & Immunology	2010 (http://www.aaaai.org/practice-resources/statements-and-practice-parameters/practice-parameters-and-other-guidelines-page.aspx)

Section 9: Evidence
Not applicable for this topic.

Section 10: Images
Not applicable for this topic.

Additional material for this chapter can be found online at:
www.mountsinaiexpertguides.com
This includes a case study, multiple choice questions, advice for patients, and ICD codes

CHAPTER 23

Adverse Reactions to Food and Drug Additives

Julie Wang

Department of Pediatrics, Division of Allergy/Immunology, Icahn School of Medicine at Mount Sinai, New York, NY, USA

OVERALL BOTTOM LINE

- The prevalence of adverse reactions to food additives ranges from 0.01–0.23%.
- A variety of food and drug additives have been reported to cause symptoms including urticaria, asthma, and anaphylaxis.
- The majority of these adverse reactions have not been confirmed with controlled challenge procedures.
- Management entails avoidance of the triggering agent and preparedness to treat reactions in case of inadvertent exposures.

Section 1: Background

Definition of disease

- Food and drug additives serve a range of functions, including coloring, flavoring, binding agent, antimicrobial, and preservative. Many of these additives have been reported to cause adverse reactions such as contact dermatitis, urticaria, asthma, and anaphylaxis.

Disease classification

Not applicable for this topic.

Incidence/prevalence

- Based on several large studies, the prevalence of adverse reactions to food additives is approximately 0.01–0.23%.
- The prevalence of adverse reactions to drug additives is unknown, but is less than that of food additives.

Economic impact

Not applicable for this topic.

Etiology

- A variety of food and drug additives have been reported to cause adverse reactions.
- Natural food colorants that have been reported to cause adverse reactions, including anaphylaxis, are annatto (extract from the seeds of the fruit of the *Bixa orellana* tree) and carmine

---

Mount Sinai Expert Guides: Allergy and Clinical Immunology, First Edition. Edited by Hugh A. Sampson.

© 2015 John Wiley & Sons, Ltd. Published 2015 by John Wiley & Sons, Ltd.

Companion website: www.mountsinaiexpertguides.com

(derived from dried female insects of the species *Dactylopius coccus*). As these are extracts of seeds and insect bodies, they are likely to contain proteins and could elicit IgE-mediated reactions.

- Synthetic food colorants such as tartrazine, sunset yellow (FD&C Yellow #6), and brilliant blue (FD&C Blue #1) have been associated with various symptoms, however, there is no compelling evidence for the involvement of these colors in urticaria, angioedema, asthma, or atopic dermatitis.
- Sulfites, which are used as food and drug additives, also occur naturally in foods. In addition, to urticaria and angioedema, sulfites can trigger severe bronchoconstriction in sensitive patients, particularly in those with more severe, persistent asthma.
- Monosodium glutamate (MSG) symptom complex (also known as Chinese restaurant syndrome) is a mild, transient, subjective syndrome characterized by a burning sensation, facial pressure or tightness, headaches, nausea, chest pain, palpitations, numbness, tingling, and weakness. MSG has also been linked to asthma, atopic dermatitis, and persistent rhinitis. These associations have not been definitively established, but seem to occur at very high levels of exposure.

Pathology/pathogenesis
- The pathology/pathogenesis of adverse reactions to food and drug additives is unknown. Mechanisms include immunologic, pharmacologic, toxic, or irritant effects. Sulfite-induced asthma may be caused by release of sulfur dioxide, an airway irritant, but other mechanisms including IgE-mediated mechanisms and cholinergic reflex mechanisms have been suggested.

Predictive/risk factors
- There are no known risk factors.
- Atopic individuals are at higher risk.
- The prevalence is 0.01–0.23% in the general population compared to 2–7% in atopic individuals.

Section 2: Prevention
No interventions have been demonstrated to prevent the development of this disease.

Screening
Not applicable for this topic.

Primary prevention
Not applicable for this topic.

Secondary prevention
Not applicable for this topic.

Section 3: Diagnosis (Algorithm 23.1)

> **BOTTOM LINE/CLINICAL PEARLS**
> - The diagnosis of adverse reactions to food and drug additives is based on medical history.
> - The clinician taking the history should inquire about the types and severity of symptoms, timing between exposure and onset of symptoms, reproducibility of symptoms, amount consumed, and association with modifying factors such as alcohol consumption or exercise.
> - There are no standardized laboratory tests to diagnose allergies to food and drug additives.

Algorithm 23.1 Diagnosis of adverse reactions to food and drug additives

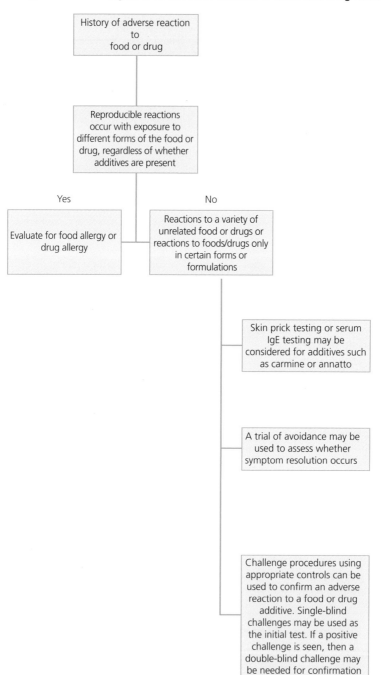

Differential diagnosis

Differential diagnosis	Features
Allergy to food	Reproducible reactions will occur with exposure to different forms of the food, regardless of whether additives are present Positive skin prick test or serum IgE to the food allergen
Allergy to drugs	More common than reactions to drug additives

Typical presentation
- Symptoms of adverse reactions to food and drug additives are varied and can range from urticaria or contact dermatitis to asthma and anaphylaxis.

Clinical diagnosis
History
- Adverse reactions to food or drug additives should be suspected if a patient has reactions to a variety of unrelated foods or reactions to foods only in certain forms (i.e. reactions to commercially packaged foods, but not home-cooked foods).
- Adverse reactions to drug additives should be suspected if symptoms arise with different medications or different formulations of medications.
- The diagnosis of adverse reactions to food and drug additives is based on history, which should include the type and severity of symptoms, timing between exposure and onset of symptoms, duration and reproducibility of symptoms, and amount consumed to trigger a reaction. Additional questions should ascertain whether reactions are associated with modifying factors such as alcohol consumption or exercise.

Physical examination
- Physical examination may reveal urticaria or dermatitis if these are the symptoms associated with the adverse reactions.
- Other signs of atopy may be observed on examination.
- For many, the physical examination will be unrevealing if the patient is not acutely reacting.

Useful clinical decision rules and calculators
Not applicable for this topic.

Disease severity classification
Not applicable for this topic.

Laboratory diagnosis
List of diagnostic tests
- There are no standardized laboratory studies available to diagnose adverse reactions to food and drug additives.
- If the history is suggestive of an adverse reaction to food or drug additive, skin prick testing or serum IgE testing may be considered for additives such as carmine or annatto.
- A trial of avoidance of the agent may be used to assess whether symptom resolution occurs.

- Challenge procedures using appropriate controls are used to confirm an adverse reaction to a food or drug additive. Single-blind challenges may be used as the initial test. If a positive challenge is seen, then a double-blind challenge may be needed for confirmation.
- The criterion for a positive challenge for inducing asthma symptoms is a 20% or greater decrease in FEV_1 from the baseline.

Lists of imaging techniques
No imaging studies are indicated for adverse reactions to food and drug additives.

Potential pitfalls/common errors made regarding diagnosis of disease
- A detailed history and testing should exclude the possibility of a food allergy to a hidden ingredient.
- Current evidence does not support routinely recommending patients with chronic urticaria to avoid foods containing additives.
- Challenges performed to determine the association between a food or drug additive with chronic urticaria can result in a false positive test if the patient is taken off antihistamines prior to the challenge. However, a false negative challenge may be seen if the patient is on chronic antihistamines.
- Similarly, for challenges to determine the association between a food or drug additive with asthma, false positive challenge results may be seen if the patient's asthma is unstable and false negative challenges can occur if the patient used a beta-agonist prior to the procedure.
- Guidelines advise against routinely instructing asthmatic patients to avoid sulfites or other food additives unless prior reactions to sulfites have occurred.
- Food additive avoidance should not be advised for the management of hyperactivity/attention deficit disorder.

Section 4: Treatment (Algorithm 23.2)
Treatment rationale
- People who experience adverse reactions to a food or drug additive should be educated on avoidance strategies for the offending agent, including label reading as additives are listed in food ingredient labels and package inserts of drugs. It is important to note that a few groups of ingredients can be declared collectively without listing individual components; these include spices, natural flavors, and artificial flavors. For those who have bronchoconstriction with sulfite exposure, use of inhaled corticosteroids that do not contain sulfites is recommended.
- As inadvertent exposures are possible, preparedness to manage reactions (i.e. anaphylaxis, asthma exacerbations) is essential.

When to hospitalize
- Adverse reactions to food and drug additives are typically managed in the outpatient setting.
- Anaphylactic reactions or severe asthma exacerbations may require management in the emergency department or inpatient admission (see Chapters 29 and 14, on Anaphylaxis and Asthma).

Managing the hospitalized patient
Not applicable for this topic.

Algorithm 23.2 Management of adverse reactions to food and drug additives

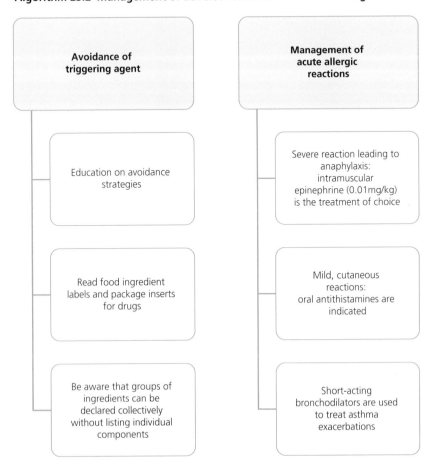

Table of treatment

Treatment	Comment
Conservative • Avoidance of the triggering agent is advised • Patients are instructed to read all ingredient labels	This is applicable to all patients
Medical Acute reactions should be managed as follows: • If a severe reaction leading to anaphylaxis occurs, intramuscular epinephrine (0.01 mg/kg) is the treatment of choice • For mild, cutaneous reactions, oral antithistamines are indicated (i.e. diphenhydramine, cetirizine, loratadine, fexofenadine) • Short-acting bronchodilators are used to treat asthma exacerbations (i.e. albuterol 2 puffs every 4 hours as needed) • Topical corticosteroids can improve symptoms of contact dermatitis	For severe allergic reactions (i.e. anaphylaxis), immediate medical attention should be sought after epinephrine is administered. These patients should be observed to ensure resolution of symptoms as biphasic reactions are possible

Prevention/management of complications
- Anaphylaxis and asthma exacerbations should be managed with physician supervision to prevent mortality.

CLINICAL PEARLS
- Avoidance of the offending agent is essential.
- Patients should be educated to read ingredient labels.
- Preparedness to manage reactions is necessary in cases of accidental exposures.

Section 5: Special populations
Not applicable for this topic.

Section 6: Prognosis

BOTTOM LINE/CLINICAL PEARLS
- With strict avoidance of the triggering agent, prognosis is good for adverse reactions to food and drug additives.

Natural history of untreated disease
Not applicable for this topic.

Prognosis for treated patients
Not applicable for this topic.

Follow-up tests and monitoring
Not applicable for this topic.

Section 7: Reading list

Ardern KD, Ram FS. Tartrazine exclusion for allergic asthma. Cochrane Database Syst Rev 2001;4:CD000460

Nowak-Wegrzyn A, Assa'ad AH, Bahna SL, Bock SA, Sicherer SH, Teuber SS; Adverse Reactions to Food Committee of American Academy of Allergy, Asthma and Immunology. Work Group report: oral food challenge testing. J Allergy Clin Immunol 2009;123(6 Suppl):S365–83

Sampson HA, Aceves S, Bock SA, James J, Jones S, Lang D, et al. Food allergy: a practice parameter update – 2014. J Allergy Clin Immunol 2014;134:1015–25

Simon RA. Update on sulfite sensitivity. Allergy 1998;53(46 Suppl):78–9

Young E, Patel S, Stoneham M, Rona R, Wilkinson JD. The prevalence of reaction to food additives in a survey population. J R Coll Physicians Lond 1987;21:241–7

Zhou Y, Yang M, Dong BR. Monosodium glutamate avoidance for chronic asthma in adults and children. Cochrane Database Syst Rev 2012;6:CD004357

Suggested websites
American Academy of Allergy, Asthma and Immunology (AAAAI). www.aaaai.org
American College of Allergy, Asthma and Immunology (ACAAI). www.acaai.org
US FDA Center for Food Safety and Nutrition. http://www.fda.gov/Food/default.htm

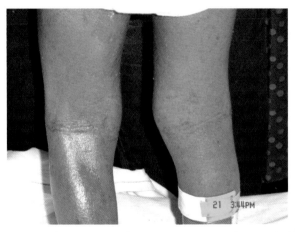

Plate 1.1 A child with multiple food allergies and severe persistent atopic dermatitis (AD) with acute exacerbation due to *Staphylococcus aureus* superinfection. Note the diffuse erythroderma and open sores.

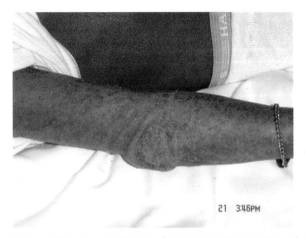

Plate 1.2 AD chronic lesions of skin hypertrophy, lichenification, hyperpigmentation, and xerosis.

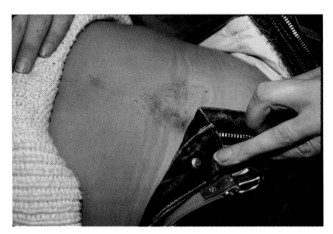

Plate 3.1 Contact dermatitis to nickel from belt buckle.

Mount Sinai Expert Guides: Allergy and Clinical Immunology, First Edition. Edited by Hugh A. Sampson.
© 2015 John Wiley & Sons, Ltd. Published 2015 by John Wiley & Sons, Ltd.
Companion website: www.mountsinaiexpertguides.com

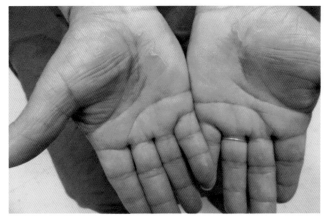

Plate 3.2 Contact dermatitis to propylene glycol, a preservative used in steroid creams. Consider this diagnosis if patient is not responding to treatment.

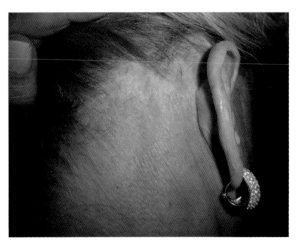

Plate 3.3 Contact dermatitis to Bronopol.

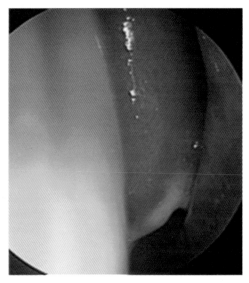

Plate 6.1 Nasal endoscopy of left middle meatus with purulent drainage noted in infundibulum. Patient had an acute maxillary sinusitis.

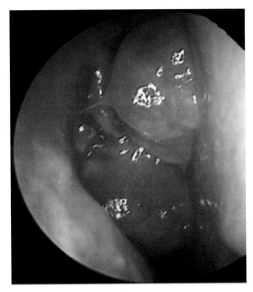

Plate 6.2 Nasal endoscopy of patient with nasal polyps and complete nasal airway obstruction. This patient had complaints of anosmia and nasal congestion.

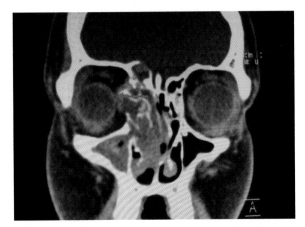

Plate 6.3 Chronic rhinosinusitis with polyposis. Non-contrast CT scan of the sinuses of patient in Plate 6.2 demonstrates expansile polyposis of the right sinonasal cavity. The arrow points to area of polyp extension from ethmoid cavity into the orbit. In these cases the periorbita of the eye is usually not violated; however, caution is needed during surgical clearance of polyps in this area to avoid risk of intraorbital injury.

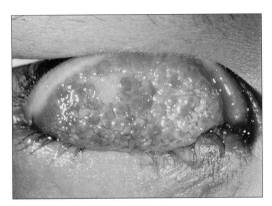

Plate 7.1 Vernal conjunctivitis – cobblestone papillae cover the superior tarsal conjunctiva. From Rubenstein JB, Tannan A. Conjunctivitis: infectious and noninfectious. In Yanoff M, Duker JS, eds. Ophthalmology. 4th ed. St. Louis, MO, Mosby Elsevier; 2013:chap 4.6. Reproduced with permission.

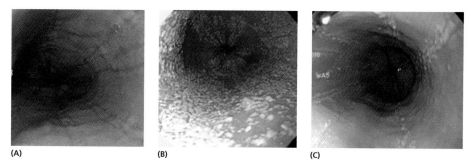

(A)   **(B)**   **(C)**

Plate 20.1 Inflammatory features of eosinophilic esophagitis (EoE) on endoscopy. Patients with EoE can present with furrows (A), white plaques (B), or white plaques aligning along the furrows (C) on endoscopy.

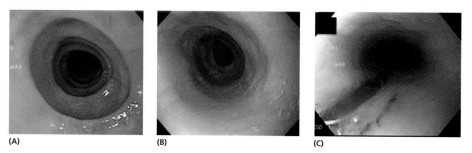

(A)   **(B)**   **(C)**

Plate 20.2 Fibrostenotic features of EoE on endoscopy. Rings (A), esophageal stricture (B), or esophageal shearing (C) can be present in patients with advanced EoE on endoscopy.

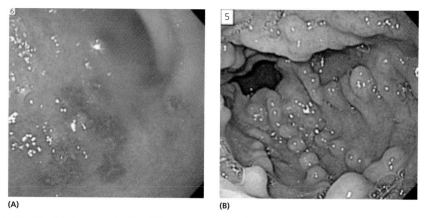

(A)   **(B)**

Plate 21.1 Possible features of eosinophilic gastroenteritis (EG) on endoscopy include multiple erosions of the gastric mucosa (A) or multiple gastric pseudopolyps in advanced cases (B).

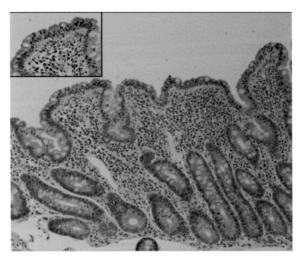

Plate 24.1 Histopathologic features of an intestinal biopsy from a patient with celiac disease (hematoxylin and eosin stain, magnification 100×): Blunted villi, crypt hyperplasia, mononuclear infiltration of the lamina propria, and intraepithelial lymphocytic infiltration. The latter is made visually clear in the inset (magnification 400×). Source: Courtesy of Margret Magid, MD, Pediatric Pathology, Icahn School of Medicine at Mount Sinai.

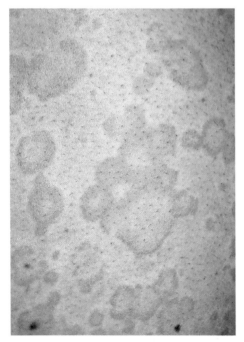

Plate 26.1 Superficial urticarial lesions often have central pallor and raised erythematous edematous borders, but can vary in size, shape, and color. From Habif TP. Clinical Dermatology: A Color Guide to Diagnosis and Therapy. 5th edition. 2010 Philadelphia, PA, Mosby/Elsevier. Reproduced with permission.

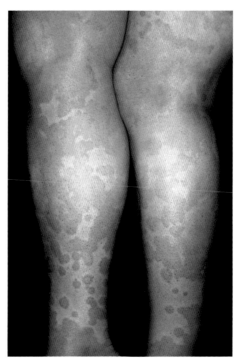

Plate 26.2 Confluent urticaria. From Habif TP. Clinical Dermatology: A Color Guide to Diagnosis and Therapy. 5th edition. 2010 Philadelphia, PA, Mosby/Elsevier. Reproduced with permission.

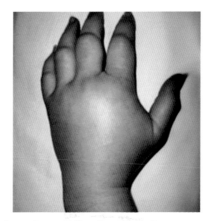

Plate 28.1 Extremity attack. Source: Bowen T. Hereditary angioedema consensus 2010. Allergy Asthma Clin Immunol 2010;6:13. Creative Commons Attribution License CC BY 4.0.

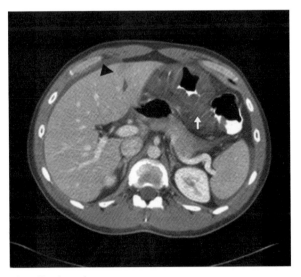

Plate 28.2 Abdominal swelling (arrow).

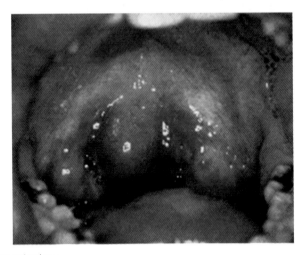

Plate 28.3 Airway angioedema.

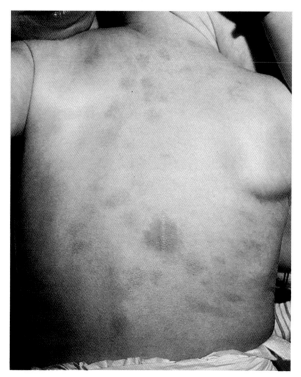

Plate 30.1 Stroking one UP lesion has caused a linear raised area (wheal) with surrounding erythema to develop (Darier's sign) on this child's back. From Habif TP. Clinical Dermatology: A Color Guide to Diagnosis and Therapy. 5th edition. 2010 Philadelphia, PA, Mosby/Elsevier. Reproduced with permission.

Section 9: Guidelines
National society guidelines

Guideline title	Guideline source	Date
Food Allergy: A practice parameter update—2014	Joint Task Force on Practice Parameters	2014 (http://www.allergyparameters.org/published-practice-parameters/alphabetical-listing/food-allergy-download/)

International society guidelines
Not applicable for this topic.

Section 9: Evidence

Type of evidence	Title, comment	Date
Cochrane Review	Tartrazine exclusion for allergic asthma **Comment:** Insufficient evidence to conclude that tartrazine induces asthma exacerbations	2001 (http://www.ncbi.nlm.nih.gov/pubmed/11687081)
Cochrane Review	Monosodium glutamate avoidance for chronic asthma in adults and children **Comment:** Insufficient evidence support avoidance of MSG for patients with asthma	2012 (http://www.ncbi.nlm.nih.gov/pubmed/22696342)

Section 10: Images
Not applicable for this topic.

Additional material for this chapter can be found online at:
www.mountsinaiexpertguides.com
This includes a case study, multiple choice questions, advice for patients, and ICD codes

CHAPTER 24

Celiac Disease

Mirna Chehade

Division of Allergy/Immunology, Department of Pediatrics, Icahn School of Medicine at Mount Sinai, New York, NY, USA

OVERALL BOTTOM LINE

- Celiac disease (CD) is a chronic, small intestinal, immune-mediated enteropathy precipitated by exposure to dietary gluten and related prolamins in genetically predisposed individuals.
- Clinical manifestations of celiac disease range from the completely asymptomatic patient to the severely affected patient with classic signs including bulky, foul-smelling, floating stools due to steatorrhea and flatulence. A number of non-gastrointestinal manifestations of CD can also be present.
- A hallmark of CD is the presence of antibodies directed against transglutaminase (anti-TTG) that can be detected in the serum. Anti-TTG antibodies (especially IgA) are highly sensitive and specific for the disease.
- Histopathologically, blunted or atrophic villi, crypt hyperplasia, mononuclear infiltration of the lamina propria, structural abnormalities in epithelial cells, and intraepithelial lymphocytic infiltration are seen in an intestinal biopsy.
- The cornerstone of treatment of CD is elimination of gluten from the patient's diet.

Section 1: Background

Definition of disease

- CD is a chronic, small intestinal, immune-mediated enteropathy precipitated by exposure to dietary gluten and related prolamins in genetically predisposed individuals.

Disease classification

Not applicable for this topic.

Incidence/prevalence

- CD is thought to occur primarily in white people of northern European ancestry. However, despite a lack of worldwide epidemiologic information, further studies in other areas of the world have shown a similar prevalence.
- Epidemiologic studies using serologic assays for CD with biopsy verification have reported a prevalence of 1 in 70–300 in most countries.
- The frequency of CD is substantially increased in patients who have a first degree family member affected with CD. The risk is highest in monozygotic twins, next in human leukocyte antigen (HLA) matched siblings, siblings, and finally parents and children of patients with CD.

Economic impact

Not applicable for this topic.

Mount Sinai Expert Guides: Allergy and Clinical Immunology, First Edition. Edited by Hugh A. Sampson.
© 2015 John Wiley & Sons, Ltd. Published 2015 by John Wiley & Sons, Ltd.
Companion website: www.mountsinaiexpertguides.com

Etiology
- Gluten (the commonly used term for the complex of water-insoluble proteins from wheat, rye, and barley) and related prolamins act as the trigger in patients with CD.

Pathology/pathogenesis
- A hallmark of CD is the presence of antibodies directed against transglutaminase (anti-TTG) that can be detected in the serum. Anti-TTG antibodies (especially IgA) are highly sensitive and specific for the disease. The mechanism of autoantibody formation remains incompletely understood.
- Immune dysregulation in CD occurs at multiple levels:
  - *Dysregulation in the adaptive immune system:* HLA-DQ2 or DQ8 bind gluten on antigen-presenting cells and present to T lymphocytes leading to anti-gluten T-cell response, which releases IFN-γ and possibly IL-21, leading to epithelial damage. In addition, up-regulation of IL-15 and IFN-α in the lamina propria induces dendritic cells to acquire a pro-inflammatory phenotype.
  - *Dysregulation in the innate immune system:* intraepithelial lymphocytes undergo reprogramming to acquire an NK phenotype characterized by up-regulation of NKG2D and CD94/NKG2C receptors that recognize major histocompatibility complex (MHC) class I-related chains A and B, and HLA-E on epithelial cells mediating tissue damage. IL-15 up-regulates NK receptors and promotes T-cell receptor-independent killing as well as blocking Foxp3 regulatory T-cell action on intraepithelial lymphocytes.
  - *Dysregulation in the humoral immune system:* the humoral immune system produces gluten-specific antibodies that mediate systemic manifestations such as dermatitis herpetiformis.
- Histopathologically, the following changes are seen in an intestinal biopsy: blunted or atrophic villi, crypt hyperplasia, mononuclear infiltration of the lamina propria, structural abnormalities in epithelial cells, and intraepithelial lymphocytic infiltration.

Predictive/risk factors

Risk factor	Estimated prevalence
First and second degree relatives of patients with CD	10% and 5%, respectively
Unexplained iron deficiency anemia	3–15%
Unexplained folic acid, iron, or vitamin B_{12} deficiency	N/A
Reduced serum albumin	N/A
Unexplained hypertransaminasemia	2–9%
Osteoporosis and osteomalacia of premature onset	2–4%
Recurrent abdominal pain or bloating	
Other autoimmune disorders:	
• Type 1 diabetes mellitus	2–15%
• Thyroid dysfunction	2–7%
• Addison's disease	N/A
• Autoimmune hepatitis	3–6%
Ataxia and idiopathic neuropathy	N/A
Down's and Turner's syndromes	6% each
Irritable bowel syndrome	3%

Section 2: Prevention
No interventions are indicated unless the diagnosis of CD is made.

Screening

- Widespread screening of asymptomatic individuals is not generally advocated at this time.
- Testing for CD is considered in the following groups of patients:
  - Those with gastrointestinal symptoms including chronic or recurrent diarrhea, malabsorption, weight loss, abdominal distension, or bloating. In addition, screening should be considered in patients with symptoms suggestive of irritable bowel syndrome or severe lactose intolerance.
  - Those without other explanations for iron deficiency anemia, folate or vitamin B_{12} deficiency, persistent elevation in hepatic transaminases, short stature, delayed puberty, recurrent fetal loss, reduced fertility, persistent aphthous stomatitis, dental enamel hypoplasia, idiopathic peripheral neuropathy, non-hereditary cerebellar ataxia, or recurrent migraine headaches.
  - Those with type 1 diabetes mellitus, autoimmune thyroiditis, Down's syndrome, Turner's syndrome, William's syndrome, and those with first degree relatives of individuals with CD if they have signs, symptoms, or laboratory evidence of CD.
- Serum immunoglobulin A (IgA) anti-TTG antibody is the single preferred test for the detection of CD in individuals over the age of 2 years. Total serum IgA should be measured, especially if IgA anti-TTG is negative, to rule out IgA deficiency that precludes accurate interpretation of the test. In patients with IgA deficiency or those with very low serum IgA, IgG-based testing (IgG anti-deamidated gliadin peptides (DGPs) and IgG anti-TTG) should be performed.

Primary prevention – bulleted pearls

Not applicable for this topic.

Secondary prevention

- Maintaining a gluten-free diet assures continued disease remission.

Section 3: Diagnosis (Algorithm 24.1)

Algorithm 24.1 Diagnosis of celiac disease

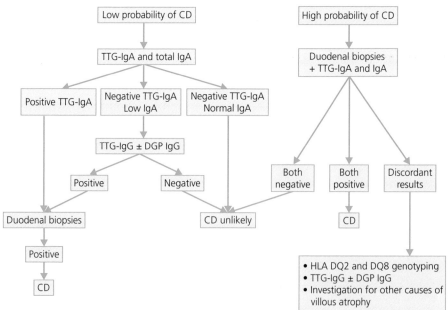

Note: CD, celiac disease; DGP IgG, deamidated gliadin peptide IgG; TTG-IgA, tissue transglutaminase IgA titer; TTG-IgG, tissue transglutaminase IgG titer.

> **BOTTOM LINE/CLINICAL PEARLS**
> - Clinical manifestations of celiac disease fall into a large spectrum, ranging from the completely asymptomatic patient to the severely affected patient with classic signs including bulky, foul-smelling, floating stools due to steatorrhea and flatulence. These symptoms can also be associated with those resulting from malabsorption, such as growth failure in children, weight loss, anemia, neurologic disorders from vitamin B deficiencies, and osteopenia from calcium and vitamin D deficiencies.
> - A number of non-gastrointestinal manifestations of CD have also been described, including neuropsychiatric disorders, rheumatologic disorders, osteomalacia, osteoporosis, and infertility. In some patients, they are the presenting symptoms and should prompt the consideration of serologic testing for CD.
> - Physical examination may reveal abnormalities related to the various clinical manifestations described above.
> - In addition to the screening serologic tests described above, the diagnosis of CD is confirmed by esophagogastroduodenoscopy (EGD) with intestinal biopsies, looking for histologic features of CD. Multiple duodenal biopsies need to be obtained, since the disease is patchy in nature. HLA DQ2 and DQ8 genotyping may be helpful in the event of biopsy/serology disagreement, if the patient is already on a gluten-free diet at the time of the diagnostic investigation, or in the case of equivocal duodenal biopsy findings in seronegative patients.

Differential diagnosis

Differential diagnosis	Features
Eosinophilic enteritis	Predominantly eosinophilic infiltration of the duodenal lamina propria
Protracted infectious enteritis	Recovery of causative infectious agent upon stool testing
Autoimmune enteropathy	
Giardiasis	Recovery of *Giardia* upon stool testing or on biopsies
Crohn's disease	No intestinal villous atrophy, no intraepithelial lymphocytosis, histological features suggestive of Crohn's disease such as granulomas may be present
Primary or acquired lactase deficiency	Failure to thrive is rare, symptoms resolve with avoidance of milk products
Irritable bowel syndrome	No histologic abnormalities are seen on intestinal biopsy

Typical presentation
- Due to increased physician awareness and screening at risk populations, most patients present with minimal to no gastrointestinal symptoms, or non-specific symptoms, such as fatigue, iron deficiency anemia, or otherwise unexplained elevation in hepatic transaminases. Some patients present with irritable bowel syndrome like symptoms. The typical patient with classic symptoms of abdominal pain and diarrhea with bulky, foul-smelling, and floating stools is becoming less frequent. Patients can also present with a variety of non-gastrointestinal manifestations, such as neuropsychiatric disorders, arthritis, and other manifestations listed above.

Clinical diagnosis
History
- The clinician should enquire about various gastrointestinal and non-gastrointestinal features, in addition to family history of celiac disease.

Physical examination
- Physical examination should include an abdominal examination for distension, increased tympanicity or tenderness, and a perianal examination that would be suggestive of other diseases such as Crohn's disease. In addition, a complete examination should be done to detect signs of anemia, neurologic deficiencies, and other non-gastrointestinal manifestations of, or associations with, CD.

Useful clinical decision rules and calculators
Not applicable for this topic.

Disease severity classification
Not applicable for this topic.

Laboratory diagnosis
List of diagnostic tests
- Immunoglobulin A (IgA) anti-TTG antibody is the single preferred test for the detection of CD in individuals over the age of 2 years. Total IgA should be measured, especially if IgA anti-TTG is negative, to rule out IgA deficiency that precludes accurate interpretation of the test. In patients with IgA deficiency or those with very low serum IgA, IgG-based testing (IgG anti-deamidated gliadin peptides (DGPs) and IgG anti-TTG) should be performed.
- HLA DQ2 and DQ8 genotyping should not be used routinely, but should be considered in the event of biopsy–serology disagreement, if the patient is already on a gluten-free diet at the time of the diagnostic investigation, or in the case of equivocal duodenal biopsy findings in seronegative patients.
- Endoscopy may reveal scalloped duodenal folds, though this finding is not common.
- Intestinal biopsies reveal the following features on hematoxylin and eosin (H&E) staining of biopsy sections to variable degrees: blunted or atrophic villi, crypt hyperplasia, mononuclear infiltration of the lamina propria, structural abnormalities in epithelial cells, and intraepithelial lymphocytic infiltration.

Lists of imaging techniques
- Radiologic tests are not routinely recommended for the diagnosis of CD.

Potential pitfalls/common errors made regarding diagnosis of disease
- To under-diagnose CD in patients because of non-specific gastrointestinal symptoms, or because of a non-gastrointestinal presentation.
- To under-diagnose CD based on negative TTG-IgA in patients with IgA deficiency.
- To over-diagnose CD based only on symptoms or symptom response to a gluten-free diet alone, because these alone do not differentiate CD from non-celiac gluten sensitivity.

Section 4: Treatment (Algorithm 24.2)
Treatment rationale
- The cornerstone of treatment of CD is elimination of gluten from the patient's diet, because CD is triggered by gluten. Treatment of the patient begins with dietary counseling by a registered dietitian who is knowledgeable in CD. Foods containing wheat, rye, and barley

Algorithm 24.2 Management of celiac disease

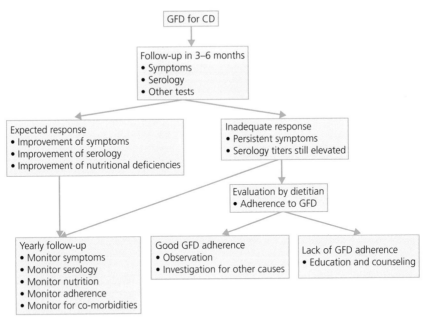

Note: CD, celiac disease; GFD, gluten-free diet.

should be avoided, as well as gluten-contaminated oats. The dietitian should also educate the patient about other sources of gluten besides food, such as certain alcoholic beverages. Education regarding food label reading and monitoring for adequate caloric intake and balance while on this restricted diet is important. In addition, early in the course of therapy, dairy products may not be tolerated because of secondary lactose intolerance, and lactose-containing foods may be avoided until intestinal villous regeneration occurs. Presence of any nutritional deficiencies should be investigated and corrected. Treatment with a gluten-free diet is life-long. Therefore, education of the patient and his/her family about the disease is important, and access to an advocacy group, if needed, should be made available. Finally, continuous long-term follow-up is important, and screening of family members at risk for CD should be carried out.

When to hospitalize
Not applicable for this topic.

Managing the hospitalized patient
Not applicable for this topic.

Table of treatment

Treatment	Comments
Dietary Gluten-free diet	Education and monitoring with the help of a dietitian with expertise in CD is important

Prevention/management of complications

- Dietary therapy with a gluten-free diet can be associated with decreased quality of life, malnutrition, or lack of adherence if not properly monitored and difficulties addressed.

CLINICAL PEARLS
- Monitor patients on a gluten-free diet to ensure adequate caloric intake and balance, and good adherence. A dietitian with expertise in CD is important for this.
- Check for any nutritional deficiencies and correct those as needed.
- Monitor patients for any decreased quality of life or coping difficulties and provide counseling when needed. A mental health professional may be needed for this.

Section 5: Special populations

Not applicable for this topic.

Section 6: Prognosis

BOTTOM LINE/CLINICAL PEARLS
- Patients with CD seem to be at a small increased risk of mortality.
- Patients with CD seem to have an increased risk of lymphoproliferative malignancy and a short-term excess risk of gastrointestinal malignancy.

Natural history of untreated disease

- In addition to nutritional complications, patients with CD have a higher risk of small bowel adenocarcinoma. The predominant celiac-associated lymphoma is the enteropathy-associated T-cell lymphoma.

Prognosis for treated patients

- A gluten-free diet to treat CD is thought to be protective against the development of malignant disease.

Follow-up tests and monitoring

Not applicable for this topic.

Section 7: Reading list

Bai J, Fried M, Corazza GR, Schuppan D, Farthing M, Catassi C, et al. World Gastroenterology Organisation global guidelines on celiac disease. J Clin Gastroenterol 2013;47:121–6

Fasano A, Araya M, Bhatnagar S, Cameron D, Catassi C, Dirks M, et al. Federation of international societies of pediatric gastroenterology, hepatology, and nutrition consensus report on celiac disease. J Pediatr Gastroenterol Nutr 2008;47:214–9

Husby S, Koletzko S, Korponay-Szabó IR, Mearin ML, Phillips A, Shamir R, et al. European Society for Pediatric Gastroenterology, Hepatology, and Nutrition guidelines for the diagnosis of coeliac disease. J Pediatr Gastroenterol Nutr 2012;54:136–60

Ludvigsson JF, Leffler DA, Bai JC, Biagi F, Fasano A, Green PH, et al. The Oslo definitions for coeliac disease and related terms. Gut 2013;62:43–52

Rubio-Tapia A, Hill ID, Kelly CP, Calderwood AH, Murray JA; American College of Gastroenterology. ACG clinical guidelines: diagnosis and management of celiac disease. Am J Gastroenterol 2013;108: 656–76

Suggested websites

Academy of Nutrition and Dietetics. www.eatright.org

American Gastroenterological Association. www.gastro.org/patient-center/digestive-conditions/celiac-disease

American Celiac Disease Alliance. www.americanceliac.org

Celiac Disease Foundation. www.celiac.org

Gluten Intolerance Group of North America. www.gluten.net

National Foundation for Celiac Awareness. www.celiaccentral.org

North American Society for the Study of Celiac Disease. www.nasscd.org

Section 8: Guidelines
National society guidelines

Guideline title	Guideline source	Date
ACG clinical guidelines: diagnosis and management of celiac disease	American College of Gastroenterology (ACG)	2013 (http://www.ncbi.nlm.nih.gov/pubmed/23609613)

International society guidelines

Guideline title	Guideline source	Date
European Society for Pediatric Gastroenterology, Hepatology, and Nutrition guidelines for the diagnosis of coeliac disease	European Society for Pediatric Gastroenterology, Hepatology, and Nutrition (ESPGHAN)	2012 (http://espghan.med.up.pt/position_papers/Guidelines_on_coeliac_disease.pdf)
World Gastroenterology Organization global guidelines on celiac disease	World Gastroenterology Organization (WGO)	2013 (http://www.worldgastroenterology.org/celiac-disease.html)

Section 9: Evidence

Type of evidence	Title, comment	Date
Clinical guidelines	ACG clinical guidelines: diagnosis and management of celiac disease **Comment:** Summary of what is known and what still needs to be investigated on CD, with evidence grading for each statement or recommendation	2013 (http://www.ncbi.nlm.nih.gov/pubmed/23609613)

Section 10: Images

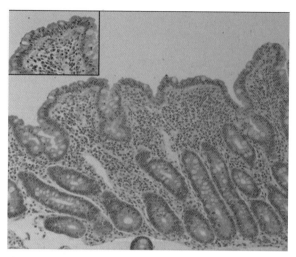

Figure 24.1 Histopathologic features of an intestinal biopsy from a patient with celiac disease (hematoxylin and eosin stain, magnification 100×): Blunted villi, crypt hyperplasia, mononuclear infiltration of the lamina propria, and intraepithelial lymphocytic infiltration. The latter is made visually clear in the inset (magnification 400×). Source: Courtesy of Margret Magid, MD, Pediatric Pathology, Icahn School of Medicine at Mount Sinai. See color plate 24.1.

**Additional material for this chapter can be found online at:
www.mountsinaiexpertguides.com**
This includes a case study, multiple choice questions, advice for patients, and ICD codes

CHAPTER 25

Oral Food Challenges (Procedure)

Hugh A. Sampson

Jaffe Food Allergy Institute, Icahn School of Medicine at Mount Sinai, New York, NY, USA

OVERALL BOTTOM LINE

- The clinical history, skin prick tests, and serum food-specific IgE antibody levels are useful for making the diagnosis of food allergy. However, without an unequivocal allergic reaction to an isolated food ingestion with supportive laboratory data, some form of oral food challenge is necessary to establish the diagnosis of a food allergy.
- The double-blind placebo-controlled oral food challenge is the "gold standard" for diagnosing food allergy. However, in the routine clinical setting, a single-blind or open challenge is more practical and often adequate.
- When the food challenge is negative, or when ingestion of a food induces the same symptoms as reported in the history, the single-blind or open challenge is sufficiently specific to confirm the diagnosis of food allergy.
- In clinical practice, oral food challenges are typically used to confirm the presence of food allergy or demonstrate that a patient, typically a child, has outgrown their food allergy.

Section 1: Indications

- Indications for oral food challenge:
  - To confirm clinical reactivity to foods suspected of inducing allergic reactions based on history, skin test results, and/or serum food-specific IgE levels;
  - To determine whether a patient has "outgrown" their food allergy; and
  - To establish a threshold of clinical reactivity (lowest eliciting dose) to a food allergen (used predominantly in clinical trials of immunotherapy for food allergy).

Section 2: Procedure

- Patient must be off antihistamine medications for approximately 5 half-lives of the specific medication.
- Oral food challenges may be performed in three basic formats: double-blind placebo-controlled (neither the physician nor the patient are aware of the contents of the challenge), single-blind (patient is unaware of the contents of the challenge), or open (both the physician and patient are aware of the contents of the challenge).
- For practical reasons, an open challenge may be the first approach when the probability of a negative challenge seems high and in infants and children <3 years of age, who are unlikely to have any psychological component influencing the outcome.
- The double-blind, placebo-controlled oral food challenge (DBPCFC) is considered the "gold standard" for diagnosing food allergy.

Mount Sinai Expert Guides: Allergy and Clinical Immunology, First Edition. Edited by Hugh A. Sampson.
© 2015 John Wiley & Sons, Ltd. Published 2015 by John Wiley & Sons, Ltd.
Companion website: www.mountsinaiexpertguides.com

- A negative DBPCFC must always be followed by an open, normal serving of the challenged food in order to avoid the rare false negative outcome due to destruction of the allergen during preparation of the blinded challenge material.
- A single-blind or open food challenge may be considered diagnostic under the following circumstances: if either of these challenges elicits no symptoms (i.e. the challenge is negative) food allergy is ruled-out; and when either challenge elicits objective symptoms (i.e. the challenge is positive) and those objective symptoms correlate with the medical history and are supported by laboratory tests.
- Before undertaking an oral food challenge, the patient should be avoiding the food to be challenged and have attained a stable baseline with regard to atopic disease. The length of time a patient needs to eliminate a food in order to improve a chronic disease (e.g. atopic dermatitis) varies by disease and individual patient, but at least 2 weeks is suggested.

Oral food challenge

- Starting dose: it is advisable to start with a dose less than the expected "threshold" dose to elicit symptoms. If unknown, it is recommended starting with a dose equivalent to 1–10 mg of food protein (e.g. 2–20 mg of peanut flour), depending on the expected degree of sensitivity.
- For investigating immediate (IgE-mediated) food allergy, an interval of 20–30 minutes between successive doses is adequate. For non-IgE-mediated food allergy, longer intervals between doses increasing the dose by ½ logs (e.g. Practall schedule – 1, 3, 10, 30, 100, 300 mg, etc.) or a doubling of the dose (e.g. 5, 10, 20, 40, 80, 160, 320, 640 mg, etc.) until a cumulative dose of 10 g food protein has been ingested. Individuals with a past history of food-induced anaphylaxis, persistent asthma, and/or reacting to trace food contaminants are at increased risk for severe reactions and should have their dosage titrated upwards cautiously.
- Vehicles (matrix) selected to mask the taste, odor, texture, and color of the challenge food are dependent upon the patient's preferences. For most challenges in infants and young children, infant formulas and applesauce are convenient vehicles. Other vehicles used for masking purposes include fruit juices, oatmeal, puddings, potato pancakes, ground lean meat patties, and fruit smoothies.
- Non-fat dried milk and egg powders, and wheat, rye, oat, rice, barley, corn, potato, and soy flours can be added to almost any food vehicle. Peanut and various nut flours must be mixed with vehicles that have strong flavors. Meats and fish can be masked in another tolerated ground meat, and fish and shellfish can be mixed with canned tuna, which is tolerated even by most tuna-allergic patients.
- If a placebo is utilized, it must consist of another food that is in similar texture, look, smell, mouth feel, and taste to the challenge food and known to be tolerated by the patient.
- When evaluating IgE-mediated reactions, the patient should not eat for at least 4 hours prior to the challenge, which enhances the absorption of the challenge material and ensures that the challenge results are caused by the food administered in the challenge. When evaluating non-IgE-mediated reactions, longer fasting times may be necessary.
- Before beginning the food challenge, baseline vital signs (respiratory rate, heart rate, and blood pressure), peak flow, and physical findings should be evaluated and documented to serve as a reference. Emergency medications must be readily accessible, including access to oxygen, intravenous fluids, and a crash cart.
- With the first symptom or sign of an allergic reaction, the physician should immediately inspect the skin and oropharynx and auscultate the chest. Vital signs should be measured, and oxygen saturation if available. The food challenge should be stopped with any objective finding of an allergic reaction, and treatment initiated immediately (see Table 25.1 for guidance on scoring

Table 25.1 Oral food challenge symptom scoring.

I. SKIN
A. Erythematous rash - % area involved_____
B. Pruritus
0 = Absent
1 = Mild, occasional scratching
2 = Moderate – scratching continuously for >2 minutes at a time
3 = Severe – hard continuous scratching – excoriations
C. Urticaria/angioedema
0 = Absent
1 = Mild – <3 hives, or mild lip edema
2 = Moderate – <10 hives but >3, or significant lip or face edema
3 = Severe – generalized involvement
D. Rash
0 = Absent
1 = Mild – few areas of faint erythema
2 = Moderate – areas of erythema
3 = Severe – generalized marked erythema (>50%)

II. UPPER RESPIRATORY
A. Sneezing/itching
0 = Absent
1 = Mild – rare bursts, occasional sniffing
2 = Moderate – bursts <10, intermittent rubbing of nose, and/or eyes or frequent sniffing
3 = Severe – continuous rubbing of nose and/or eyes, periocular swelling and/or long bursts of sneezing, persistent rhinorrhea

III. LOWER RESPIRATORY
A. Wheezing
0 = Absent
1 = Mild – expiratory wheezing to auscultation
2 = Moderate – inspiratory and expiratory wheezing
3 = Severe – use of accessory muscles, audible wheezing
B. Laryngeal
0 = Absent
1 = Mild – >3 discrete episodes of throat clearing or cough, or persistent throat tightness/pain
2 = Moderate – hoarseness, frequent dry cough
3 = Severe – stridor

IV. GASTROINTESTINAL
A . Subjective complaints
0 = Absent
1 = Mild – complaints of nausea or abdominal pain, itchy mouth/throat
2 = Moderate – frequent c/o nausea or pain with normal activity
3 = Severe–notably distressed due to GI symptoms with decreased activity
B . Objective complaints
0 = Absent
1 = Mild – 1 episode of emesis or diarrhea
2 = Moderate – 2–3 episodes of emesis or diarrhea or 1 of each
3 = Severe – >3 episodes of emesis or diarrhea or 2 of each

V. CARDIOVASCULAR/NEUROLOGIC
0 = normal heart rate or BP for age/baseline
1 = Mild-subjective response (weak, dizzy), or tachycardia
2 = Moderate-drop in blood pressure and/or >20% from baseline, or significant change in mental status.
3 = Severe-cardiovascular collapse, signs of impaired circulation (unconscious)

⬜ - Not usually an indication to alter dosing. Not generally sufficient to consider a challenge positive.

◼ - Caution, dosing could proceed, be delayed, have a dose repeated rather than escalated. If clinically indicated, dosing is stopped. Symptoms that recur on 3 doses, or persist (e.g., 40 minutes) are more likely indicative of a reaction than when such symptoms are transient and not reproducible. 3 or more scoring areas in orange more likely represent a true response.

◼ - Objective symptoms likely to indicate a true reaction. Usually an indication to stop dosing.

Color coding provides guidance on when to discontinue an oral food challenge and designate it as "positive."

Source: adapted from Practall Guidelines; Sampson et al. J Allergy Clin Immunol 2012;130:1260–74.

the outcome of oral food challenges). Patients should be checked prior to each successive food challenge dose and every 15 minutes thereafter for approximately 2 hours, or at the first symptom or sign of a possible reaction.

- A challenge may also be considered positive if subjective symptoms follow three successive doses of the test food, but not the placebo. In non-verbal children, clues to the onset of a reaction may be subtle signs such as ear picking, scratching at the tongue, inside of the mouth, or neck; or a change in general behavior (e.g. becoming quiet, withdrawn, or insisting on being held by the parent). Similarly, isolated subjective symptoms in older patients (e.g. complaints of throat tightness or pruritus, nausea, abdominal pain, or general malaise) may represent early signs of a more severe reaction.
- When an oral food challenge results in an allergic reaction, treatment should be initiated promptly according to guidelines for anaphylaxis treatment (see Chapters 22 and 29).
- When patients experience a reaction during the oral food challenge (i.e. a "positive challenge"), they should remain under observation following the resolution of symptoms with treatment based on the clinical judgment of the physician conducting the challenge. However, 2–4 hours following the resolution of symptoms for immediate hypersensitivity reactions and about 4–6 hours for food protein-induced enterocolitis syndrome are usually recommended.

Section 3: Management of complications
- Systemic allergic reactions from oral food challenges are fairly common. Consequently, physicians must have the appropriate expertise, equipment, and medical personnel to treat anaphylactic reactions (see Chapters 22 and 29).
- Patients should be observed for at least 2 hours following a food challenge to ensure that the challenged food has not provoked an allergic reaction. Follow-up may need to be longer if the clinical history suggests a more prolonged period between ingestion and the development of symptoms.

Section 4: Follow-up
- Physicians should discuss the relevance, implications, and associated treatment instructions of positive and negative food challenges in the context of the patient's medical history.
- Physicians should discuss the need for and timing of follow-up food challenges in children who are likely to "outgrow" their food allergy (e.g. milk and egg allergy).

Section 5: Reading list

Bernhisel-Broadbent J, Strause D, Sampson HA. Fish hypersensitivity. II: Clinical relevance of altered fish allergenicity caused by various preparation methods. J Allergy Clin Immunol 1992; 90:622–9

Bindslev-Jensen C, Ballmer-Weber BK, Bengtsson U, Blanco C, Ebner C, Hourihane J, et al. Standardization of food challenges in patients with immediate reactions to foods: position paper from the European Academy of Allergology and Clinical Immunology. Allergy 2004;59:690–7

Bock SA, Sampson HA, Atkins FM, Zeiger RS, Lehrer S, Sachs M, et al. Double-blind placebo-controlled food challenge (DBPCFC) as an office procedure: a manual. J Allergy Clin Immunol 1988;82:986–97

Boyce JA, Assa'ad A, Burks AW, Jones SM, Sampson HA, Wood RA, et al. Guidelines for the diagnosis and management of food allergy in the United States: report of the NIAID-sponsored expert panel. J Allergy Clin Immunol 2010;126(Suppl):S1–58

Niggemann B, Beyer K. Pitfalls in double-blind, placebo-controlled oral food challenges. Allergy 2007;62: 729–32

Nowak-Wegrzyn A, Assa'ad AH, Bahna SL, Bock SA, Sicherer SH, Teuber SS. Work Group report: oral food challenge testing. J Allergy Clin Immunol 2009;123:S365–83

Sampson HA, Gerth van Wijk R, Bindslev-Jensen C, Sicherer S, Teuber SS, Burks AW, et al. Standardizing double-blind, placebo-controlled oral food challenges: American Academy of Allergy, Asthma and Immunology–European Academy of Allergy and Clinical Immunology PRACTALL consensus report. J Allergy Clin Immunol 2012;130:1260–74

Suggested websites

www.foodallergy.org

www.aaaai.org

www.acaai.org

Section 6: Guidelines
National society guidelines

Guideline title	Guideline source	Date
Standardizing double-blind, placebo-controlled oral food challenges: American Academy of Allergy, Asthma and Immunology–European Academy of Allergy and Clinical Immunology PRACTALL consensus report	American Academy of Allergy, Asthma and Immunology (AAAI); European Academy of Allergy and Clinical Immunology (EAACI)	2012 (http://www.ncbi.nlm.nih.gov/pubmed/23195525)

Section 7: Evidence
Not applicable for this topic.

Section 8: Images
Not applicable for this topic.

Additional material for this chapter can be found online at:
www.mountsinaiexpertguides.com
This includes a case study, multiple choice questions, advice for patients, and ICD codes

CHAPTER 26

Acute Urticaria

Amanda L. Cox

Division of Pediatric Allergy/Immunology, Icahn School of Medicine at Mount Sinai, New York, NY, USA

OVERALL BOTTOM LINE

- Urticarial lesions ("hives" or "welts") are vascular skin reactions characterized by extremely pruritic, circumscribed, raised, erythematous plaques or papules, often with a pale center. Individual lesions are transient and generally resolve within 24 hours.
- The majority of cases of new onset urticaria are acute (<6 weeks in duration) and self-limited.
- The lesions of acute and chronic urticaria are identical, so when they first develop it is not possible to differentiate acute from chronic urticaria by physical examination.
- There are numerous possible causes of acute urticaria, and for many patients no specific etiology can be identified.
- In some cases, urticaria may be a presenting feature of a systemic disorder or may persist and represent the beginning of chronic urticaria.
- Non-sedating second generation H1 antihistamines are the mainstay of therapy for acute urticaria.

Section 1: Background
Definition of disease

- Urticaria is characterized by skin findings of spontaneously erupting, pruritic, short-lived wheals (or hives), which may be caused by a variety of triggers or may be idiopathic, and may be associated with angioedema. Acute urticaria refers specifically to urticaria that does not exceed 6 weeks in duration.

Disease classification

- Urticaria may be classified as: (i) acute urticaria; (ii) chronic urticaria; (iii) physical urticaria (reproduced by specific stimuli); or (iv) contact urticaria (secondary to skin contact with allergens or chemicals). Underlying diseases such as urticarial vasculitis and autoinflammatory syndromes, or acute infections may also present with acute or chronic urticaria.

Incidence/prevalence

- Acute urticaria affects up to 20% of the population at some point in their lives and occurs across all ages.

Mount Sinai Expert Guides: Allergy and Clinical Immunology, First Edition. Edited by Hugh A. Sampson.
© 2015 John Wiley & Sons, Ltd. Published 2015 by John Wiley & Sons, Ltd.
Companion website: www.mountsinaiexpertguides.com

- Acute urticaria is most commonly seen in the pediatric population, and is often associated with atopy; boys are affected at the same rates as girls.
- Atopy seems to be more prevalent in individuals with urticaria than in the general population.
- Acute urticaria is less likely to progress to chronic urticaria in children, but overall, 20–30% of patients with acute urticaria will progress to chronic or recurrent urticaria.

Economic impact
- The economic impact of acute urticaria has not been determined.

Etiology
- There are many potential causes of new onset acute urticaria, and in some cases no etiology can be identified.
- Common causes include viral and bacterial infections, parasitic infections, IgE-mediated reactions to medication, vaccination, stinging or biting insects, latex exposure, blood product transfusion, skin contact with allergens, and ingestion of foods. Non-IgE-mediated reactions to medications and transfusions can also cause urticaria. In children, infectious causes are believed to be by far the most common etiology for acute urticaria.
- Urticaria can also be triggered by specific physical stimuli as in physical urticarial disorders, which include dermatographism, delayed pressure urticaria, cholinergic urticaria, adrenergic urticaria, solar urticaria, aquagenic urticaria, and vibratory urticaria/angioedema.
- Food-dependent exercise-induced urticaria/anaphylaxis is a unique IgE-mediated allergic condition that presents with acute hives (or systemic allergic reaction) only when exercise follows ingestion of a specific food that is otherwise tolerated.
- Serum sickness and hormone-associated disorders can cause acute urticaria.
- Urticaria is often an early manifestation of a systemic disorder such as urticarial vasculitis, autoimmune disease, mastocytosis/mast cell disorder, or malignancy.

Pathology/pathogenesis
- Cutaneous mast cells in the superficial dermis are primarily responsible for the appearance of urticaria (or hives), although basophils may be involved in some lesions. Mast cells express high-affinity IgE receptors (FcϵRIs), which interact with the constant domain of IgE antibodies. Mast cells degranulate when IgE forms a complex with FcϵRI on the mast cell, when adjacent FcϵRIs cross-link, or if receptor-bound IgE binds to allergen, anti-IgE, or anti-FcϵRI antibodies. Opioids, complement, anaphylatoxin, stem cell factor, and neuropeptides can cause direct mast cell degranulation without interacting with the FcϵRIs. Immune complexes can also cause acute urticaria, although the mechanism for this is unclear.
- Mast cell degranulation ultimately involves fusion of intercellular storage granules with the mast cell membrane, such that granule contents including histamine, prostaglandin D2 (PGD2), leukotrienes, tumor necrosis factor α (TNF-α), and other cytokines are released from the cell into surrounding tissues. Histamine and leukotriene C4 (LTC4) mediate a wheal-and-flare skin reaction, itching, and vasodilatation that causes swelling in the upper layers of skin. Histamine, TNF-α, and IL-8 also up-regulate adhesion molecule expression on endothelial cells and promote inflammatory cell migration into urticarial lesions. Angioedema is similar to urticarial lesion formation, but involves mast cells of the deeper dermis and subcutaneous tissues.

Predictive/risk factors
Not applicable for this topic.

Section 2: Prevention

- No interventions have been demonstrated to prevent the development of acute urticaria, because acute new onset urticaria is spontaneous and generally unpredictable.
- In the majority of cases, which are infection-related or idiopathic, acute urticaria resolves without recurrence.
- No intervention has been shown to prevent acute urticaria from progressing to chronic urticaria.

Screening

Not applicable for this topic.

Primary prevention

Not applicable for this topic.

Secondary prevention

- Avoidance of food/inhalant/contact allergens, medications, or physical stimuli will prevent further episodes of acute or recurrent urticaria in individuals for whom these triggers have been identified.
- Specific allergen immunotherapy may be indicated in patients with inhalant, contact, or insect venom allergy, especially when there is a risk of anaphylaxis.

Section 3: Diagnosis

BOTTOM LINE/CLINICAL PEARLS
- The appearance of urticaria on physical examination does not provide clues about the etiology.
- History should be positive for the sudden appearance of hives with or without angioedema. Patients report wheals on any area of the skin surface, of variable size, surrounded by erythema and associated with itching, and occasionally a burning sensation. No individual hive should persist more than 24 hours, and no hive or wheal should leave any residual ecchymosis, bruising, or pigmentation.
- History should also focus on any potential inciting factors or triggers for hives, such as recent medications, illnesses, food exposures, exercise, insect stings, travel, and sexual history.
- The clinician must ask about associated signs or symptoms of a generalized allergic reaction or anaphylaxis including respiratory, gastrointestinal, or circulatory symptoms (see Chapter 29). The clinician should also enquire about signs and symptoms such as fever, weight loss, arthralgia, and arthritis, which might suggest an underlying systemic disorder.
- Skin lesions should be visualized directly in order to make a diagnosis of urticaria, as the term "hives" is used often by patients to describe any rash or exanthem.
- For patients who have acute urticaria (<6 weeks' duration), laboratory testing is not absolutely necessary unless there is a suspicion of an underlying disorder or urticarial vasculitis.
- Laboratory studies may be used to investigate an IgE-mediated (allergic) cause for acute urticaria. If an allergic cause is suspected, the patient should be referred to an allergist or immunologist for evaluation.

Differential diagnosis

Differential diagnosis	Features
Viral exanthem	Fixed, non-pruritic, maculopapular eruption that persists for days, often with fever, common in children, caused by many different viruses
Auriculotemporal syndrome	Transient post-prandial non-pruritic flushing of skin over cheeks and jawline, generally unilateral
Sweet's syndrome	Recurrent episodic painful rash of papules and plaques associated with fever, arthralgia, and peripheral leukocytosis
Atopic dermatitis	Intensely pruritic erythematous patches with papules and scaling, lasting in patches for days to weeks or longer
Contact dermatitis	Irritant or allergic dermatitis arising from direct skin exposure to a substance, erythematous or papular, and sometimes maculopapular
Drug eruptions	Maculopapular rash with lesions that become larger and confluent over time, associated with a medication exposure, may or may not be pruritic
Bullous pemphigoid	Pruritus with or without urticarial lesions that progresses to blistering lesions, occurs in older adults
Erythema multiforme	Erythematous macules, vesiculobullous lesions with a target appearance, may be painful or pruritic, distributed on extensor surfaces of extremities, and individual lesions last for several days, associated with fever and malaise
Serum sickness	Pruritic urticarial, macular, or raised serpiginous rash, associated with fever, polyarthralgias, polyarthritis, and malaise. Individual urticarial lesions may last for several days to weeks

Typical presentation
- The presenting feature of acute urticaria is hives, which are circumscribed, raised, pink–red edematous plaques with central pallor that are intensely pruritic. Hives may be round, oval, or serpiginous, and range from millimeters to centimeters in diameter. Hives may also become confluent. Individual lesions are transient, and can appear and enlarge over minutes to hours. Surrounding erythema should blanch with pressure. Individual hives disappear within 24 hours and leave no residual skin marking. Urticaria can appear on any area of the body, and may be found where clothing compresses the skin or where skin rubs another skin surface (e.g. axillae). There may be associated angioedema, or swelling of the lower dermis and subcutaneous layer, usually of the face, lips, extremities, or genitals.

Clinical diagnosis
History
- Acute urticaria arises spontaneously, with or without angioedema. Acute urticaria may be isolated to one eruption, may occur continuously, or may be intermittent over the course of a 6-week (or shorter) period. Patients describe extreme pruritus, and, occasionally, burning, but should not report pain. It is important to ask about symptoms suggesting anaphylaxis or an acute systemic allergic reaction. Patients may complain that the pruritus disrupts their daily activities and sleep, and that it is most intense at night. In some cases, the history reveals a temporal relationship to a suspected eliciting trigger, such as a food ingestion, insect sting, medication exposure, environmental exposure, recent/concurrent illness, or physical stimulus. Past history and family history of urticaria should also be noted.

Physical examination

- For a patient presenting with acute urticaria, vital signs, circulatory, neurologic, respiratory, and gastrointestinal systems should be fully evaluated to differentiate acute urticaria from anaphylaxis.
- A comprehensive physical examination is essential, with close examination of the skin. Urticarial lesions are pruritic, circumscribed, raised, erythematous plaques of a few millimeters to several centimeters in diameter. Wheals may arise in crops on any area of the body, enlarge, develop central pallor, and/or coalesce with other wheals. Each lesion is usually short-lived and resolves within a few hours, leaving no residual skin marks.
- If a patient is currently taking H1-blocking antihistamine, the lesions may appear flat.
- Angioedema, defined as deep dermal, subcutaneous tissue, or mucous membrane swelling, may also be present.
- Note any non-urticarial exanthem, other rash, pigment changes, ecchymosis, or purpura, as these findings suggest other underlying conditions.
- As individual hives are evanescent, the patient may have no urticaria at the time of examination and photographs may be helpful.
- If a patient states individual hives persist for days or longer, a single lesion may be circled with pen and monitored for resolution or persistence beyond 24–48 hours.

Useful clinical decision rules and calculators

Not applicable for this topic.

Disease severity classification

Scoring system for severity of acute urticaria. Total score of severity is sum of grades for wheals and pruritus (0–4).

Symptom	Grade	Criteria
Wheals	0	None
	1	<20 wheals/24 hours
	2	>20 wheals/24 hours
Pruritus	0	No pruritus
	1	Mild–moderate: tolerable, does not interfere with activities or sleep
	2	Severe: intolerable, interferes with activities and/or sleep

Source: Frigas E, Park MA. Acute urticaria and angioedema: diagnostic and treatment considerations. Am J Clin Dermatol 2009;10:239–50. Reproduced with permission of Elsevier.

Laboratory diagnosis

List of diagnostic tests

- Laboratory tests are not required for most cases of acute spontaneous urticaria without other symptoms or signs of illness, but may be considered for chronic urticaria of over 6 weeks' duration (see Chapter 27).
- Physical provocation tests may be used to evaluate physical urticaria:
  - Assess for dermatographism by stroking the skin with a firm object;
  - Conduct physical testing with suspected stimuli (e.g. ice, heat, pressure) if feasible in the clinical setting.
- Specific allergen IgE levels (for foods, latex, insect venom, select medications, and inhalant allergens) may be measured or allergy skin testing pursued if an allergic trigger is strongly suspected or if clinical history suggests an allergic cause.

- Laboratory tests to confirm a suspected infection may be performed if clinically indicated.
- If a single wheal persists >24 hours, does not respond to antihistamine, leaves pigmentary changes, or is associated with petechiae, or palpable purpura, a skin biopsy should be performed.

Lists of imaging techniques
Imaging studies are not indicated for acute spontaneous urticaria.

Potential pitfalls/common errors made regarding diagnosis of disease
- For a patient with acute urticaria, it is essential that anaphylaxis is not overlooked. Anaphylaxis is a potentially life-threatening condition and requires emergency medical intervention.
- The skin lesions of acute and chronic urticaria are identical so, at initial onset, it is not possible to differentiate acute from chronic forms of urticaria.
- Urticaria that is recurrent or persistent for 6 weeks or longer is considered to be chronic urticaria and warrants further diagnostic evaluation.
- Angioedema without urticaria requires a different course of evaluation and management (see Chapter 28).

Section 4: Treatment (Algorithm 26.1)

Algorithm 26.1 Treatment of acute urticaria

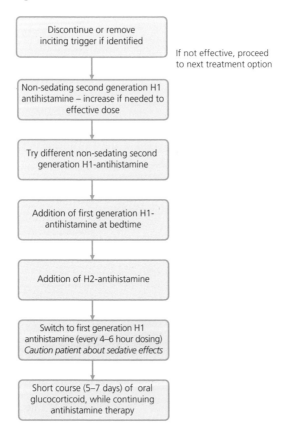

Note: Evaluate for chronic urticaria if ≥6 weeks of symptoms

Treatment rationale

- Acute management of anaphylaxis is critical if systemic symptoms such as hypotension/shock, syncope, bronchospasm, or severe gastrointestinal distress are also present. If acute urticaria is not associated with a systemic allergic reaction, begin with elimination or discontinuation of the causative agent, if identified, as this may result in rapid resolution of urticaria as well as prevent recurrence. Appropriate and prompt treatment should be considered for any underlying infection or illness if suspected.
- Acute urticaria without anaphylaxis or underlying illness is generally benign, and not life-threatening. Treatment is focused on providing short-term symptom relief of pruritus and urticaria. The first line pharmacotherapeutic agents are non-sedating oral antihistamines, titrated to the lowest effective recommended daily dosage. In some cases urticaria will occur once without recurrence, or resolve after a few days, and the antihistamine may be discontinued. If urticaria persists despite this regimen, a first generation sedating oral antihistamine may be added to the regimen, starting with a low dose at bedtime and increased gradually, if needed, to the dosage that controls symptoms. An H2 receptor antagonist may also be added to the antihistamine regimen. An effective antihistamine regimen should be continued for 4–6 weeks before being tapered or discontinued. When antihistamines alone are not effective, a short course of systemic oral glucocorticoids (5–7 days) may be added to the antihistamine regimen.

When to hospitalize

- Emergent stabilization and possible hospitalization is required for acute urticaria with life-threatening symptoms of anaphylaxis including:
  - Syncope;
  - Rapid onset of unresponsiveness or lethargy;
  - Hypotension and/or hypovolemic shock;
  - Bronchospasm, stridor, wheezing, or respiratory distress;
  - Hypotonia;
  - Severe vomiting, diarrhea, abdominal pain.

Managing the hospitalized patient

- Acute urticaria associated with anaphylactic shock may require all or some of the following treatment measures (see Chapter 29):
  - Intramuscular epinephrine (multiple doses may be required);
  - Rapid and continuous intravascular volume replacement;
  - Continuous intravenous pressor administration;
  - H2 antihistamine (PO, IM, or IV);
  - Systemic glucocorticoid (PO or IV);
  - Inhaled beta-agonist;
  - H1 antihistamine (PO or IV).

Table of treatment

Treatment	Comment
Conservative Avoidance, removal or discontinuation of causative agent or physical trigger	May be sufficient treatment for patients who have an identifiable allergen trigger (food, medication, latex) or pseudoallergen trigger, or for patients who have physical urticaria with known physical stimulus (e.g. dermatographism, cold, cholinergic, pressure)

Treatment	Comment
Medical (oral dosing only) *Second generation H1 antihistamines* • Cetirizine (children 6 months–2 years, 2.5 mg QD; children 2–5 years, 5 mg QD; children 6 years and older, 5–10 mg QD; adults, 10 mg QD to BID) • Levocetirizine (children 6–11 years, 2.5 mg QD; 12 years and older, 5 mg QD; adults, up to 5 mg BID) • Loratadine (children 2–5 years, 5 mg QD; 6 years and older, 10 mg QD) • Desloratadine (children 6 months–1 year, 1 mg QD; 1–5 years, 1.25 mg QD; 6–11 years, 2.5 mg QD; 12 years and older, 5 mg QD up to 5 mg BID in adults) • Fexofenadine (children 6 months–2 years, 15 mg BID; 2–11 years, 30 mg BID; 12 years and older, 180 mg QD up to 180 mg BID in adults)	• Second-generation H1 antihistamines are the recommended first line therapy for acute urticaria • Evidence for effectiveness of second generation • H1 antihistamines is very high, and these are safe and well tolerated by most patients, with minimal sedation and anticholinergic side effects, and minimal interaction with other medications • Response to and tolerance of individual H1 antihistamine agents varies between patients • Drowsiness can be experienced at higher doses • Dosage adjustments for all H1 antihistamines are necessary for patients with renal or hepatic insufficiency
First generation H1 antihistamines • Diphenhydramine (children, 5 mg/kg/24 hr ÷ every 6 hr, max dose 300 mg/24 hr; adults, 10–50 mg/dose every 4–8 hr, max dose 400 mg/24 hr) • Chlorpheniramine (children 2–6 years, 1 mg every 4–6 hr; 6–11 years, 2 mg every 4–6 hr; 12 years and older, 4 mg every 4–6 hr, max dose 24 mg/24 hr) • Hydroxyzine (children, 2 mg/kg/24 hr ÷ every 6–8 hr PRN; adult, 25–100 mg/dose every 4–6 hr PRN, max dose 600 mg/24 hr)	• First generation H1 antihistamines are second line agents, but may be helpful at bedtime in combination with a non-sedating agent taken during the day, or when second generation agent is not effective • Many patients experience sedative and anticholinergic side effects with first generation antihistamines • Diphenhydramine or hydroxyzine can be given intravenously
H2 antihistamines • Ranitidine HCL (infants/children 1 month–16 years, 5–10 mg/kg/24 hr ÷ every 12 hr, max dose 300 mg/24 hr; adults, 150 mg/dose BID or 300 mg QHS) • Famotidine (children, 1 mg/kg/24 hr ÷ every 12 hr, max dose 80 mg/24 hr; adolescent and adult, 20 mg BID) • Cimetidine (children, 20–40 mg/kg/24 hr ÷ every 6 hr; adult, 300 mg/dose QID or 400 mg BID or 800 mg/dose QHS)	• Combination of H1 and H2 antihistamine may be more effective than H1 antihistamine alone, although data are limited • H2 antihistamines are generally well tolerated • Cimetidine can increase circulating levels of other medications so should be used with caution
Glucocorticoids • Prednisone (adults, 30–60 mg QD, tapered over 5–7 days) • Prednisolone (children, 0.5–1 mg/kg/day, max 60 mg QD, tapered over 5–7 days)	• A short course of glucocorticoid may be added to antihistamine for severe or persistent symptoms, or when angioedema is present • Repeat courses of oral glucocorticoids should be avoided • Optimal dosing and duration of glucocorticoid therapy has not been established • Tapering or withdrawal of glucocorticoids can result in resurgence of urticaria; antihistamine should be continued for duration of glucocorticoid course and for several days after glucocorticoid course is complete
Other Referral to an allergist or immunologist	• Appropriate when allergic etiology is suspected

Prevention/management of complications

- First generation H1 antihistamines have sedative and anticholinergic side effects, to which very young and elderly patients may be more susceptible.
- Anticholinergic effects of first generation H1 antihistamines include dry mouth, diplopia, blurred vision, urinary retention, and vaginal dryness. Sedative effects can cause fine motor skills, driving skills, and reaction times to be impaired.
- First generation H1 antihistamines can cause cognitive impairment and sleep disturbance in children.
- First generation H1 antihistamines are contraindicated in patients with gastrointestinal (GI) or urinary obstruction.
- For second generation H1 antihistamines, dose adjustments (lower doses and decreased frequency of administration) are required in patients with renal or hepatic impairment.
- All H1 antihistamines should be used with caution in patients with glaucoma and prostatic hyperplasia.
- Prolonged use of glucocorticoids is associated with osteopenia, adrenal suppression, Cushingoid effects, cataracts, diabetes, and GI bleeding. Short-term use may cause mood changes, appetite changes, hyperglycemia, diarrhea, nausea, and abdominal distension.

CLINICAL PEARLS

- The physician must assess a patient who presents with acute spontaneous urticaria for possible anaphylaxis because this is a life-threatening emergency that requires prompt and specific treatment.
- Urticaria may present as a single acute episode for which no treatment or only a limited course of treatment is indicated.
- Medical treatment for acute urticaria is intended to provide relief from symptoms, predominantly pruritus.
- Non-sedating oral second generation H1 antihistamines are the first line treatment, while first generation H1 antihistamines may be added or substituted if second generation H1 antihistamines are not effective. H2 antihistamines may be helpful in combination with H1 agents for some patients.
- A short course of glucocorticoids is a last resort, but may be considered if symptoms are severe and if H1 and H2 antihistamines are not effective.
- Acute urticaria is by definition a temporary condition (≤6 weeks) with a benign course, so chronic therapy is not necessary.

Section 5: Special populations

Pregnancy

- Avoidance of all antihistamines is generally recommended during the first trimester, even though none has been proven to be teratogenic. There are no oral antihistamines with a Category A listing for pregnancy. Hydroxyzine is specifically contraindicated during the early stages of pregnancy. Chlorpheniramine, loratadine, cetirizine, and levocetirizine are listed by the US FDA as Category B medications. Chlorpheniramine or diphenhydramine (first generation H1 antihistamines) are most often recommended, followed by second generation agents, loratadine and cetirizine, for which there is some evidence of safety when used in pregnancy. However, antihistamines should only be given as needed, and at the lowest effective dose. Short courses of glucocorticoids can be given during pregnancy, but should be avoided during the first trimester, and should always be closely monitored. Glucocorticoids are given for other conditions during pregnancy. Areas of concern include congenital malformations, neonatal adrenal insufficiency, and low birth weight, although the risks are low for short courses of low-dosage glucocorticoids during pregnancy.

Children

- In children, the most common cause of acute urticaria is viral infection, and may be associated with only transient urticaria.
- Food allergy is also more prevalent in children, and should be considered in the evaluation of any child presenting with acute urticaria, as dietary restrictions may be essential to preventing recurrence and repeat exposure may trigger severe allergic reactions.
- Treatment of children with first generation H1 antihistamines can lead to cognitive impairment and sleep disturbances, and parents should be told to observe for these changes.

Elderly

- Elderly patients may be more susceptible to the anticholinergic and sedative effects of H1 antihistamines and should be monitored closely for these symptoms. Dosage adjustments may be necessary for these patients.

Others

- If acute urticaria progresses to chronic urticaria, further diagnostic evaluation and additional medical therapies may be indicated.
- For patients with treatable infectious causes of acute urticaria, treatment of the underlying infection should result in resolution of urticaria.
- Urticaria associated with systemic disorders is often persistent, chronic, and more difficult to treat.

Section 6: Prognosis

BOTTOM LINE/CLINICAL PEARLS
- The overall prognosis for acute urticaria, without associated underlying disease, is excellent. Most cases resolve spontaneously or within days.
- For those for whom an allergic cause of acute urticaria is identified, symptoms resolve with removal or avoidance of the trigger, and do not recur if there is no further exposure.
- Acute urticaria is by definition self-limited, resolves within 6 weeks, with no residual or permanent skin changes, and no adverse health sequelae.
- Acute urticaria may be a manifestation of an underlying condition, for which the prognosis depends on the specific diagnosis.

Natural history of untreated disease

- Regardless of treatment, some cases (20–30%) of acute urticaria will persist or recur for >6 weeks, and thus progress to chronic urticaria. This is more common for adults than for children.

Prognosis for treated patients

- As treatment of acute urticaria is meant only to control appearance of urticaria and relieve pruritus, and is a not a cure, the prognosis for treated patients does not differ from that of untreated patients.

Follow-up tests and monitoring

- Patients with acute urticaria should be followed to determine whether there is recurrence or persistence of urticaria. Clinical response and tolerance of medical therapy should be assessed, as the medication regimen may require adjustment. For those who have urticaria due to an infectious etiology, resolution of infection should be assessed. If an allergic or physical trigger is suspected, the patient should be referred to an allergy/immunology specialist for additional testing and management. Diagnostic and treatment considerations differ for patients who progress to develop chronic urticaria, and are not reviewed here.

Section 7: Reading list

Frigas E, Park MA. Acute urticaria and angioedema: diagnostic and treatment considerations. Am J Clin Dermatol 2009;10:239–50

Greaves M. Chronic urticaria. J Allergy Clin Immunol 2000;105:664–72

Kanani A, Schellenberg R, Warrington R. Urticaria and angioedema. Allergy Asthma Clin Immunol 2011;7(Suppl 1):S9.

Poonawalla T, Kelly B. Urticaria: a review. Am J Clin Dermatol 2009;10: 9–21

Saini S. Urticaria and angioedema. In: Adkinson F, Bochner B, Burks AW, et al. (eds). Middleton's Allergy: Principles and Practice, 8th edn, Vol 1. St. Louis, MO: Mosby, 2014, pp. 575–87

Sánchez-Borges M, Asero R, Ansotegui IJ, Baaiardini I, Bernstein JA, Canonica GW, et al. Diagnosis and treatment of urticaria and angioedema: worldwide perspective. World Allergy Organ J 2012; 5:125–47

Winters M. Initial evaluation and management of patients presenting with acute urticaria or angioedema. American Academy of Emergency Medicine (AAEM); 2006, Position Statement. Available at: http://www.aaem.org/em-resources/position-statements/2006/clinical-practice-guidelines (accessed October 17, 2014)

Zuberbier T, Balke M, Worm M, Edenharter G, Maurer M. Epidemiology of urticaria: a representative cross-sectional population survey. Clin Exp Dermatol 2010;35:869–73

Zuberbier T, Asero R, Bindslev-Jensen C, Walter Canonica G, Church MK, Giménez-Amau A, et al. EAACI/GA2LEN/EDF/WAO guideline: definition, classification and diagnosis of urticaria. Allergy 2009;64:1417–26

Suggested websites

www.aaaai.org

www.acaai.org

www.aad.org

www.uptodate.com/new-onset-urticaria (Note: uptodate membership to access required)

Section 8: Guidelines
National society guidelines

Guideline title	Guideline source	Date
Initial evaluation and management of patients presenting with acute urticaria or angioedema	American Academy of Emergency Medicine (AAEM)	2006 (http://www.aaem.org/em-resources/position-statements/2006/clinical-practice-guidelines)

International society guidelines

Guideline title	Guideline source	Date
Guidelines for definition, classification and diagnosis of urticaria	European Academy of Allergology and Clinical Immunology (EAACI), Global Allergy and Asthma European Network (GA2LEN), European Dermatology Forum (EDF), and the World Allergy Organization (WAO)	2009 (http://www.ncbi.nlm.nih.gov/pubmed/19772512)
Diagnosis and Treatment of Urticaria and Angioedema: a Worldwide Perspective	World Allergy Association (WAO)	2012 (http://www.waojournal.org/content/5/11/125)

Section 9: Evidence
Not applicable for this topic.

Section 10: Images

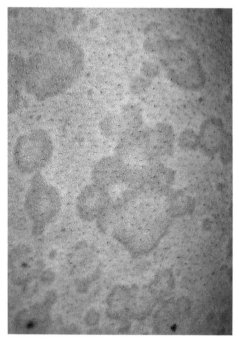

Figure 26.1 Superficial urticarial lesions often have central pallor and raised erythematous edematous borders, but can vary in size, shape, and color. See color plate 26.1. From Habif TP. Clinical Dermatology: A Color Guide to Diagnosis and Therapy. 5th edition. 2010 Philadelphia, PA, Mosby/Elsevier. Reproduced with permission.

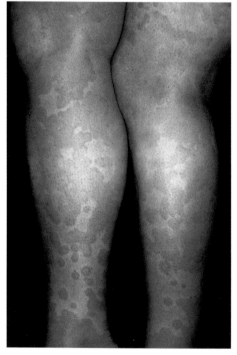

Figure 26.2 Confluent urticaria. See color plate 26.2. From Habif TP. Clinical Dermatology: A Color Guide to Diagnosis and Therapy. 5th edition. 2010 Philadelphia, PA, Mosby/Elsevier. Reproduced with permission.

Additional material for this chapter can be found online at:
www.mountsinaiexpertguides.com
This includes a case study, multiple choice questions, advice for
patients, and ICD codes

CHAPTER 27

Chronic Urticaria

Julie Wang

Department of Pediatrics, Division of Allergy/Immunology, Icahn School of Medicine at Mount Sinai, New York, NY, USA

OVERALL BOTTOM LINE

- Chronic urticaria (CU) is defined as recurrent, spontaneous hives persisting for at least 6 weeks.
- CU impacts people of any age, with peak incidence at 20–40 years of age.
- CU has a significant negative impact on quality of life.
- In many cases, no identifiable triggers are found.
- The main goal of management is symptom relief to improve quality of life.

Section 1: Background

Definition of disease

- Urticaria is characterized by erythematous, blanching, circumscribed, pruritic lesions that wax and wane, and individual lesions do not persist in any given location for more than 24 hours. Chronic urticaria (CU) is defined as persistent or recurring urticaria for at least 6 weeks in duration.

Disease classification

- Chronic urticaria may be caused by physical stimuli (physical urticaria), infections, autoreactive mechanisms, or may be idiopathic.

Incidence/prevalence

- Lifetime prevalence rate of CU is estimated to be 1.8%.
- More women develop CU than men.
- Peak age is 20–40 years in most studies.

Economic impact

- The mean estimated annual costs of chronic urticaria patients conventionally treated with antihistamines are >$2000 per patient per year.
- In addition to medical costs, indirect costs are also accrued as a result of absence from work and/or reduced productivity and efficiency at work.

Mount Sinai Expert Guides: Allergy and Clinical Immunology, First Edition. Edited by Hugh A. Sampson.
© 2015 John Wiley & Sons, Ltd. Published 2015 by John Wiley & Sons, Ltd.
Companion website: www.mountsinaiexpertguides.com

Etiology

- CU may be caused by physical triggers, infections, or autoreactive mechanisms; however, for many patients there is no identifiable trigger.
- Thyroid auto-antibodies are often found in patients with CU, but their clinical relevance is not clear.
- 30–50% of patients with CU produce IgG antibodies against the FcεR1α subunit of the high affinity IgE receptor.

Pathology/pathogenesis

- Urticarial lesions are characterized by pruritic, erythematous, blanching, circumscribed, raised lesions involving the epidermis and dermis. Biopsy typically shows non-necrotizing peri-vascular mononuclear cell infiltrates. Mast cells in the skin have a key role and histamine is the predominant mediator, but other cells and mediators are also involved. A predominantly lymphocytic infiltrate with a Th0 pattern can be found in urticarial lesions.
- Autoreactive mechanisms have been implicated because nearly one-quarter of patients with CU have thyroid autoantibodies, 30–50% have anti-IgE receptor antibodies, and 10% have anti-IgE antibodies. The pathogenesis of autoantibody associated urticaria is still unclear, but studies suggest that T cells, soluble CD40 ligand, and basophil histamine responsiveness are involved.

Predictive/risk factors

- There are no known risk factors.
- Female : male ratio ranges from 7 : 3 to 4 : 1.

Section 2: Prevention

No interventions have been demonstrated to prevent the development of this disease.

Screening

Not applicable for this topic.

Primary prevention

Not applicable for this topic.

Secondary prevention

Not applicable for this topic.

Section 3: Diagnosis (Algorithm 27.1)

> **BOTTOM LINE/CLINICAL PEARLS**
> - The diagnosis of CU is based on the episodic appearance of characteristic urticarial lesions for 6 weeks or longer.
> - Physical examination will typically reveal urticaria affecting any part of the body.
> - Extensive laboratory testing is not indicated for patients with CU who present with an otherwise unremarkable history and physical examination because no identifiable trigger is found in most cases; it is not cost-effective and it does not improve patient outcomes.

- Guidelines suggest initial limited testing with complete blood count with differential, C-reactive protein (CRP) or erythrocyte sedimentation rate (ESR) and thyroid stimulating hormone (TSH) level.
- Utility of testing for autoantibodies for IgE or the IgE receptor has not been established.

Algorithm 27.1 Diagnosis of chronic urticaria

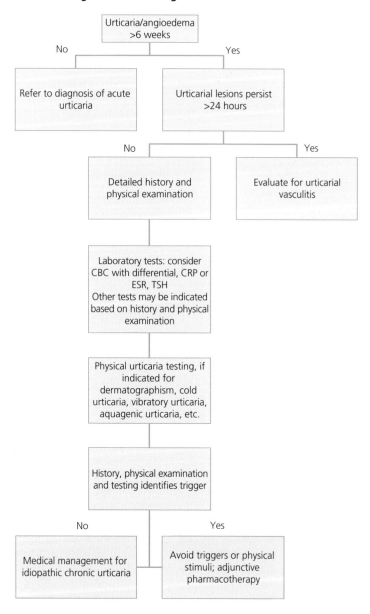

Differential diagnosis

Differential diagnosis	Features
Hereditary angioedema	Angioedema without urticaria, can have episodic abdominal pain. Unresponsive to antihistamines
Mast cell releasability syndromes (e.g. urticaria pigmentosa)	Pigmented papules with positive Darier's sign (urtication when lesions of urticarial pigmentosa are stroked). Biopsy reveals focal collection of mast cells
Erythema multiforme minor	Preceded by prodromal symptoms such as malaise, fever, sore throat, and arthralgia. Cutaneous symptoms are frequently target-like, non-pruritic, have a dusky center, and are fixed
Urticarial vasculitis	Individual lesions persist >24 hours, may be palpable and purpuric, are painful rather than pruritic, leave residual pigmentation, and may be accompanied by systemic symptoms (i.e. fever, chills, arthralgias). Diagnosis confirmed with skin biopsy
Hypereosinophilic syndrome	Urticaria can be seen; however, angioedema and erythroderma are more common
Systemic lupus erythematosus (SLE)	Urticaria is one of the dermatologic manifestations of SLE. Often, these patients have other systemic symptoms, such as fever, weight loss, arthritis, lymphadenopathy, renal disease, pulmonary disease, or cardiac disease
Cryoglobulinemia	Urticarial and vasculitis can be seen in hepatitis B or C infection. Lesions are primarily on the buttocks and lower back

Typical presentation
- Urticaria (hives) are circumscribed, raised, erythematous lesions, often with central pallor.
- Lesions are pruritic and can affect any area of the body. Individual lesions resolve within 24 hours.
- Exacerbating factors may include physical stimuli (e.g. cold, pressure, vibration), stress, anti-inflammatory medications, and alcohol.

Clinical diagnosis
History
- History is important for the diagnosis of CU. Patients should be asked about the onset of symptoms, frequency and duration of individual lesions, chronicity of symptoms (6 weeks or longer), potential physical triggers (e.g. cold, vibration, pressure), exacerbating factors (e.g. medications, stress, physical factors), signs and symptoms associated with the lesions (e.g. angioedema, systemic symptoms), and personal and family history of urticaria and atopy.
- History should exclude other types of urticaria (acute urticaria), as well as the possibility of systemic disease (e.g. SLE, thyroid disorder).
- Treatments used and response to treatment should also be recorded.

Physical examination
- Physical examination may reveal urticaria on any part of the body.

Useful clinical decision rules and calculators
Not applicable for this topic.

Disease severity classification
Not applicable for this topic.

Laboratory diagnosis
List of diagnostic tests
- The most common physical urticaria is dermatographism. Stroking the skin with a tongue blade will elicit wheal formation within 1–3 minutes.
- Methacholine intradermal challenge or partial immersion using hot water (42°C) is used for the diagnosis of cholinergic urticaria.
- Other challenge procedures for physical urticarias include ice cube test for cold-induced urticaria, applying vortex to forearm for vibratory urticaria, and water compress for aquagenic urticaria.
- If the clinical history is not suggestive of an underlying allergic etiology or systemic disease, then it is unlikely that routine laboratory tests would be informative.
- Guidelines suggest initial limited testing with complete blood count with differential, CRP or ESR and TSH levels.
- Complete blood count with differential may reveal eosinophilia, which suggests evaluation for atopic disorder or parasitic disease is indicated.
- Significantly elevated CRP or ESR should prompt investigations for systemic disease (i.e. autoimmunity, rheumatologic, infectious, or neoplastic disease).
- Abnormal TSH level would be suspicious for thyroid disease.
- Investigational tests include the autologous serum skin test and anti-FcεRIα antibodies, which are used to screen for autoimmunity.
- Expanded laboratory testing and/or skin biopsy may be considered if CU is not responsive to therapy.
- Skin testing and serum IgE testing to foods or other allergens are not recommended for the routine investigation of CU.

Lists of imaging techniques
No imaging studies are indicated for chronic urticaria.

Potential pitfalls/common errors made regarding diagnosis of disease
- IgE-mediated food allergies do not typically cause CU.
- *Helicobacter pylori* infection does not cause CU.
- If individual lesions persist beyond 24 hours, are painful, have associated petechiae or purpura, leave residual pigmentation, or are associated with elevated CRP/ESR and/or systemic symptoms, then skin biopsy is recommended to exclude urticarial vasculitis.

Section 4: Treatment (Algorithm 27.2)
Treatment rationale
- The goal of pharmacotherapy is to provide symptom relief to improve quality of life while minimizing side effects of therapy. Avoidance of triggers or physical stimuli for physical urticaria is advised. First line medical treatment of CU is with non-sedating second generation antihistamines (e.g. cetirizine, fexofenadine, loratadine). First generation antihistamines are not routinely used given their major side effects of sedation and anticholinergic effects. For patients who do not respond adequately to standard doses of H1 antihistamines, guidelines suggest increasing the dosage up to fourfold. Modest improvements may be seen for some with the addition of H2

Algorithm 27.2 Managment of chronic urticaria

Non-sedating H1 antihistamine
- Should be taken daily rather than as needed
- Doses can be increased up to fourfold
- e.g. cetirizine, fexofenadine, loratadine

Sedating H1 antihistamine
- Dosing is based on severity of urticaria and sedation effects
- e.g. diphenhydramine, hydroxyzine, doxepine

Omalizumab
- Indicated for those refractory to H1 antihistamines
- Dosing is not dependent on serum IgE or body weight

H2 antihistamine
- Can provide additional relief for some
- e.g. ranitidine or cimetidine

Leukotriene receptor antagonist
- Can be used as add-on therapy

Systemic corticosteroids
- Used for short-term relief of severe symptoms
- Should be tapered as rebound of symptoms can occur when corticosteroids discontinued

Anti-inflammatory or immunosuppressive agents
- Limited data regarding use of these agents for CU
- Reserved for cases where antihistamines are insufficiently effective

antihistamines. Those who experience exacerbations of CU with aspirin or NSAIDs may derive the benefit from leukotriene modifiers.

- Omalizumab has been shown to be effective in treating CU refractory to H1-antihistamine therapy. Significant improvements in itching and hives are observed after a 12-week treatment period, with effects seen as early as 1–2 weeks. It is now FDA approved for patients 12 years and older.
- Systemic glucocorticoids are generally reserved for short-term relief of severe symptoms or CU refractory to antihistamines. Prolonged use is not advised given the known adverse effects of systemic glucocorticoids and, in many cases, rebound symptoms are seen as glucocorticoids are tapered or discontinued.
- Although evidence of efficacy is limited for anti-inflammatory agents (i.e. dapsone, sulfasalazine, colchicine, hydroxychloroquine), these medications may be considered given their favorable cost and safety profile.
- For patients with CU unresponsive to antihistamines and anti-inflammatory agents or who are glucocorticoid dependent, immunosuppressive agents are used (i.e. cyclosporine, tacrolimus, sirolimus, mycophenolate).

When to hospitalize
- Chronic urticaria is managed in the outpatient setting.

Managing the hospitalized patient
Not applicable for this topic.

Table of treatment

Treatment	Comment
Medical • Non-sedating H1 antihistamines: cetirizine 10 mg/day), fexofenadine (180 mg/day), loratadine (10 mg/day) – doses can be increased up to fourfold • Sedating H1 antihistamines: diphenhydramine or hydroxyzine (200 mg/day divided into 3–4 doses) • Doxepine is particularly sedating, but can be considered because it has H1 and some H2 receptor activity (25–50 mg at bedtime) • Omalizumab: 150 or 300 mg subcutaneous injection every 4 weeks. Unlike for allergic asthma, dosing for CU is not dependent on serum IgE level or body weight • H2 antihistamines can provide additional relief for some: ranitidine (150 mg twice a day) or cimetidine (300–400 mg twice a day) • Leukotriene receptor antagonists can be used as add-on therapy: montelukast, zafirlukast • Systemic corticosteroids are used for short-term relief of severe symptoms • Anti-inflammatory agents: dapsone, sulfasalazine, colchine, hydroxychloroquine • Immunosuppressive agents: cyclosporine, tacrolimus, sirolimus, mycophenolate	• Medications should be taken daily rather than as needed • Dosing of sedating antihistamines is based on severity of urticaria and sedation effects • Systemic corticosteroids should be tapered as rebound of symptoms can occur when corticosteroids discontinued • Few data are available regarding the use of anti-inflammatory and immunosuppressive agents. These are reserved for cases where antihistamines are insufficiently effective

Prevention/management of complications
- Corticosteroids may be considered for short-term use to gain control of severe symptoms; however, rebound of urticaria may occur as corticosteroids are withdrawn.

CLINICAL PEARLS
- The goal of therapy is to improve quality of life while minimizing side effects of therapy.
- Non-sedating second generation antihistamines are first line therapy and can be increased in dosage up to fourfold.
- Omalizumab is indicated for those with symptoms refractory to H1 antihistamine therapy.
- Long-term use of systemic glucocorticoids should be avoided; short-term use for the management of severe symptoms may be considered, but rebound symptoms may occur when it is discontinued.
- Anti-inflammatory or immunosuppressive agents can be considered for refractory cases.

Section 5: Special populations
Pregnancy
- Pruritic urticarial plaques and papules of pregnancy can occur in the third trimester and can cause severe pruritus. Symptoms commonly resolve within 2 weeks of delivery, but may also resolve beforehand. Management entails antihistamines and topical steroids to relieve symptoms. In severe cases, systemic corticosteroids may be needed.
- Gestational pemphigoid is the abrupt onset of pruritic urticaria that starts on the trunk and then becomes generalized.
- Prurigo of pregnancy is characterized by pruritic papules and nodules that primarily affect the extensor surfaces. Lesions start in the latter half of the pregnancy and can last for weeks to months after delivery.

Section 6: Prognosis

BOTTOM LINE/CLINICAL PEARLS
- CU is a self-limited disorder for most, with the average duration being 2–5 years.
- 30–50% of patients have spontaneous resolution within 1 year and another 20% resolve within 5 years.
- More severe disease tends to be associated with a longer duration.
- In those with moderate to severe symptoms, up to 30% have symptoms that persist >5 years.

Natural history of untreated disease
- Natural history of CU is not altered by treatment.
- Patients with evidence of autoimmunity are more likely to have severe disease that responds poorly to H1 antihistamines.

Prognosis for treated patients
Not applicable for this topic.

Follow-up tests and monitoring
Not applicable for this topic.

Section 7: Reading list

Bernstein JA, Lang DM, Khan DA, Craig T, Dreyfus D, Hsieh F, et al. The diagnosis and management of acute and chronic urticaria: 2014 update. J Allergy Clin Immunol 2014;133:1270–7

Joint Task Force on Practice Parameters. The diagnosis and management of urticaria: a practice parameter Part I: acute urticaria/angioedema Part II: chronic urticaria/angioedema. Ann Allergy Asthma Immunol 2000; 85:521–44

Maurer M, Weller K, Bindslev-Jensen C, Giménez-Arnau A, Bousquet PJ, Bousquet J, et al. Unmet clinical needs in chronic spontaneous urticaria. A GA²LEN task force report. Allergy 2011; 66:317–30

Sánchez-Borges M, Asero R, Ansotegui IJ, Baiardini I, Bernstein JA, Canonica GW, et al. Diagnosis and treatment of urticaria and angioedema: a worldwide perspective. World Allergy Organ J 2012;5:125–47

Suggested websites

American Academy of Allergy, Asthma and Immunology (AAAAI). www.aaaai.org

American College of Allergy, Asthma and Immunology (ACAAI). www.acaai.org

Section 8: Guidelines
National society guidelines

Guideline title	Guideline source	Date
The diagnosis and management of urticaria: a practice parameter Part I: acute urticaria/angioedema Part II: chronic urticaria/angioedema	Joint Task Force on Practice Parameters	2000 (http://www.allergyparameters. org/published-practice-parameters/ alphabetical-listing/urticaria-download/)

International society guidelines

Guideline title	Guideline source	Date
Diagnosis and treatment of urticaria and angioedema: a worldwide perspective	World Allergy Organization (WAO)	2012 (http://www.waojournal.org/ content/5/11/125)

Section 9: Evidence

Type of evidence	Title, comment	Date
Cochrane Review	Histamine H2-receptor antagonists for urticaria	2012 (http://www.ncbi.nlm.nih.gov/ pubmed/22419335)
Phase 3, multicenter, randomized, double-blind study	Omalizumab for the treatment of chronic idiopathic or spontaneous urticaria **Comment:** Omalizumab significantly reduced itch-severity scores in patients unresponsive to antihistamine therapy	2013 (http://www.nejm.org/doi/ full/10.1056/NEJMoa1215372)

Section 10: Images

Not applicable for this topic.

Additional material for this chapter can be found online at:
www.mountsinaiexpertguides.com
This includes a case study, multiple choice questions, advice for
patients, and ICD codes

CHAPTER 28

Hereditary Angioedema

Paula J. Busse

Department of Medicine, Division of Clinical Immunology, Icahn School of Medicine at Mount Sinai, New York, NY, USA

OVERALL BOTTOM LINE

- Hereditary angioedema (HAE) is a rare and potentially life-threatening disease characterized by recurrent episodes of angioedema (without urticaria – hives) typically involving the extremities (e.g. hands, feet), abdomen, face, larynx, and genitourinary track.
- HAE is secondary to mutations in the C1-inhibitor gene (C1-INH) which results in excess generation of bradykinin, subsequent vascular leak, and swelling.
- Approximately 75% of patients with HAE have an inherited form (transmitted in an autosomal dominant fashion) and 25% of patients have a spontaneous mutation in the C1-INH gene.
- Although some triggers of HAE may be identified (estrogens, ACE-I, trauma, surgery, stress, infection), many episodes of angioedema in HAE occur unpredictably.
- Treatment of angioedema due to HAE with antihistamines and corticosteroids is not effective. Treatment of HAE is directed at replacement of C1-INH and inhibition of the bradykinin pathway.
- All patients with HAE must have easy access to an on-demand medication to treat an acute attack.

Section 1: Background
Definition of disease

- Hereditary angioedema is a disease characterized by recurrent non-pruritic and non-pitting swelling of subcutaneous or submucosal tissues (without hives) typically affecting the face, extremities, abdomen, genitals, and larynx due to dysfunction of the C1-inhibitor protein. Episodes of angioedema do not respond to antihistamine and corticosteroid treatment and, without appropriate medication, may lead to asphyxiation if swelling occurs in the larynx. The underlying mechanism of HAE is unregulated C1-INH function leading to excess bradykinin generation.

Disease classification

- HAE is classified as either type I or II, although the clinical presentations and treatment do not differ significantly. HAE type I is seen in approximately 85% of patients and is a result of under-production of *functional* C1 INH. HAE type II is seen in approximately 15% of patients and is

---

Mount Sinai Expert Guides: Allergy and Clinical Immunology, First Edition. Edited by Hugh A. Sampson.
© 2015 John Wiley & Sons, Ltd. Published 2015 by John Wiley & Sons, Ltd.
Companion website: www.mountsinaiexpertguides.com

due to the expression of *dysfunctional* C1 INH. The severity of HAE is variable, both between patients and with a patient over time, and there are no standardized definitions to classify disease severity.

Incidence/prevalence
- HAE is estimated to occur in 1 in 30 000–80 000 individuals (approximately 4000–10 000 people in the United States).
- There are no known ethnic or gender differences.
- Patients' first symptoms of HAE typically present before the age of 10 years; however, the time between symptom onset and diagnosis of HAE may be closer to 9 years.

Economic impact
- Total average annual per-patient cost is estimated at $42 000.
- The total average annual per-patient cost in patients with severe disease is > $100 000.

Etiology
- HAE is an inherited autosomal dominant disease in 75% of patients; a spontaneous mutation in the C1 INH gene accounts for the remaining 25% of patients.
- >280 mutations in the C1-INH have been identified.

Pathology/pathogenesis
- C1-INH is a serine protease inhibitor that has key regulatory functions in the activation of the complement system (inhibiting C1r and C1s proteases) and contact system (activated factor XII (factor XIIa) and kallikrein), and to a lesser extent regulation of factor XI in the coagulation system, and the fibrinolytic pathway.
- Factor XIIa activates additional factor XII, cleaving prekallikrein to kallikrein, which then cleaves high molecular weight kininogen, generating the vasoactive peptide bradykinin.
- Bradykinin binds to the BK2 receptor inducing vascular permeability, vasodilatation, and contraction of non-vascular smooth muscle, resulting in the pain and swelling associated with an HAE attack.

Predictive/risk factors
Not applicable for this topic.

Section 2: Prevention

BOTTOM LINE
- No interventions have been demonstrated to prevent the development of the disease in genetically predisposed individuals; however, education about HAE and its possible triggers must be discussed with the patient and his/her family and/or caregivers.
- There is no evidence to suggest that early treatment of HAE alters the natural history of disease.
- Patients with HAE (whether symptomatic or asymptomatic) should avoid the use of estrogens and angiotensin-converting enzyme inhibitors (ACE-I) as these can exacerbate angioedema.
- Patients undergoing invasive dental work or surgery should receive short-term prophylaxis prior to the procedure to reduce the risk of an episode of angioedema.

Screening

- A serum C4 level is an initial screening test for HAE, and if low, measurement of C1-INH protein and function should be obtained (if clinically indicated).
- Offspring of patients with HAE (whether inherited or due a spontaneous mutation in C1-INH) have a 50% chance of inheriting HAE. Screening of HAE in first degree relatives should be offered.
- Cord blood is not reliable to measure complement levels to screen newborn infants; by age 1 year of life, screening can be performed reliably.
- Genetic studies may be performed on amniotic fluid or chronic villus samples to screen for HAE, but is not standard of care.

Primary prevention

Not applicable for this topic.

Secondary prevention

- A critical factor for management of patients with HAE is education about potential triggers and coordination of care with their other health care providers. The following are potential triggers of HAE attacks:
  - Estrogen containing medications. Patients may safely receive progesterone for oral birth control;
  - ACE-I;
  - Surgery, invasive dental work (general cleaning is generally not a trigger), and oral surgery can trigger an attack of angioedema. If patients have a planned procedure, they should receive short-term prophylaxis (see Section 4). They must also have access to a rescue medication at the time and for several days after procedure as attacks typically develop 24 hours after procedures;
  - Trauma may trigger attacks and, for some patients, administration of C1-INH after trauma is advisable to prevent a possible attack.

Section 3: Diagnosis

> **BOTTOM LINE/CLINICAL PEARLS**
> - A history of one or more of the following may suggest HAE:
>   - Recurrent swelling (without urticaria) of the extremities (hands, feet), abdomen, face, oropharynx, genitourinary;
>   - Angioedema not improving with antihistamines and corticosteroids;
>   - Unexplained recurrent abdominal pain;
>   - A history of laryngeal edema.
> - The diagnosis of HAE I or II is confirmed with at least two sets of complement testing with similar results, ideally carried out without recent use of HAE medications and separated by 1 month.
> - Results of laboratory testing for complement studies takes >24 hours; an immediate diagnosis of HAE with initial presentation may be difficult.

Differential diagnosis

Differential diagnosis	Features
Allergic angioedema	Often presents with hives and itching Swelling onset more rapid than HAE Responds to antihistamines and corticosteroids, epinephrine Frequently a clear trigger such as food, drug, insect bite
ACE-I induced angioedema	Angioedema usually involves the face and airway only History of ACE-I use
Autoimmune diseases (systemic lupus erythematosus, scleroderma)	Swelling is usually persistent
Superior vena cava syndrome	Edema of neck, face that does not resolve
Acquired C1-INH deficiency	Due to consumption of C1-INH; typically associated with underlying malignancy or autoimmune disease. Patients should have screen for malignancy and MGUS (monoclonal gammopathy of unknown significance) Presents later in life No family history of HAE Decreased C1q
Edema secondary to hydrostatic changes from cardiac or liver failure, or protein losing enteropathy	Pitting edema Usually symmetric distribution in dependent areas of the body
HAE with normal C1-INH deficiency	Family history with a first relative with symptoms Usually in women only with estrogen exacerbation Angioedema typically in face or upper airway
Hypothyroidism	Skin changes that develop and resolve slowly, mimicking angioedema
Idiopathic angioedema	Diagnosis of exclusion May be histamine or bradykinin mediated

Typical presentation

- HAE frequently presents with recurrent and unexplained episodes of angioedema (without hives) that occur in the extremities, abdomen (mimicking a "surgical abdomen"), face (can be disfiguring), larynx (risk of death), or genitals.
- An attack usually involves one site of the body, although it can migrate; abdominal and peripheral attacks are the most common sites.
- The frequency and location of attacks is variable in patients and in family members with the same mutation of C1-INH. Onset of swelling is prolonged (over 24 hours) and, if untreated, resolves in 2–5 days.

Clinical diagnosis

History

- Angioedema often severe and unpredictable.
- Recurrent abdominal pain.
- Attacks without urticaria; some patients may have a "prodromal" rash described as serpentine, resembling erythema marginatum, prior to an attack.

- Family history present approximately 75% of the time.
- Angioedema frequently worse at puberty, menses, estrogen-containing medications, and ACE-I.

Physical examination
- Normal physical examination during asymptomatic periods.
- During an attack, angioedema is non-pitting and in non-dependent areas of the body.
- No hives.
- Careful examination to check for airway patency if the patient is having an airway attack.
- Abdomen may be distended (lack of this finding *does not* exclude the presence of an abdominal attack).

Laboratory diagnosis
- A diagnostic algorithm is presented in Algorithm 28.1. Results of complement studies may be inaccurate if not performed by a certified laboratory and if not carried out on fresh serum, or serum frozen shortly after collection:
  - *C4:* a low C4 suggests HAE and is the initial screening test. C4 is also low during asymptomatic periods;
  - *C1-INH function:* low in both HAE I and II. Requires special handling of serum. Two assays can be used: ELISA (commercially available) and chromogenic (higher sensitivity and lower variability, available at National Jewish Laboratories);
  - *C1-INH protein:* low in HAE I;
  - *C1q:* low in acquired C1-INH deficiency.

Lists of imaging techniques
- CT: rarely used unless documenting the extent of angioedema or evaluating other causes of abdominal pain in a patient with known HAE is required.

Potential pitfalls/common errors made regarding diagnosis of disease
- HAE may be confused with allergic or histamine-mediated angioedema. Hives, onset of symptoms within less than 60 minutes, and/or pruritus suggest allergic or histamine-mediated angioedema.
- HAE is frequently not in a symmetric distribution or in dependent areas of the body (to distinguish from edema secondary to hydrostatic etiologies including heart failure, protein loss).
- Family history of angioedema is not always present; 25% of patients have a new onset mutation in C1-INH.

Interpretation of complement testing (Table 28.1)

Type	C1-INH Level	C1-INH Function	C4 Level	C1q Level
HAE type I	<30%	<30%	Low	Normal
HAE type II	Normal	<30%	Low	Normal
HAE with normal C1-INH	Normal	Normal	Normal	Normal
Acquired C1-INH I/II	Low	Low	<30%	Low
ACE inhibitor	Normal	Normal	Normal	Normal
Idiopathic angioedema	Normal	Normal	Normal	Normal

Algorithm 28.1 Diagnosis of hereditary angioedema

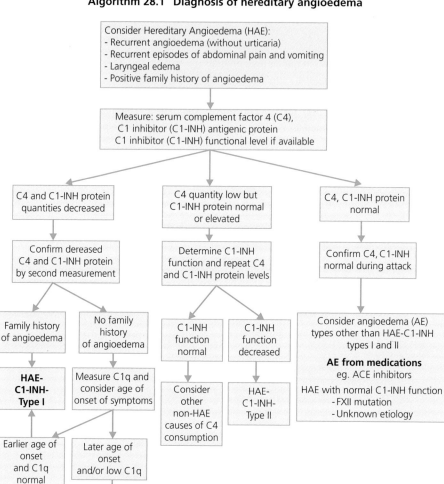

Source: Modified from Bowen. Allergy Asthma Clin Immunol 2010;6:24.

Section 4: Treatment
Treatment rationale

- Treatment of HAE is generally classified as:
  - *Treatment of acute attacks:* needed by *all* patients regardless of severity and attack frequency;
  - *Prophylactic therapy:* not needed by all patients, depends upon frequency of attacks, severity, and patient preference; and
  - *Short-term prophylaxis:* to prevent attacks prior to procedures.
- Some patients treat each attack as they occur, which is called "on-demand" therapy.
- The medication options for acute therapy include plasma-derived (pd) C1-INH replacement (given intravenously; many patients self-infuse or have a family member infuse via a butterfly

needle), a bradykinin receptor antagonist (icatibant, subcutaneous), or a kallikrein inhibitor (ecallantide, subcutaneous).
- Options for prophylactic therapy include C1-INH administered every 3–4 days, anabolic androgens, or antifibrinolytics.
- Options for short-term prophylaxis include C1-INH (administered 1–6 hours prior to procedure), fresh frozen plasma (2 units, 1–2 hours prior), or high dose androgens (started 5 days before and continued 5 days after).
- Many patients will be initially treated with on-demand therapy. However, based upon attack frequency, severity, and patient preference, they may be changed to prophylactic therapy. Patients may be treated prophylactically for periods of time and later changed to on-demand therapy depending upon their symptoms.

When to hospitalize
- The goal of HAE treatment is to prevent hospitalizations and decrease morbidity and mortality.
- If patients are treated in the emergency room for an acute attack, they can be discharged if stable after a few hours. They do not need to be kept overnight for observation if they respond to administration of 1–2 doses of acute therapy within approximately 2 hours.
- Intubation for airway attacks.
- Hemodynamically unstable (some patients will develop hypovolemia due to fluid shifts).
- Lack of response to two doses of acute therapy.
- Severe abdominal attacks with protracted vomiting and complications such as pancreatitis and ascites.

Table of treatment
Acute attacks

Treatment	Comment
Conservative Fluid replacement	Hemodynamic instability
Medical pdC1-INH (20 U/kg IV) Ecallantide (30 mg SC) Icatibant (30 mg SC) Fresh frozen plasma (2 units) Analgesics	Can be self-administered Must be administered by a health care professional; approx. 3% risk of anaphylaxis Medication can be kept at room temperature; pre-loaded into syringe Use with caution; may exacerbate ongoing attack
Surgical Preparation for intubation or tracheostomy	Airway attacks

Prophylactic treatment

Treatment	Comment
Medical pd C1-INH (1000 units IV every 3–4 days) Anabolic androgens • Danazol (50–600 mg/day) • Stanozolol (1–6 mg/day) Antifibrinolytics • Aminocaproic acide (1 g po TID) • Tranexamic acid (0.25 g BID–1.5 g TID)	Can be self-administered Not effective in an acute attack; contraindications (see Prevention/management of complications section), side effects (see Prevention/management of complications section), therapeutic goal is lowest possible dose May be less effective than pd C1-INH or androgens; aminocaproic acid may be particularly useful for acquired C1-INH deficiency

Short-term prophylaxis

Treatment	Comment
Medical C1-INH (20 U/kg IV) Fresh frozen plasma (2 units) High dose androgens	Administer 1–6 hours prior to procedure Administer 1–2 hours prior to procedure Start 5 days prior and continue 5 days post procedure
Other Coordination of care with other providers about HAE care	Discuss with provider of procedure management of an acute attack and have plan in place

Prevention/management of complications
- *Androgens:* contraindicated in pregnancy, lactating women, liver disease, children (before Tanner stage V), cancer, nephrotic syndrome. Follow LFTs, lipid panel every 6 months, and abdominal ultrasound every 12 months. Side effects include virilization, weight gain, mood changes, headache, generalized ache, and hepatocellular adenoma.
- *Plasma derived C1-INH:* low risk potential for blood-borne pathogens, care of IV access, concern for use of ports (infection, clotting), possible administration of hepatitis B vaccination prior to starting pd C1-INH.
- *Fresh frozen plasma:* small risk of blood-borne pathogens.
- *Antifibrinolytics:* may cause nausea, vertigo, muscle cramps, fatigue.
- *Ecallantide:* small risk of allergic reaction – should be administered by a health care provider with epinephrine on hand.
- *Icatibant:* burning or pain at injection site.

CLINICAL PEARLS
- All patients require easy access to on-demand therapy for acute attacks, some of which can be self-administered.
- Patients must be educated that, regardless of past HAE history or family HAE history, they may experience a life-threatening airway attack, highlighting the importance of on-demand treatment for all patients.
- HAE does not respond clinically to treatment with antihistamines or corticosteroids. Epinephrine may cause a transient benefit in airway symptoms, but should not be considered standard of care.

Section 5: Special populations
Pregnancy
- One-third of patients have worsening of HAE during pregnancy, one-third have improvement of symptoms, and one-third are without change.
- Androgens are contraindicated.
- Cesarean section may trigger an attack. Administer C1-INH prior to C-section delivery. If C-section is emergent, administer C1-INH after delivery as attacks may develop 24 hours after the procedure.

Children
- Androgens are contraindicated.
- C1-INH can be safely given to children.

- Puberty often worsens disease.
- Education of school and caregivers on administration of rescue medication.

Section 6: Prognosis

> **BOTTOM LINE/CLINICAL PEARLS**
> - Most patients are healthy, although slightly increased rates of autoimmune diseases.
> - 50% of subjects may have an airway attack; without treatment there is a 30% chance of mortality.
> - Prognosis is variable and the frequency and severity of attacks can change through life.
> - At present, there is no cure for HAE and it is a lifetime disease.

Natural history of untreated disease
- Without appropriate treatment, mortality from laryngeal edema is approximtely 30%.
- HAE may produce a substantial effect on quality of life.

Prognosis for treated patients
- Education for patients about HAE and easy access to on-demand treatments (including self-administration of medication) for acute attacks significantly improves quality of life.
- Goals of HAE treatment include decreasing morbidity and mortality and improving quality of life.

Follow-up tests and monitoring
- For patients prescribed androgens, LFTs and lipid panel every 6 months, and yearly abdominal ultrasound scanning.
- Once the diagnosis of HAE has been established, it is not necessary to repeat complement testing; these levels do not generally reflect disease activity or control by medications. Treatment based upon clinical symptoms and response to medications.
- Ongoing education about disease triggers.
- Review of self-administration techniques.
- Follow-up of frequency of on-demand therapy; frequent use may suggest a patient to be treated with prophylactic therapy.

Section 7: Reading list

Bowen T. Hereditary angioedema consensus 2010. Allergy Asthma Clin Immunol 2010;6:13

Bowen T, Brosz J, Brosz K, Hebert J, Ritchie B. Management of hereditary angioedema: 2010 Canadian approach. Allergy Asthma Clin Immunol 2010;6:20

Caballero T, Farkas H, Bouillet L, Bowen T, Gompel A, Fagerberg C, et al. International consensus and practical guidelines on the gynecologic and obstetric management of female patients with hereditary angioedema caused by C1 inhibitor deficiency. J Allergy Clin Immunol 2012;129:308–20

Cicardi M, Bork K, Caballero T, Craig T, Li HH, Longhurst H, et al. Evidence-based recommendations for the therapeutic management of angioedema owing to hereditary C1 inhibitor deficiency: consensus report of an International Working Group. Allergy 2012;67:147–57

Craig T, Aygoren-Pursun E, Bork K, Bowen T, Boysen H, Farkas H, et al. WAO Guideline for the Management of Hereditary Angioedema. World Allergy Organ J 2012;5:182–99

Lang DM, Aberer W, Bernstein JA, Chng HH, Grumach AS, Hide M, et al. International consensus on hereditary and acquired angioedema. Ann Allergy Asthma Immunol 2012;109:395–402

Wahn V, Aberer W, Eberl W, Fasshauer M, Kuhne T, Kurnik K, et al. Hereditary angioedema (HAE) in children and adolescents: a consensus on therapeutic strategies. Eur J Pediatr 2012;171:1339–48

Zuraw BL. Clinical practice: hereditary angioedema. N Engl J Med 2008;359:1027–36

Zuraw BL, Banerji A, Bernstein JA, Busse PJ, Christiansen SC, Davis-Lorton M, et al. Hereditary Angioedema Association Medical Advisory Board 2013 recommendations for the management of hereditary angioedema due to C1 inhibitor deficiency. J Allergy Clin Immunol Pract 2013;5:458–67

Suggested websites

Hereditary Angioedema Association. www.haea.org

Section 8: Guidelines

Guideline title	Guideline source	Date
Consensus Report of Hereditary Angioedema Working Group	Allergy	2012 (http://www.ncbi.nlm.nih.gov/pubmed/22126399)
WAO Guideline for Management of HAE	World Allergy Organization	2012 (http://www.waojournal.org/content/pdf/1939-4551-5-12-182.pdf)
International Consensus Algorithm on HAE	Allergy, Asthma and Clinical Immunology	2010 (http://www.aacijournal.com/content/6/1/24)
Recommendations for the management of hereditary angioedema due to C1 inhibitor deficiency	Journal of Allergy and Clinical Immunology	2013 (http://www.jaci-inpractice.org/article/S2213-2198(13)00296-1/pdf)

Section 9: Evidence

See guidelines in Section 8.

Section 10: Images

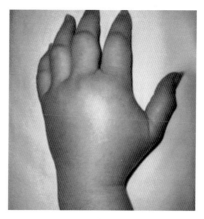

Figure 28.1 Extremity attack. Source: Bowen T. Hereditary angioedema consensus 2010. Allergy Asthma Clin Immunol 2010;6:13. Creative Commons Attribution License CC BY 4.0. See color plate 28.1.

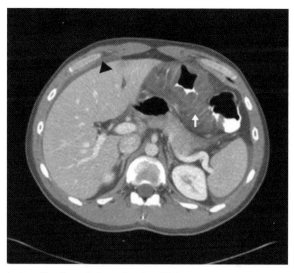

Figure 28.2 Abdominal swelling (arrow). See color plate 28.2.

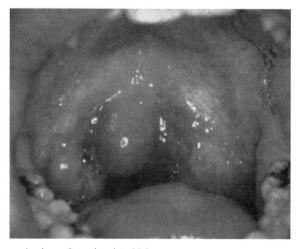

Figure 28.3 Airway angioedema. See color plate 28.3.

Additional material for this chapter can be found online at:
www.mountsinaiexpertguides.com
This includes a case study, multiple choice questions, advice for patients, and ICD codes

CHAPTER 29

Anaphylaxis

Jacob D. Kattan

Division of Allergy/Immunology, Department of Pediatrics, Icahn School of Medicine at Mount Sinai, New York, NY, USA

OVERALL BOTTOM LINE
- Anaphylaxis is an acute, life-threatening, systemic allergic reaction that typically occurs suddenly after contact with an allergy-causing substance, and has varied causes, mechanisms, clinical presentations, and severity.
- The history and physical examination are the most important tools in making the diagnosis of anaphylaxis, as well as the cause of the episode.
- In the outpatient setting, food is the most common cause of anaphylaxis.
- Epinephrine is the initial drug of choice in the treatment of anaphylaxis and should be administered as soon as the diagnosis is suspected.
- Patient education is an important preventative strategy and should be individualized. Allergen avoidance measures may not always be successful, and education should include instruction in self-management of anaphylaxis.

Section 1: Background
Definition of disease
- Anaphylaxis has been defined as a serious allergic reaction that typically occurs suddenly after contact with an allergy-causing substance, is rapid in onset, and may cause death.
- A meeting of experts in the field of allergy and immunology developed a definition of anaphylaxis in 2006, describing it as one of three clinical scenarios:
  - The acute onset of a reaction (minutes to hours) with involvement of the skin, mucosal tissue, or both, and at least one of the following: (i) respiratory compromise; (ii) reduced blood pressure or symptoms of end-organ dysfunction;
  - Two or more of the following that occur rapidly after exposure to a likely allergen for that patient: involvement of the skin/mucosal tissue, respiratory compromise, reduced blood pressure or associated symptoms, and/or persistent gastrointestinal symptoms; or
  - Reduced blood pressure after exposure to a known allergen.

Disease classification
Not applicable for this topic.

Mount Sinai Expert Guides: Allergy and Clinical Immunology, First Edition. Edited by Hugh A. Sampson.
© 2015 John Wiley & Sons, Ltd. Published 2015 by John Wiley & Sons, Ltd.
Companion website: www.mountsinaiexpertguides.com

Incidence/prevalence

- The lifetime prevalence of anaphylaxis in the general US population is at least 1.6% and probably higher.
- Numerous studies have reported that the prevalence of anaphylaxis appears to be increasing worldwide.

Economic impact

- While data for costs of anaphylaxis alone are lacking, food allergy and anaphylaxis in the United States was estimated to cost $225 million in direct medical costs, and $115 million in indirect costs in 2007; 43.5% of this cost was due to emergency department visits (20%), inpatient hospitalizations (11.8%), ambulance runs (3%), and epinephrine devices (8.7%).

Etiology

- The etiology of anaphylaxis is often due to allergic reactions to food, drugs, biologics, insect sting, radiocontrast media, and so on.

Pathology/pathogenesis

- Anaphylaxis can be classified as immunologic or non-immunologic.
- In immunologic IgE-mediated anaphylaxis, the activation of mast cells, eosinophils, and basophils results in the release of preformed inflammatory mediators, including histamine, tryptase, heparin, platelet activating factor, histamine releasing factor, and chymase. Cellular activation also stimulates the production of lipid-derived mediators such as prostaglandins and cysteinyl leukotrienes.
- In non-immunologic anaphylaxis, agents or events induce sudden, massive mast cell or basophil degranulation in the absence of immunoglobulins.

Predictive/risk factors

Risk factors for the development of anaphylaxis are unknown.

Section 2: Prevention

> **BOTTOM LINE/CLINICAL PEARLS**
> - No interventions have been demonstrated to prevent the development of the disease.
> - Avoidance of known allergens is the mainstay of prevention of anaphylaxis, but even when the allergen is known, avoidance measures are not always successful.
> - Education may be the most important preventive strategy.

Screening

Not applicable for this topic.

Primary prevention

Not applicable for this topic.

Secondary prevention

- Avoidance of known allergens is the mainstay of anaphylaxis prevention.
- Desensitization to a medication that is known to have caused anaphylaxis can temporarily prevent reoccurrence, if the medication is required in the future.

- Venom immunotherapy is successful in preventing anaphylaxis in up to 98% of patients who have previously experienced venom-induced anaphylaxis.
- Pharmacologic prophylaxis with glucocorticoids and H1 antihistamines can prevent recurrent anaphylactic reactions in idiopathic anaphylaxis.

Section 3: Diagnosis

> **BOTTOM LINE/CLINICAL PEARLS**
> - The history is the most important tool in determining whether or not a patient has had anaphylaxis and the cause of the episode.
> - The most common symptoms seen in anaphylaxis include urticaria and angioedema, flushing, dyspnea, wheezing, rhinitis, dizziness, syncope, hypotension, nausea, vomiting, and diarrhea.
> - Anaphylaxis may be confirmed by measurement of elevated concentrations of plasma and urinary histamine or serum tryptase levels, although elevations in these mediators are transient and samples for measuring histamine require special handling. The serum tryptase is seldom elevated in food-induced anaphylaxis.
> - In addition to the history, skin testing, serum testing for allergen-specific IgE, and challenge tests may help to identify the cause of anaphylaxis.

Differential diagnosis

Differential diagnosis	Features
Generalized urticaria	Limited to the skin Circumscribed, raised erythematous plaques that are intensely itchy Lesions are transient
Angioedema	Localized swelling of the skin or mucosal tissues Patients with non-allergic hereditary or acquired angioedema typically have intermittent swelling episodes that are unilateral and not associated with itching or urticaria C4 is low and C1 esterase inhibitor is deficient or functionally absent in most patients with hereditary angioedema
Acute asthma exacerbation	Intermittent dyspnea, cough, and wheezing Symptoms often occur in a pattern with exposure to triggers such as exercise or viral infection Symptoms other than wheeze, cough, or shortness of breath, such as urticaria, angioedema, vomiting or diarrhea, are more likely to occur with anaphylaxis
Vasovagal syncope	Syncope is typically preceded by stress or standing Usually relieved by recumbency Patient may have a history of syncope Associated with pallor while anaphylaxis is more likely to be associated with flushing Heart rate is typically bradycardic
Panic disorder	Episodes of intense fear that begin suddenly and last several minutes to an hour Symptoms include chest pain or shortness of breath Can occur in other anxiety disorders

(Continued)

Differential diagnosis	Features
Vocal cord dysfunction	Stridor that may be inspiratory, expiratory, or both, accompanied by respiratory distress Albuterol typically has little or no beneficial effect In a symptomatic patient, direct observation of the adducted vocal cords by laryngoscopy is diagnostic Patients will lack uvular edema often associated with anaphylaxis
Myocardial infarction	Chest pain may be associated with radiation to shoulders/arms and may be preceded by exertion Similar to anaphylaxis, tryptase level may be elevated May see findings on electrocardiogram such as pathologic Q waves, ST elevation, new left bundle branch block, or T wave inversions Troponin or the MB isoenzyme of creatinine kinase (CK-MB) are elevated in an acute myocardial infarction

Typical presentation

- Patients typically present with symptoms within minutes to 4–6 hours after exposure to a food, drug, insect bite or sting, or other allergen, although signs and symptoms often develop within minutes of exposure to the offending agent. A total of 85–90% of patients with anaphylaxis will have urticaria or angioedema, so a lack of cutaneous symptoms may put the diagnosis in doubt. Other common symptoms include flushing, dyspnea, wheezing, upper airway angioedema, rhinitis, dizziness, syncope, nausea, vomiting, diarrhea, or crampy abdominal pain.

Clinical diagnosis

History

- In making a clinical diagnosis of anaphylaxis, one should ask about manifestations that the patient may be aware of, such as urticaria, angioedema, flushing, pruritus, difficulty breathing, gastrointestinal symptoms, syncope, or dizziness. It is important to obtain a detailed history of all medications and foods consumed within 6 hours of the episode, as well as any stings or bites that occurred. The activities that the patient was participating in, such as exercise, should be reviewed. One should also obtain a detailed history of any known allergies or past allergic reactions, other allergic disorders such as atopic dermatitis, asthma, or allergic rhinitis, as well as a family history of any known allergic disorders.

Physical examination

- On physical examination, attention should initially be paid to airway, breathing, and circulation, along with the patient's level of consciousness.
- Patients with anaphylaxis may have physical examination findings related to upper and lower airway impairment including stridor, cough, or wheezing, cardiovascular dysfunction, including hypotension or cardiac arrhythmias, and skin involvement, including erythema, urticaria, or angioedema.
- While not every patient will have cutaneous symptoms, 85–90% of patients with anaphylaxis will have urticaria or angioedema, so a lack of these symptoms may put the diagnosis in doubt.

Useful clinical decision rules and calculators

See Algorithm 29.1.

Algorithm 29.1 Diagnosis of anaphylaxis

Do the history and physical examination fit one of the following criteria for anaphylaxis?

Criteria 1: Acute onset of an illness with involvement of the skin and/or mucosal tissue (generalized hives, pruritus, swollen tongue or lips) and at least one of the following:
(a) Respiratory compromise (dyspnea, wheeze/bronchospasm, stridor, hypoxemia)
(b) Reduced blood pressure or associated symptoms of end organ dysfunction (hypotonia, collapse, syncope, incontinence)

Criteria 2: Two or more of the following that occur rapidly after exposure to a likely allergen for that patient (within minutes to several hours):
(a) Involvement of the skin/mucosal tissue (generalized hives, itch/flush, swollen lips/tongue/uvula)
(b) Respiratory compromise (dyspnea, wheeze/bronchospasm, stridor, hypoxemia)
(c) Reduced blood pressure or associated symptoms (hypotonia, collapse, syncope, incontinence)
(d) Persistent gastrointestinal symptoms (crampy abdominal pain, vomiting)

Criteria 3: Reduced blood pressure after exposure to a known allergen for that patient (within minutes to several hours).
(a) Infants and children: low systolic BP (age specific) or greater than 30% decrease in systolic BP for that patient
(b) Adults: systolic BP of less than 90 mmHg or greater than 30% decrease from that patient's baseline

---

Is the cause readily identifiable by history, allergy skin tests, in vitro tests, or challenge tests?

Yes / **No**

Diagnosis made for specific cause of anaphylaxis

Reconsider clinical diagnosis
Consider idiopathic anaphylaxis
Consider other triggers
Consider further testing

Disease severity classification
- Allergic reactions are defined as mild when features are limited to the skin and subcutaneous tissues.
- Moderate reactions have features suggesting respiratory, cardiovascular, or gastrointestinal involvement.
- Severe reactions involve hypoxia, hypotension, or neurologic compromise, including cyanosis or oxygen saturation ≤92%, hypotension, confusion, loss of consciousness, or incontinence.

Laboratory diagnosis
List of diagnostic tests
- An elevated serum or plasma total tryptase can support the clinical diagnosis of anaphylaxis. It needs to be obtained from 15 minutes to 3 hours after symptom onset. The tryptase level is often not elevated in individuals with food-induced anaphylaxis.
- An elevated plasma histamine level can also support the clinical diagnosis of anaphylaxis. Due to the short half-life, it is usually only elevated within 60 minutes of the onset of symptoms. Samples require special handling.
- The tryptase and histamine levels are not necessary for making the diagnosis of anaphylaxis, but may help to confirm it if the diagnosis is unclear.

Lists of imaging techniques
Not applicable for this topic.

Potential pitfalls/common errors made regarding diagnosis of disease

- While many physicians do not diagnose anaphylaxis when hypotension is absent, a drop in blood pressure is not required to make the diagnosis.
- Skin symptoms and signs, such as hives, itching, or angioedema, can be missed if an individual is not undressed or fully examined, and may be lacking if the patient has taken an H1 antihistamine.
- Many patients experiencing anaphylaxis may also have known asthma, and the episode may be mistaken for an asthma exacerbation if other signs and symptoms are missed.

Section 4: Treatment (Algorithm 29.2)

Treatment rationale

- Epinephrine is the treatment of choice for anaphylaxis. It is best delivered intramuscularly into the lateral thigh (vastus lateralis muscle). The administration of epinephrine may be repeated every 5 minutes if necessary to control symptoms.
- In addition to epinephrine, a patient who presents with anaphylaxis should receive an H1 antagonist such as diphenhydramine, an H2 antagonist such as ranitidine, fluid resuscitation with normal saline, and a systemic corticosteroid such as methylprednisolone. While the use of steroids is not helpful acutely, it may help prevent recurrent or protracted anaphylaxis.
- Supplemental oxygen should be administered by face mask and the patient should be placed in a recumbent position with the lower extremities elevated.
- Other treatments that patients may require include an inhaled beta-agonist, a vasopressor, and glucagon. Glucagon may be required in patients taking beta-blockers who have treatment-refractory anaphylaxis.

When to hospitalize

- Observation periods must be individualized to each patient. The minimum observation period should be 4–6 hours.
- In general, those with severe anaphylaxis involving hypoxia, hypotension, or neurologic compromise, or moderate reactions that do not respond promptly to epinephrine should be admitted to a hospital.

Managing the hospitalized patient

- Monitoring of airway, breathing, and circulation
- As up to 23% of patients may have a biphasic reaction, epinephrine should be readily available.
- Continue H1 antagonist for 48–72 hours.
- Continue H2 antagonist for 48–72 hours.
- Continue corticosteroids for 48–72 hours.
- Provide patient education on allergen avoidance, recognition and management of future reactions, and proper use of the epinephrine auto-injector.

Algorithm 29.2 Treatment of anaphylaxis

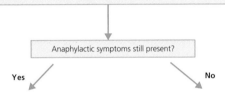

Immediate administration of epinephrine and assessment of airway, breathing and circulation

- Epinephrine 0.01 mg/kg up to 0.5 mg IM every 5–15 minutes as necessary
- Place patient on continuous cardiorespiratory monitor
- High-flow oxygen should be administered
- Obtain IV access
- Place patient in recumbent position with lower extremities elevated unless precluded by emesis or shortness of breath

Additional medications

- **H1 antagonist** (diphenhydramine), IV, IM or, for mild symptoms, orally, at 1–2 mg/kg up to 50 mg
- **H2 antagonist** (ranitidine) 50 mg IV in adults, 1 mg/kg up to 50 mg IV in children
- **Corticosteroid** (methylprednisolone) loading dose of 2 mg/kg IV, up to 125 mg
- **Glucagon** 20–30 μg/kg IV, (maximum dose 5 mg in adults, 1 mg in children) over 5 minutes, followed by an infusion of 5–15 μg/min, titrated to clinical response, for patients on beta-blockers who may be refractory to treatment
- **Bronchodilator** (albuterol) 2.5–5 mg via nebulizer for bronchospasm refractory to epinephrine
- **Normal saline bolus** 1–2 L in adults, 20 mL/kg in children

Anaphylactic symptoms still present?

Yes

No

Reassess airway, breathing, and circulation

Contact critical care medicine department for possible further management in the ICU

IV epinephrine is an option in the setting of severe hypotension or cardiac arrest unresponsive to IM doses of epinephrine and fluid resuscitation

Potent vasopressors, such as norepinephrine or vasopressin may be required if unable to maintain adequate BP

Observation (minimum 4–6 hours)

Maintenance or discharge medications

- Continue H1 antagonist every 6–8 hours for 48–72 hours
- Continue H2 antagonist twice daily for 48–72 hours
- Continue corticosteroids twice daily for 48–72 hours
- Epinephrine auto injector, 0.15 mg for children below 25 kg, 0.3 mg for children weighting 25 kg or more, as needed

Discharge plan

- Prescribe an anaphylaxis action plan; a sample can be downloaded at http://www.foodallergy.org
- Education on allergen avoidance
- Follow-up with an allergist or immunologist

Table of treatment

Treatment	Comment
Medical Epinephrine (0.01 mg/kg up to 0.5 mg IM every 5–15 minutes as necessary)	Rarely, and especially after overdose or IV administration, may lead to ventricular arrhythmias, myocardial infarction, pulmonary edema, or a sharp increase in blood pressure
H1 antagonist (diphenhydramine 1–2 mg/kg up to 50 mg)	Often causes drowsiness

Treatment	Comment
H2 antagonist (ranitidine 50 mg IV in adults, 1 mg/kg up to 50 mg IV in children)	
Corticosteroid (methylprednisolone 2 mg/kg up to 125 mg IV)	Although unproven, some believe it may help prevent a protracted or biphasic reaction
Glucagon (20–30 μg/kg over 5 minutes, maximum dose 5 mg in adults, 1 mg in children IV, followed by an infusion of 5–15 μg/min, titrated to clinical response)	Must protect the airway as glucagon frequently causes emesis
Normal saline bolus (1–2 L in adults, 20 mL/kg in children)	
Bronchodilator (2.5–5 mg albuterol via nebulizer)	

Prevention/management of complications

- Particular attention should be paid to the dosage of epinephrine that is administered. Incorrect dosing can occur when an inappropriate dilution (1:1000) is injected IV (as opposed to the 1:10 000 dilution). This can lead to ventricular arrhythmias, myocardial infarction, a sharp increase in blood pressure, angina, or pulmonary edema.
- Glucagon can induce nausea and vomiting. One should make sure to take steps to protect the airway when administering this medication.

CLINICAL PEARLS
- Epinephrine is the medication of choice for anaphylaxis.
- Individuals taking beta-blockers may not respond to epinephrine. If the patient does not respond, glucagon should be administered.
- Glucocorticoids may help prevent a biphasic reaction, but onset of action takes several hours. Steroids should not be administered as the first line therapy for the initial signs and symptoms of anaphylaxis.

Section 5: Special populations

Pregnancy

- During labor and delivery, the patient should be positioned on her left side.
- It is important to maintain a systolic blood pressure of at least 90 mmHg, and supplemental oxygen should be administered by face mask.
- There should be continuous fetal monitoring. Even when maternal outcome is favorable, maternal hypoxemia and hypotension in anaphylaxis are associated with a high risk of fetal asphyxia or death.

Children

- It may be difficult to make the diagnosis of anaphylaxis in infants as they cannot describe symptoms such as difficulty swallowing, chest tightness, or pruritus; symptoms may be similar to those seen in healthy infants, such as spitting up or loss of sphincter control; and the episode may only manifest with sudden onset of lethargy or clinging to a caregiver.

Others

- Patients who are taking beta-blockers may be resistant to treatment with epinephrine. In these cases, glucagon should be administered.
- While there may be reluctance to administer epinephrine to patients with cardiovascular disease, there are no absolute contraindications to the use of epinephrine in anaphylaxis.

Section 6: Prognosis

> **BOTTOM LINE/CLINICAL PEARLS**
> - Prompt use of epinephrine is vital in the management of anaphylaxis. In the majority of anaphylaxis deaths, epinephrine was either not administered or was administered after respiratory or cardiac arrest.
> - Patients who have experienced anaphylaxis are at risk for future episodes, which can be limited with risk reduction measures.
> - Avoidance measures are the most effective treatment for preventing recurrent episodes of anaphylaxis.

Follow-up tests and monitoring

- Consultation with an allergist or immunologist for diagnosis of allergies, prevention, and treatment should occur for individuals who have experienced anaphylaxis. The allergist or immunologist can identify possible triggers of anaphylaxis using a detailed history and allergy diagnostic testing including skin testing, serum IgE levels, and/or oral food challenges. They can also help assess the risks and benefits of potential therapies, provide counseling on avoidance measures, and train the patient and his or her family on how to administer epinephrine.

Section 7: Reading list

Bock SA, Muñoz-Furlong A, Sampson HA. Further fatalities caused by anaphylactic reactions to food, 2001–2006. J Allergy Clin Immunol 2007;119:1016–18

Lieberman P, Nicklas RA, Oppenheimer J, Kemp SF, Lang DM, Bernstein DI, et al. The diagnosis and management of anaphylaxis practice parameter: 2010 update. J Allergy Clin Immunol 2010;126:477–80

Patel DA, Holdford DA, Edwards E, Carroll NV. Estimating the economic burden of food-induced allergic reactions and anaphylaxis in the United States. J Allergy Clin Immunol 2011;128:110–5

Sampson HA, Muñoz-Furlong A, Campbell RL, Adkinson NF Jr, Bock SA, Branum A, et al. Second symposium on the definition and management of anaphylaxis: summary report. Second National Institute of Allergy and Infectious Disease/Food Allergy and Anaphylaxis Network symposium. J Allergy Clin Immunol 2006; 117:391–7

Simons FE, Gu X, Simons KJ. Epinephrine absorption in adults: intramuscular versus subcutaneous injection. J Allergy Clin Immunol 2001;108:871–3

Simons FE, Schatz M. Anaphylaxis during pregnancy. J Allergy Clin Immunol 2012;130:597–606

Simons FE. Anaphylaxis. J Allergy Clin Immunol 2010;125:S161–81

Wood RA, Camargo CA Jr, Lieberman P, Sampson HA, Schwartz LB, Zitt M, et al. Anaphylaxis in America: the prevalence and characteristics of anaphylaxis in the United States. J Allergy Clin Immunol 2014;133:461–7

Suggested websites

American Academy of Allergy Asthma and Immunology. www.aaaai.org

American College of Allergy, Asthma and Immunology. www.acaai.org

Food Allergy Research and Education. www.foodallergy.org

Section 8: Guidelines
National society guidelines

Guideline title	Guideline source	Date
The diagnosis and management of anaphylaxis practice parameter: 2010 update	Joint Task Force on Practice Parameters representing the American Academy of Allergy, Asthma and Immunology (AAAAI), the American College of Allergy, Asthma and Immunology (ACAAI)	2010 (http://www.jacionline.org/article/S0091-6749(10)01004-3/abstract)
Second Symposium on the definition and management of anaphylaxis: summary report—Second National Institute of Allergy and Infectious Disease/Food Allergy and Anaphylaxis Network symposium	National Institute of Allergy and Infectious Disease (NIAID)	2006 (http://www.ncbi.nlm.nih.gov/pubmed/16546624)

International society guidelines

Guideline title	Guideline source	Date
World Allergy Organization anaphylaxis guidelines: summary	World Allergy Organization (WAO)	2011 (http://www.worldallergy.org/anaphylaxis/)
2012 Update: World Allergy Organization Guidelines for the assessment and management of anaphylaxis	World Allergy Organization (WAO)	2012 (http://www.bsaci.org/guidelines/wao_anaphylaxis_guideline_2012.pdf)

Section 9: Evidence
See guidelines of the Joint Task Force (AAAAI and ACAAI) and the NIAID

Type of evidence	Title, comment	Date
Guidelines	Food allergy: a practice parameter update—2014	2014 (http://www.jacionline.org/article/S0091-6749(14)00672-1/abstract)
Guidelines	Food allergy: a practice parameter update—2014 Practice Parameters and Other Guidelines (AAAAI)	2014 (http://www.aaaai.org/practice-resources/statements-and-practice-parameters/practice-parameters-and-other-guidelines-page.aspx)
Guidelines	Guidelines for the Diagnosis and Management of Food Allergy in the United States (NIAID)	2011 (http://www.niaid.nih.gov/topics/foodallergy/clinical/Pages/default.aspx)

Section 10: Images

Not applicable for this topic.

Additional material for this chapter can be found online at: www.mountsinaiexpertguides.com
This includes a case study, multiple choice questions, advice for patients, and ICD codes

---

CHAPTER 30

Mastocytosis

Amanda L. Cox

Division of Pediatric Allergy/Immunology, Icahn School of Medicine at Mount Sinai, New York, NY, USA

OVERALL BOTTOM LINE
- Chemical mediators released from mast cells are responsible for the symptoms of mast cell disorders which often manifest as allergic and anaphylactic reactions.
- Mastocytosis is a primary mast cell disorder characterized by excessive mast cell proliferation and infiltration of one or several tissues.
- There are several subtypes of mastocytosis. Classification is based on the tissues and cell-lines involved.
- Cutaneous mastocytosis describes forms of mastocytosis limited to the skin without other organ involvement, whereas systemic mastocytosis involves bone marrow and other extracutaneous tissues.
- Activating mutations of *KIT* (the gene for the c-kit receptor protein) are strongly associated with and involved in the pathogenesis of mastocytosis.

Section 1: Background

Definition of disease
- Mastocytosis is a primary mast cell disorder in which there is an abnormal accumulation of tissue mast cells in one or more organ systems.

Disease classification
- Mastocytosis falls into the category of primary mast cell activation syndromes (MCAS), which also includes monoclonal MCAS. Cutaneous mastocytosis (CM) subtypes include urticaria pigmentosa (UP), telangiectasia macularis eruptiva perstans (TMEP), diffuse cutaneous mastocytosis (DCM), and solitary mastocytoma. Systemic mastocytosis (SM) subtypes include indolent systemic mastocytosis (ISM), systemic mastocytosis with an associated hematologic non-mast cell lineage disorder (SM-AHNMD), aggressive systemic mastocytosis (ASM), and mast cell leukemia (MCL).

Incidence/prevalence
- All forms of mastocytosis are rare disorders, and the exact incidence is not known.
- In children, onset occurs in the first year of life in 80% of cases, and most are limited to cutaneous forms that resolve by adolescence.
- In adults, systemic forms of mastocytosis are more common, and tend to be persistent disorders.

Economic impact
Not applicable for this topic.

Mount Sinai Expert Guides: Allergy and Clinical Immunology, First Edition. Edited by Hugh A. Sampson.
© 2015 John Wiley & Sons, Ltd. Published 2015 by John Wiley & Sons, Ltd.
Companion website: www.mountsinaiexpertguides.com

Etiology

- Primary mast cell disorders, including mastocytosis, are caused by intrinsic defects of mast cells that affect mast cell proliferation and activation.
- The basis for disease is due most often to a somatic genetic mutation in a mast cell surface receptor.
- The tissues and organs where these activated mast cells accumulate result in various disease manifestations, severities, and complications.

Pathology/pathogenesis

- The molecular pathogenesis of mastocytosis is not completely understood and is an area of ongoing investigation. Stem cell factor (SCF), or kit ligand, is a growth factor required for expansion of mast cells from hematopoietic progenitors. Mast cells express the surface receptor c-kit (CD 117), a tyrosine kinase, which is a receptor for SCF. Many molecular defects associated with mastocytosis are secondary to gain-of-function mutations in the gene encoding the c-kit receptor. The most common *KIT* mutation, Asp816Val, is present in most patients with systemic mastocytosis. This mutation leads to clonal expansion and apoptotic defects of mast cells, and results in accumulation of mast cells in tissues.

Predictive/risk factors

Not applicable for this topic.

Section 2: Prevention

No interventions have been demonstrated to prevent the development of mastocytosis.

Screening

Not applicable for this topic.

Primary prevention

Not applicable for this topic.

Secondary prevention

Not applicable for this topic.

Section 3: Diagnosis

> **BOTTOM LINE/CLINICAL PEARLS**
> - Consider a mast cell disorder in any individual with a constellation of symptoms suggestive of mast cell activation or who has recurrent allergic reactions/anaphylaxis without an identifiable trigger.
> - Examination should include skin inspection for UP or mastocytomas. Darier's sign may be elicited upon rubbing a small UP skin lesion.
> - Examination should also include palpation for organomegaly (spleen, liver) and lymphadenopathy.
> - Skin biopsy should be considered for patients with cutaneous mastocytosis lesions and specimens should be stained for tryptase and c-kit (CD117).
> - CBC, liver function tests (LFT), and serum tryptase should be drawn.
> - Bone marrow biopsy and/or aspiration with staining for mast cells should be ordered for any adult with UP, or any patients with signs and symptoms of SM or elevated serum tryptase levels.

Differential diagnosis

Differential diagnosis	Features
Monoclonal mast cell activation syndrome (MMAS)	Mast cell activation symptoms +1 or 2 minor diagnostic criteria for systemic mastocytosis
Anaphylaxis, idiopathic anaphylaxis	Elevated beta tryptase during acute events but normal baseline serum tryptase
Mast cell activation syndrome (MCAS)	Recurrent mast cell activation symptoms affecting ≥2 organ systems, with no *KIT* mutations or mast cell CD25 expression, and favorable response to medications that counteract mast cell mediators
Hereditary/acquired angioedema	Episodic angioedema of skin, larynx, bowel walls Abnormal complement studies
Carcinoid syndrome	Episodic flushing and diarrhea with elevated 24-hr urine 5-HIAA
Pheochromocytoma	Flushing, paroxysmal hypotension without other signs of mast cell activation
Vasoactive intestinal peptide-secreting tumors	Flushing episodes and significant diarrhea, associated with increased levels of VIP

Typical presentation

- Presentations of mastocytosis and other mast cell disorders vary and depend on the specific disorder and tissues involved. Individuals typically present with manifestations of mast cell activation, including episodic flushing, tachycardia, hypotension, abdominal pain, nausea, vomiting, diarrhea, fatigue, musculoskeletal pain, or syncope. They may present with recurrent allergic reactions or anaphylaxis without any identifiable or consistent trigger.
- Cutaneous mastocytosis (CM) presents most often in children, with maculopapular hyperpigmentated lesions that urticate when rubbed (urticaria pigmentosa, or UP), as well as symptoms of dermatographism.
- UP lesions may also be found in patients who have systemic mastocytosis. Patients with UP may have pruritus especially with certain triggers, as well as flushing, blistering skin, or urticaria.
- In diffuse cutaneous mastocytosis (DCM) there are no discrete skin lesions, but skin may be yellowish-brown and thick. DCM may present with bullous eruptions that can hemorrhage. Additional symptoms in systemic forms of mastocytosis are associated with specific organ infiltration and hematologic abnormalities.
- MMAS presents with recurrent episodes of mast cell activation symptoms, including anaphylaxis, but without UP or increase in mast cell numbers in tissues.

Clinical diagnosis

History

- Mastocytosis involves dermatologic symptoms arising from mediator release (in CM, SM, solid mast cell tumors, MCAS), and non-cutaneous symptoms secondary to organ infiltration (SM only). Patients may complain of pruritus, flushing, or blister formation with certain physical triggers (e.g. irritation or heat) with or without the presence of UP. CM and SM may present with the above sporadic symptoms of mast cell mediator release, or with hypotensive syncope, or anaphylaxis, in association with certain triggers (medications, exercise, massage, temperature changes, surgical procedures, alcohol ingestion, infections, stress, hymenoptera stings). Patients with CM and SM may have chronic gastrointestinal (GI) symptoms such as abdominal pain, diarrhea, nausea, vomiting, peptic ulcer disease, and GI bleeding, all of which are secondary to release of mast cell mediators. Neuropsychiatric symptoms and neurologic symptoms such as headache, dizziness, and memory problems are often reported. Diffuse musculoskeletal pain and a fibromyalgia-like pain syndrome occur in some patients with SM. A history of anemia or thrombocytopenia, organomegaly, intestinal malabsorption, and pathologic fractures suggests specific organ infiltration (bone marrow, liver, spleen, GI tract, lymph node, skeletal system) by mast cells in SM.

Physical examination

- *Skin inspection:* evaluate skin for UP lesions, bullous lesions, or mastocytomas. UP lesions are fixed, small, yellow–tan to reddish-brown macules or slightly raised papules, and occasionally form raised nodules or plaque-like lesions. UP lesions most commonly affect extremities and trunk, and tend to spare palms and soles. While children may have scalp and face involvement, adults rarely do. Darier's sign (urtication and erythema upon rubbing lesions) may be elicited. Petechiae, ecchymoses, or telangiectasias may be present in or next to UP lesions. Solitary or multiple mastocytomas may present in childhood, and are similar to UP lesions but are larger and may have yellow–orange coloration. Flushing can occur after irritation of the tumor, so rubbing these lesions is *not* recommended. Yellowish brown, thickened skin may be noted in DCM, along with generalized erythroderma or edema. Telangiectasia macularis eruptiva perstans (TMEP) is observed in <1% of CM patients. TMEP lesions are telangiectatic, red macules on a tan–brown base, 2–6 mm in diameter and without sharp borders. TMEP is not associated with blistering or pruritus.
- *Abdominal and lymph node evaluation:* in systemic forms of mastocytosis with organ infiltration by mast cells, hepatomegaly, splenomegaly, or lymphadenopathy may be noted.

Laboratory diagnosis

List of diagnostic tests

- CM is diagnosed by punch biopsy of skin lesions, with specific histopathologic stains. Mast cells may form perivascular infiltrates in papillary and upper dermis, sheet-like infiltrates in the papillary body and upper reticular dermis, interstitial infiltrates, or nodular infiltrates. Mast cells in UP lesions may have irregular shapes or bi-lobated nuclei.
- Recommended laboratory tests: CBC with differential, LFTs (including serum aminotransferases and alkaline phosphatase), and baseline serum tryptase. These laboratory studies are typically normal in CM, and more often abnormal in SM.
- Consider coagulation studies in patients with SM.
- A thorough allergy evaluation, with skin testing and *in vitro* allergen-specific IgE testing, should be completed for any patients with unexplained anaphylaxis.
- Metabolites of mast cell activation (24-hour urine *N*-methyl histamine and 11-beta-prostaglandin F2) may be measured.
- Histologic evaluation of other organs (other than bone marrow) is generally not recommended.
- Bone marrow core biopsy and aspiration is needed to differentiate CM from SM, and should be completed in all adults with UP-like skin lesions, or those who have mast cell activation symptoms and tryptase >20 ng/mL.
- Bone marrow core biopsy examination includes evaluation of histology, immunohistochemical staining with antibodies to tryptase and/or CD117 (c-kit receptor) to identify mast cells, and CD25 staining, as CD25 is pathologically expressed by mast cells in mastocytosis.

- Bone marrow aspirate sample should be evaluated for morphology of mast cells (i.e. spindle-shaped mast cells) as well as undergo flow cytometry analysis, with assessment of surface markers CD2 and CD25 on CD117(c-kit) expressing cells:
  - D816V KIT mutational analysis of bone marrow aspirates should be completed;
  - In patients who also have leukocytosis, eosinophilia, or both, examine for *BCR/ABL* and *FIP1L1-PDGFRA* fusion genes and perform routine karyotype.

Lists of imaging techniques

- Bone scans or skeletal surveys, abdominal radiography, computed tomography (CT) scan, magnetic resonance imaging (MRI), or endoscopy may be helpful in evaluating systemic disease and may be indicated depending upon the extent of organ infiltration and patient's presenting symptoms.
- DEXA (bone densitometric) scan should be performed to monitor osteoporosis when there is skeletal system involvement.

WORLD HEALTH ORGANIZATION (WHO) DIAGNOSTIC CRITERIA FOR CUTANEOUS AND SYSTEMIC MASTOCYTOSIS

Cutaneous mastocytosis: typical clinical findings and cutaneous lesions of UP, DCM, or solitary mastocytoma, with infiltrates of mast cells in a multifocal or diffuse pattern on skin biopsy.

Systemic mastocytosis: diagnosis is made if one major+one minor *or* three minor criteria are met:

- Major criterion: multifocal, dense infiltrates of mast cells (≥15 in aggregates) detected in sections of bone marrow and/or other extracutaneous organ and confirmed by tryptase immunohistochemistry stain or other special stain.
- Minor criteria:
  - In bone marrow biopsy or other organ biopsy sections >25% mast cells in infiltrate are spindle-shaped or have atypical morphology, or >25% of mast cells in aspirate spear are immature or atypical;
  - Detection of an activating point mutation at codon 816 of *KIT* in bone marrow, blood, or other extracutaneous organ;
  - Mast cells in bone marrow, blood, or other extracutaneous organ express CD117 with CD2 and/or CD25;
  - Serum total tryptase persistently >20 ng/mL in the absence of an associated clonal myeloid disorder.

Variants of systemic mastocytosis

- *Indolent systemic mastocytosis (ISM):* meets criteria for systemic findings, no "C" findings (below), no evidence of an associated clonal, hematologic non-mast cell lineage disease, mast cell burden is low, skin lesions usually present:
  - Bone marrow mastocytosis: ISM with marrow involvement, no skin lesions;
  - Smoldering systemic mastocytosis: ISM, but with ≥2 "B" findings, and no "C" findings.
- *Systemic mastocytosis with associated clonal, hematologic non-mast cell lineage disease (SM-AHNMD):* meets criteria for SM and criteria for an associated AHNMD disorder (MDS, MPN, AML, lymphoma or other hematologic neoplasm).
- *Aggressive systemic mastocytosis (ASM):* meets criteria for SM with one or more "C" findings, with no evidence of mast cell leukemia, and usually no skin lesions.
  - *Lymphadenopathic mastocytosis with eosinophilia:* progressive lymphadenopathy with peripheral blood eosinophilia, often extensive bone involvement, hepatosplenomegaly, without skin lesions. Cases with PDGFRA rearrangement are excluded.
- *Mast cell leukemia (MCL):* meets criteria for SM, usually without skin lesions, bone marrow biopsy with diffuse infiltration by atypical, immature mast cells, BM aspirate with 20% or more mast cells. In typical MCL mast cells also account for 10% or more of peripheral white blood cells. In aleukemic MCL, <10% of peripheral white blood cells are mast cells.

(Continued)

- *Mast cell sarcoma (MCS):* unifocal mast cell tumor, no evidence of SM, destructive growth pattern with high grade histology.
- *Extracutaneous mastocytoma:* unifocal mast cell tumor, no evidence of SM, no skin lesions. Non-destructive growth pattern with low grade cytology.

"B" findings

- Bone marrow biopsy showing >30% infiltration by mast cells (focal, dense aggregates) and/or serum total tryptase level >200 ng/mL.
- Signs of dysplasia or myeloproliferation, in non-mast cell lineages, but insufficient criteria for definitive diagnosis of a hematopoietic neoplasm with normal or slightly abnormal blood counts.
- Hepatomegaly without impairment of liver function and/or palpable splenomegaly without hypersplenism, and/or lymphadenopathy.

"C" findings

- Bone marrow dysfunction manifested by one or more cytopenia but no obvious non-mast cell hematopoietic malignancy.
- Palpable hepatomegaly with impairment of liver function, ascites, and/or portal hypertension.
- Skeletal involvement with large osteolytic lesions and/or pathological fractures.
- Palpable splenomegaly with hypersplenism.
- Malabsorption with weight loss due to gastrointestinal mast cell infiltrates.

Source: Horny HP, et al. Mastocytosis. In Swerdlow SH, et al. (eds). WHO classification of tumors of haematopoietic and lymphoid tissues. Lyon: IARC Press; 2008.

Potential pitfalls/common errors made regarding diagnosis of disease

- It is difficult to distinguish CM from SM based on clinical evaluation alone, as CM patients often have systemic symptoms due to mast cell mediator release.
- Skin biopsy does not provide any information about systemic involvement.
- Mast cell numbers can be elevated in skin biopsies in other inflammatory and neoplastic skin conditions.
- Bone marrow biopsy is generally unnecessary in children with UP unless there are CBC or peripheral smear abnormalities, or other signs of an aggressive form of mastocytosis.
- The absolute level of total tryptase does not determine the category of mastocytosis.
- Elevated tryptase can also occur in other conditions, including myeloproliferative or myelodysplastic disease, chronic renal failure, liver failure, and chronic eosinophilic leukemia.
- *KIT* mutational analysis (specifically for AsP816Val mutation) can also be performed on peripheral white blood cells or cells from skin or other organs, but this is much less sensitive than bone marrow analysis.

Section 4: Treatment

Treatment rationale

- There is currently no cure for mastocytosis, and treatment depends upon the classification and symptoms of disease.
- In CM, ISM treatment is aimed at reducing symptoms and blocking effects of mast cell mediator release.
- Patients with diagnosed SM should avoid triggers for mast cell degranulation, including physical triggers, alcohol, certain medications, emotional stress, and known allergens.
- Patients should be trained and prepared to treat anaphylaxis, and should have self-injectable epinephrine (at least two doses) available at all times.

- SM patients with reactions to Hymenoptera stings should be tested for venom allergy and treated with venom immunotherapy.
- Those with inhalant allergies should be managed with allergen avoidance and typical medications for allergic rhinitis, allergic conjunctivitis, or allergic asthma.
- *Antihistamines:* H1 antihistamines are administered to prevent and treat flushing and pruritus. H2 antihistamines may help control abdominal pain, heartburn, cramping, and diarrhea.
- *Antileukotriene drugs* may be added in patients with flushing, itching, and abdominal cramping that does not improve with H1 and H2 antihistamines.
- *Aspirin* (if patient is ASA-tolerant) may be considered to control flushing not responsive to antihistamines.
- Oral cromolyn sodium, H2 antihistamines, and proton pump inhibitors may be used to treat GI symptoms.
- Patients with recurrent anaphylaxis should be treated with maximal doses of H1 and H2 antihistamines as well as antileukotriene drugs. Low-dose maintenance glucocorticoids, IFN-α, cladribine, or tyrosine kinase inhibitor (depending upon c-kit mutational status) can be considered as second line treatments.
- *Tyrosine kinase inhibitors* (such as imatinib) are appropriate for some patients with SM who have an associated hematologic non-mast cell lineage disorder (SM-AHNMD), aggressive systemic mastocytosis (ASM), or MCL. SM patients with the D816V KIT mutation are *not* candidates for tyrosine kinase inhibitor therapy.
- Mastocytosis with an associated clonal, non-mast cell hematologic disorder should be treated as two separate diseases, and specific hematologic disorder and may require management by a hematologist.
- Patients with ASM with "C" findings are candidates for mast cell cyto-reductive therapies including INF-α-2b, cladribine, glucocorticoids, or hydroxyurea. Tyrosine kinase inhibitor (imatinib) may also be considered in ASM patients who do not have a D816V KIT mutation.
- MCL is treated with cyto-reductive polychemotherapy, similar to treatment for acute leukemia.
- Surgical treatment may be considered for benign mast cell tumors that cause excessive mast cell mediator release symptoms. Radiation and polychemotherapy, and tyrosine kinase inhibitor, may be indicated for mast cell sarcomas.

When to hospitalize
- Patients with life-threatening mast cell mediator-related symptoms, blistering of skin, or bullous skin lesions may require hospitalization.
- Hospitalization is also necessary for any patient with acute hematologic complications, or organ failure in systemic forms of mastocytosis.

Table of treatment

Treatment	Comment
Conservative Mast cell activation trigger avoidance	Isolated cutaneous mastocytosis, indolent mastocytosis and UP in children may not require treatment, or may be managed with topical local/lesional skin care Isolated CM in adults, without systemic involvement, may also be observed, but should be closely followed for development of SM signs or symptoms

(Continued)

Treatment	Comment
Medical (with adult dosing where applicable) H1 antihistamines (oral) • Hydroxyzine (25 mg every 6 hours) • Diphenhydramine (25–50 mg PRN up to QID) • Doxepin (10–100 mg/day) • Loratidine (10 mg/day) • Fexofenidine (180–360 mg/day) • Cetirizine (10–40 mg/day) H2 antihistamines (oral) • Ranitidine (150 mg BID) • Cimetidine (400 mg BID) • Famotidine (10–20 mg BID) Leukotriene receptor antagonist • Monteleukast (10 mg/day) • Zafirleukast (20 mg/day) • Zileuton (1200 mg BID) Oral cromolyn sodium (100–200 mg up to 4 times per day PRN) Aspirin (up to 650 mg BID) Self-injectable epinephrine (0.15–0.3 mg per dose) Tyrosine kinase inhibitor (imatinib) Oral prednisone (20–60 mg/day for 2–3 weeks, then slowly tapered) Interferon alpha 2b (initiated at 1 million units 3 times weekly subcutaneously) Cladribine (0.10–0.13 mg/kg/day for 5 days every 4–8 weeks up to six cycles) Cytoreductive chemotherapy	Self-injectable epinephrine is for treatment of anaphylaxis (not reviewed here) When considering aspirin, if patient's tolerance of NSAID is not known, a first dose of aspirin should be administered in a supervised setting Most patients with systemic mastocytosis are not candidates for imatinib because they have the D816V *KIT* mutation which results in imatinib resistance INFα-2b, cladribine, and oral glucocorticoids are therapeutic options for ASM requiring cytoreductive therapy Chemotherapy is not a treatment for indolent mastocytosis
Surgical Excision of benign mast cell tumors or extracutaneous mastocytomas Surgical excision of mast cell sarcomas Splenectomy	Surgical excision of benign mast cell tumors should be considered if they cause excessive mast cell mediator release and related symptoms Mast cell sarcomas may also require radiation, chemotherapy, and imatinib therapy as well Splenectomy may be considered for hypersplenism in ASM with severe anemia and thrombocytopenia
Radiological	Bone densitometry imaging should be used to monitor patients with mastocytosis-related osteopenia/osteoporosis Imaging should be used to monitor for recurrence of metastases in patients treated for mast cell sarcomas
Other considerations Venom immunotherapy should be considered for those with SM who have Hymenoptera sting allergy Pre-treatment with diphenhydramine, ranitidine, montelukast, and prednisone for invasive surgical procedures should be considered	

Prevention/management of complications

- Aspirin can precipitate mast cell mediator release in some patients, and prolonged therapy can result in gastric irritation.
- While venom immunotherapy is recommended in SM patients with documented Hymenoptera venom allergy, adverse reactions during venom immunotherapy can occur, and should be considered especially during the build-up phase.
- IFNα-2b adverse effects include flu-like symptoms, thrombocytopenia, cardiac toxicity, and depression.
- Cladribine side effects are related to bone marrow suppression.

CLINICAL PEARLS

- Patients with isolated CM and ISM do not require cyto-reductive therapy and may be treated for mast cell activation symptoms only. However, monitoring should occur yearly (tryptase, CBC, LFTs) as abnormalities or changes may indicate disease progression.
- There is currently no cure for SM. Treatment is intended to reduce symptoms and improve quality of life.
- All patients should be educated to avoid potential triggers for mast cell activation, as well as be prepared with self-injectable epinephrine to treat anaphylaxis should it occur.
- Medical treatments are guided by mastocytosis classification and severity of manifestations.
- Patients with SM and an associated hematologic disorder should be treated as if there are two discrete diseases, and should be treated appropriately for the hematologic disorder.
- Patients with ASM and MCL may benefit from cyto-reductive therapy, although this is rarely curative.

Section 5: Special populations

Not applicable for this topic.

Section 6: Prognosis

BOTTOM LINE/CLINICAL PEARLS

- Prognosis depends upon the specific type of mastocytosis and differs for each disease category.
- Patients with CM and ISM have the best prognoses.
- UP may convert to a systemic form of mastocytosis, while in children with isolated UP, 50–70% will experience complete resolution by 21 years of age. Progression to mast cell sarcoma and MCL has been reported in some pediatric patients with UP.
- In 1–5%, ISM will convert to a more severe form of SM, such as ASM, MCL, or SM-AHNMD. The prognosis then depends upon the specific hematologic disorder and/or response to therapy.
- The prognoses for MCL and ASM are generally poor. MCL progresses to multiple organ failure in weeks to months, with mean survival time of 12–24 months. Prognosis for ASM is generally poor, with an average of 2–4 years survival from onset of systemic disease.
- Poor prognostic indicators in patients with SM include older age of onset, weight loss, thrombocytopenia, hypoalbuminemia, elevated lactic dehydrogenase, high alkaline phosphatase, qualitative changes in red and/or white blood cells, organomegaly, ascites, and excess bone marrow blasts.

Natural history of untreated disease
Not applicable for this topic.

Prognosis for treated patients
Not applicable for this topic.

Follow-up tests and monitoring
- Patients with CM and ISM should be monitored for development of systemic disease.
- For patients with uncomplicated ISM, yearly monitoring should include physical examination, serum tryptase level, CBC with differential, serum chemistry, and LFTs, and yearly bone densitometry if there is osteopenia or osteoporosis. Testing may be performed more frequently if symptoms worsen or if new symptoms develop.
- Patients with SM-AHNMD should be monitored for mast cell activation symptoms during therapy for hematologic disorder.
- Patients with ASM and organ tissue infiltration should be monitored for organ failure, as well as for side-effects of mast cell cyto-reductive therapy, if treated.
- Patients with mast cell sarcomas and extracutaneous mastocytomas should be monitored periodically with imaging (CT, MRI, or PET scan) for recurrence or metastases.

Section 7: Reading list

Akoglu G et al. Cutaneous mastocytosis: demographic aspects and clinical features of 55 patients. J Eur Acad Dermatol Venereol 2006;20:969

Castells M, Metcalfe DD, Escribano L. Diagnosis and treatment of cutaneous mastocytosis in children: practical recommendations. Am J Clin Dermatol 2011;12:259

Gotlib J, Akin C. Mast cells and eosinophils in mastocytosis, chronic eosinophilic leukemia, and non-clonal disorders. Semin Hematol 2012;49:128

Horny H-P, Metcalfe DD, Bennett JM, et al. Mastocytosis. In: Swerdlow SH, Campo E, Harris NL, et al. (eds) WHO Classification of Tumors of Haematopoietic and Lymphoid Tissues. Lyon: IARC Press, 2008: pp. 54–63

Pardanani A. Systemic mastocytosis in adults: 2012 update on diagnosis, risk stratification, and management. Am J Hematol 2012;87:401

Parker RI. Hematologic aspects of systemic mastocytosis. Hematol Oncol Clin North Am 2000;14:557

Valent P, Akin C, Arock M, Brockow K, Brockow K, Butterfield JH, Carter MC, et al. Definitions, criteria and global classification of mast cell disorders with special reference to mast cell activation syndromes: a consensus proposal. Int Arch Allergy Immunol 2012;157:215–25

Wolff K, Komar M, Petzelbauer P. Clinical and histopathological aspects of cutaneous mastocytosis. Leuk Res 2001;25:519–28

Suggested websites
American Academy of Allergy Asthma and Immunology. www.aaaai.org
The Mastocytosis Society. www.tmsforacure.org

Section 8: Guidelines
National society guidelines
Not applicable for this topic.

International society guidelines

Guideline title	Guideline source	Date
World Health Organization Diagnostic Criteria for Cutaneous and Systemic Mastocytosis	IARC	2008 (Lyon: IARC Press; 2008:54–63)

Section 9: Evidence
Not applicable for this topic.

Section 10: Images

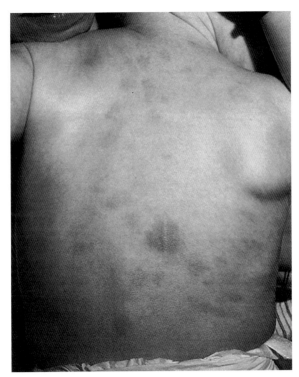

Figure 30.1 Stroking one UP lesion has caused a linear raised area (wheal) with surrounding erythema to develop (Darier's sign) on this child's back. See color plate 30.1. From Habif TP. Clinical Dermatology: A Color Guide to Diagnosis and Therapy. 5th edition. 2010 Philadelphia, PA, Mosby/Elsevier. Reproduced with permission.

Additional material for this chapter can be found online at:
www.mountsinaiexpertguides.com
This includes a case study, multiple choice questions, advice for patients, and ICD codes

CHAPTER 31

Insect Sting Allergy

Scott H. Sicherer

Department of Pediatrics, Division of Allergy/Immunology, Mount Sinai Hospital, New York, NY, USA

OVERALL BOTTOM LINE

- Allergy to stinging insect venom can result in allergic reactions that may be fatal.
- The risk for severe anaphylaxis on subsequent stings is low for persons with large local reactions, or for children with reactions isolated to urticaria, but is high for adults with any systemic symptoms or children with systemic symptoms beyond the skin.
- Venom immunotherapy is highly effective in reducing the risk of subsequent anaphylaxis and is indicated for those at risk.
- Patients at risk for anaphylaxis should be instructed on prompt self-injection of epinephrine, to seek emergency care if stung, to wear medical identification jewelry, and to take measures to avoid insect stings.

Section 1: Background

Definition of disease

- Stinging insect allergy is an IgE-mediated response against proteins in insect venoms that may result in symptoms ranging from marked localized swelling to serious anaphylactic reactions that can be fatal.

Disease classification

- Reactions are categorized into three types that carry prognostic significance:
  1. Large local reactions (swelling to more than 10 cm in diameter contiguous to the sting site);
  2. Systemic reaction isolated to the skin (urticaria and angioedema); and
  3. Systemic reaction not isolated to the skin (e.g. including respiratory, gastrointestinal, cardiac, and/or neurologic symptoms).

Incidence/prevalence

- Potentially life-threatening systemic allergic reactions occur in approximately 3% of adults and 0.4–0.8% of children.
- Anaphylactic sting reactions account for approximately 40 deaths/year in the United States.

Economic impact

Not applicable for this topic.

Mount Sinai Expert Guides: Allergy and Clinical Immunology, First Edition. Edited by Hugh A. Sampson.
© 2015 John Wiley & Sons, Ltd. Published 2015 by John Wiley & Sons, Ltd.
Companion website: www.mountsinaiexpertguides.com

Etiology

- Stinging insects of relevance are in the order Hymenoptera and include the families Apidae (honeybee, bumblebee, sweatbee), Vespidae (yellow jacket, yellow hornet, white-faced hornet, paper wasp), and Formicidae (fire ant, jack jumper ant, harvester ant).
- Insect venom contains vasoactive amines, acetylcholine and kinins responsible for pain and swelling, and proteins that can trigger allergic responses.
- Allergy to salivary proteins of biting insects (e.g. mosquitos, kissing bugs, horsefly) is uncommon.

Pathology/pathogenesis

- Significant allergic reactions to stinging insect venoms are type 1 hypersensitivity responses (IgE-mediated) where exposure to the allergen results in release of preformed mediators (e.g. histamine) from mast cells and basophils, resulting in rapid onset of symptoms.

Predictive/risk factors

Risk factor	Percentage risk within 10 years if re-stung
Systemic reaction in an individual who experienced a large local reaction	10
Systemic reaction in a child (age 16 years and under) who experienced a cutaneous systemic reaction	10
Systemic reaction in an adult who experienced a cutaneous systemic reaction	20
Systemic reaction in a child who experienced a systemic reaction	40
Systemic reaction in an adult who experienced a systemic reaction	60

Section 2: Prevention

BOTTOM LINE/CLINICAL PEARLS
- No interventions have been demonstrated to be effective for primary prevention. However, venom immunotherapy (VIT) is extremely effective and is indicated to prevent recurrence of severe anaphylactic reactions in patients who qualify for this treatment. VIT may also be considered for selected patients who experience large local reactions. Avoidance of insect stings is encouraged as a means of prevention.

Screening

- Routine screening tests are not recommended. Testing is recommended for patients who have experienced a reaction that could qualify for VIT.

Primary prevention

Not applicable for this topic.

Secondary prevention

- VIT is 95–98% effective in preventing systemic reactions.
- VIT may reduce the risk of large local reactions.

• Avoidance of stings is recommended (remove nests from vicinity of patient's home; avoid wearing bright colors and scents; avoid walking barefoot or with open shoes; wear clothing that covers skin well and gloves when working outdoors; be cautious near bushes, eaves, attics, garbage containers, and other nesting and activity areas; have insecticides nearby that can be sprayed to kill insects at a distance; caution when eating and drinking outdoors, especially drinking from opaque containers).

Section 3: Diagnosis (Algorithm 31.1)

BOTTOM LINE/CLINICAL PEARLS
• The patient history should include the symptoms (especially whether there was a systemic reaction), possibility of an insect sting triggering the reaction (e.g. outdoor activity, observation of insects nearby), and information that may indicate the type of stinging insect.
• If the patient presents having recently been stung, the size of the localized reaction should be evaluated, or signs and symptoms of anaphylaxis should be sought (e.g. hives, wheezing, decreased blood pressure).
• For patients who may qualify for VIT, skin and/or serum testing to insect venom should be performed.
• Skin testing is optional for patients who do not qualify for VIT.

Differential diagnosis

Differential diagnosis	Features
Anaphylaxis from another cause	No clear insect sting, other likely triggers such as a food or medication identified from the history
Mastocytosis	Patients experiencing anaphylaxis from insect stings with or without evidence of IgE antibodies to insect venom may have an underlying mast cell disorder identifiable with testing for serum tryptase
Toxic reactions to insect stings	Multiple simultaneous insect stings may result in toxic reactions with renal failure, seizures, adult respiratory distress syndrome, hemolysis, or diffuse intravascular coagulation

Typical presentation
• Most insect stings result in transient, local reactions that resolve without treatment. Such responses are normal and do not indicate an increased risk of future allergic reactions.
• Patients may experience large local reactions, where the sting site swells over 24–48 hours to more than 10 cm in diameter. Large local reactions are allergic in nature and may take 5–10 days to resolve but there are no reactions that are non-contiguous to the sting.
• Systemic reactions occur soon following the sting and may include any symptoms of anaphylaxis.

Algorithm 31.1 Diagnosis of insect sting allergy

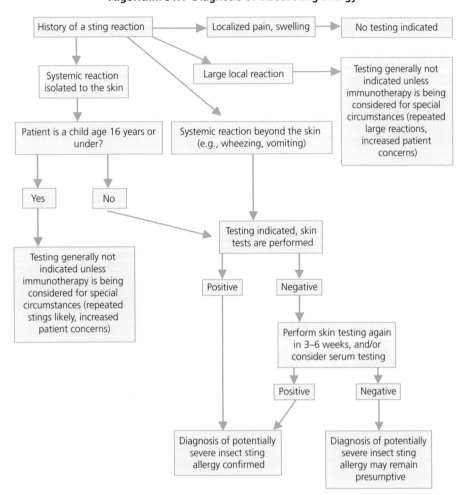

Clinical diagnosis

History

- The history should identify if an insect sting was likely a trigger, the exact symptoms (to grade the type of reaction, see below), number of stings, and, if possible, the likely culprit insect (to facilitate treatment advice). Anaphylaxis can be triggered by many allergens and, if a sting was not noted, a history of possible triggers should be sought (e.g. exercise, food, drug). In the absence of a known sting, the patient's activities and time of year might provide circumstantial evidence of a sting (e.g. warm weather outdoor activities, cutting hedges, proximity to nesting locations). If the patient can bring the insect in a jar, identification can be achieved. Otherwise, questions about nests and activities may help identification: yellow jackets (ground nesting, gardening, picnics, garbage cans), hornets (large tree/shrub nests), wasps (honeycombed nests in eaves, shrubs, scavenge like yellow jackets), honeybees (tree hollows), fire ants (mounds in the ground).

Physical examination

- If a patient is presenting acutely, emergency management may be needed to treat an allergic reaction or anaphylaxis. A thorough examination to identify skin, respiratory, or cardiovascular signs and symptoms is required. If symptoms are present, the clinician can directly confirm if the response is localized or systemic, including whether it is systemic but isolated to the skin (e.g. solely urticaria), as these determinations may have consequences for deciding upon VIT. Stingers should be removed by scraping rather than grasping the venom sac, which could squeeze more venom into the patient. If fire ant stings are suspected, a ring of pseudopustules might be identifiable.

Laboratory diagnosis

List of diagnostic tests

- Diagnostic testing is generally reserved for situations where VIT is or may be indicated (see Treatment section).
- Skin tests (prick, possibly followed by intracutaneous) should be used for initial measurement of venom-specific IgE. Extracts of honeybee, yellow jacket, white-faced hornet, yellow hornet, and wasp venom are available for testing. Cross-sensitization and cross-reactivity are high between hornet and yellow jacket, less for hornet and yellow jacket with wasp, and even less between honeybee and the others. Bumblebee venom has unique allergens with variable cross-reactivity to honeybee. Skin prick tests may be performed with concentrations of up to 100 µg/mL, and if negative followed by intracutaneous tests starting at 0.001 or 0.01 µg/mL and increasing 10-fold up to 1.0 µg/mL. Skin tests should be repeated at another time if they are initially negative and there was a severe reaction. Positive tests (with appropriate negative and positive controls) of any size indicate potential allergy of any severity. Whole body extracts of fire ant are available for evaluating fire ant hypersensitivity. There is limited cross-reactivity between fire ant venom and other Hymenoptera venom. Fire ant testing may begin with full strength extract and if negative proceed to intracutaneous testing of 1 : 1 million wt/vol up to 1 : 1000 or 1 : 500. If the history clearly indicates a fire ant reaction, tests for flying Hymenoptera are generally not pursued. If there was a reaction to a sting, even from an identified flying Hymenoptera, testing to multiple Hymenoptera is generally pursued.
- In vitro testing for venom-specific IgE is indicated if skin tests are negative in selected patients, particularly the patient who has experienced a severe reaction.
- Serum tryptase levels should be obtained in persons with negative tests and severe reactions, and considered in patients with severe reactions.

Potential pitfalls/common errors made regarding diagnosis of disease

- Testing may be negative during a "refractory period" following a sting reaction; consider retesting in 3–6 weeks.
- A patient who had a serious sting reaction and then tolerated a subsequent sting may still be at risk for insect sting anaphylaxis and should be tested.
- Large local reactions might be misdiagnosed as cellulitis.

Section 4: Treatment (Algorithm 31.2)

Treatment rationale

- Mild local (non-allergic) reactions can be approached with symptomatic treatment for pain, using cold compresses and analgesics. Large local reactions can be treated similarly, with

Algorithm 31.2 Treatment of insect sting allergy

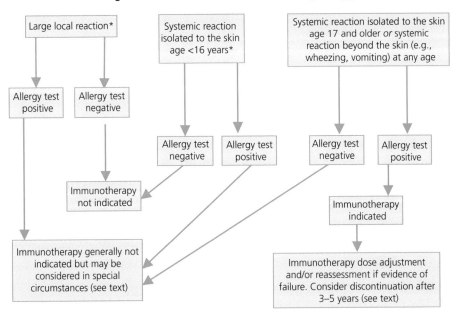

*Testing generally not indicated (see algorithm 31.1).

antihistamines as additional therapy for itch and consideration of using oral corticosteroids (proof of efficacy with controlled studies is lacking). Insect sting-induced anaphylaxis is treated like anaphylaxis from any cause with injectable epinephrine and supportive therapy. Delayed treatment with epinephrine has been associated with fatal reactions. Cutaneous systemic reactions can be treated with antihistamines.

- Immunotherapy is indicated for patients older than 16 years with isolated cutaneous systemic reactions, all patients with systemic reactions including organ systems other than skin when testing is positive because these patients are at higher risk for recurrence of a severe reaction upon re-sting. VIT may be considered for other circumstances, including patients with large local reactions who are likely to sustain frequent stings, and children who experienced isolated cutaneous systemic reactions but are likely to experience frequent subsequent stings (especially if the trigger was fire ants). Controversy exists as to whether all venoms eliciting positive tests should be used for treatment, or fewer venoms based on insect identification and known cross-reactivity.
- Treatment includes instruction on allergen avoidance, carrying self-injectable epinephrine, and wearing medical identification jewelry.

When to hospitalize
- Patients with anaphylaxis who require supportive care may require hospitalization.

Table of treatment

Treatment	Circumstances
Conservative Cold compresses, analgesics	Local and large local reactions, pain
Antihistamines	Itch
Medical Venom immunotherapy	VIT is typically started at a dose of 0.1–1 µg weekly and incrementally increased to a treatment dose of 100 µg of each venom (similar to two stings). Rapid schedules are an option. Dosing eventually may be every 6–8 weeks. VIT may elicit allergic reactions. Treatment doses might be increased if subsequent stings result in a reaction. Treatment is typically continued for 3–5 years, but may be extended depending on particular patient circumstances
Fire ant immunotherapy	Immunotherapy maintenance dose goals are 0.5 mL of 1 : 100 wt/vol or possibly a 1 : 10 concentration. Immunotherapy may elicit allergic reactions. Treatment duration is less well studied than VIT but is typically continued for 3–5 years; but it may be extended depending on particular patient circumstances
Prescription of epinephrine auto-injector to self-carry	Recommended for all patients who experienced a life-threatening reaction (even if testing is negative) and may be considered for any patient with prior allergic reactions (e.g. those with large local reactions, children with isolated cutaneous systemic reactions)
Antihistamines	For treatment of allergic reactions (itch, swelling)

Prevention/management of complications

- Immunotherapy can induce allergic reactions, including anaphylaxis. Patients are kept under observation for 30 minutes following an injection and should carry self-injectable epinephrine. Premedication with antihistamines can be considered to reduce local reactions. Rarely, VIT can induce a serum sickness type reaction.
- Although typical duration of therapy is 3–5 years, it may be extended for circumstances such as: high risk patients (near fatal reactions, honeybee allergy, increased baseline tryptase, underlying medical conditions, frequent exposures), quality of life considerations, and the fact that optimal treatment duration before any hypersensitivity is unknown.

CLINICAL PEARLS
- Indications for treatment with immunotherapy are based upon the clinical history and test results indicating an increased subsequent risk of anaphylaxis.
- For patients at risk of anaphylaxis, VIT is up to 98% effective in reducing the risk of subsequent severe sting reactions.
- Patients should be educated about allergen avoidance, carrying self-injectable epinephrine, and wearing medical identification jewelry.

Section 5: Special populations

Pregnancy
- Treatment of insect sting anaphylaxis is no different from treatment of anaphylaxis in pregnancy.
- VIT may be continued at the previously tolerated dose, but is generally not initiated or escalated during pregnancy.

Children
- The natural history of insect sting anaphylaxis in children is different from adults in that isolated cutaneous systemic reactions in children are not likely to portend future severe reactions. Therefore, indications for VIT differ between children and adults.

Elderly
Not applicable for this topic.

Others
- Concomitant medications: patients taking beta-blockers or angiotensin converting enzyme inhibitors may be at greater risk for anaphylaxis to insect stings and VIT, and should be switched to an alternative medication if possible.

Section 6: Prognosis

BOTTOM LINE/CLINICAL PEARLS
- Treatment with VIT is highly effective to prevent subsequent sting anaphylaxis.
- The risk of subsequent anaphylaxis generally decreases with time.
- The prognosis for children is generally better than for adults.

Natural history of untreated disease
- For children with cutaneous systemic reactions, the risk of subsequent anaphylaxis decreases from 10% to 5% after 10 years.
- For adults with cutaneous systemic reactions, the risk of subsequent anaphylaxis decreases from 20% to 10% after 10 years.
- For children with systemic anaphylaxis, the risk of subsequent anaphylaxis decreases from 40% to 30% after 10 years.
- For adults with systemic anaphylaxis, the risk of subsequent anaphylaxis decreases from 60% to 40% after 10 years.

Prognosis for treated patients
- Immunotherapy is up to 98% effective in reducing the risk of anaphylaxis upon subsequent stings.

Follow-up tests and monitoring
- Repeat testing may be considered because the prognosis after 3–5 years of VIT may be better if tests have become negative.

Section 7: Reading list

Bernstein IL, Li JT, Bernstein DI, Hamilton R, Spector SL, Tan R, et al. Allergy diagnostic testing: an updated practice parameter. Ann Allergy Asthma Immunol 2008;100(Suppl 3):S1–148

Bonadonna P, Zanotti R, Caruso B, Castellani L, Perbellini O, Colarossi S, et al. Allergen specific immunotherapy is safe and effective in patients with systemic mastocytosis and Hymenoptera allergy. J Allergy Clin Immunol 2008;121:256–7

Bonadonna P, Perbellini O, Passalacqua G, Caruso B, Colarossi S, Dal Fior D, et al. Clonal mast cell disorders in patients with systemic reactions to Hymenoptera stings and increased serum tryptase levels. J Allergy Clin Immunol 2009;123:680–6

Boyle RJ, Elremeli M, Hockenhull J, Cherry MG, Bulsara MK, Daniels M, et al. Venom immunotherapy for preventing allergic reactions to insect stings. Cochrane Database Syst Rev 2012;10:CD008838

Cox L, Nelson H, Lockey R, Calabria C, Chacko T, Finegold I, et al. Allergen immunotherapy: a practice parameter third update. J Allergy Clin Immunol 2011;127(Suppl):S1–55

Golden DB, Kelly D, Hamilton RG, Craig TJ. Venom immunotherapy reduces large local reactions to insect stings. J Allergy Clin Immunol 2009;123:1371–5

Golden DB, Moffitt J, Nicklas RA, Freeman T, Graft DF, Reisman RE, et al. Stinging insect hypersensitivity: a practice parameter update 2011. J Allergy Clin Immunol 2011;127:852–4

Incorvaia C, Frati F, Dell'Albani I, Robino A, Cattaneo E, Mauro M, et al. Safety of hymenoptera venom immunotherapy: a systematic review. Expert Opin Pharmacother 2011;12:2527–32

Tracy JM. Insect allergy. Mt Sinai J Med 2011;78:773–83

Tracy JM, Khan FS, Demain JG. Insect anaphylaxis: where are we? The stinging facts 2012. Curr Opin Allergy Clin Immunol 2012;12:400–5

Suggested websites

www.aaaai.org
www.acaai.org

Section 8: Guidelines
National society guidelines

Guideline title	Guideline source	Date
Stinging insect hypersensitivity: a practice parameter update 2011	Joint Council	2011 (http://www.aaaai.org/conditions-and-treatments/allergies/stinging-insect-allergy.aspx)
Allergy diagnostic testing: an updated practice parameter	Joint Council	2008 (http://www.aaaai.org/Aaaai/media/MediaLibrary/PDF%20Documents/Practice%20and%20Parameters/allergydiagnostictesting.pdf)
Allergen immunotherapy: a practice parameter third update	Joint Council	2011 (http://www.aaaai.org/Aaaai/media/MediaLibrary/PDF%20Documents/Practice%20and%20Parameters/Allergen-immunotherapy-Jan-2011.pdf)

Section 9: Evidence
See Boyle et al. 2012 (see reading list).

Section 10: Images
Not applicable for this topic.

Additional material for this chapter can be found online at:
www.mountsinaiexpertguides.com
This includes a case study, multiple choice questions (provided by
Hugh Sampson), advice for patients, and ICD codes

CHAPTER 32

Latex Allergy

Jennifer S. Kim

NorthShore University HealthSystem, Evanston, IL, USA

OVERALL BOTTOM LINE

- Latex allergy prevalence peaked in the 1990s when universal precautions were instituted.
- Contact irritant (not allergic) dermatitis is the most common adverse reaction to latex medical glove wear.
- History is the most reliable indicator of latex allergy supported by a serologic test. Other confirmatory tests are limited by reagent availability in the United States and lack of standardization.
- Cross-reactivity between latex and certain fruits (i.e. avocado, banana, chestnut, kiwi) may have clinical implications.

Section 1: Background

Definition of disease

- Clinical manifestations of latex allergy include non-IgE-mediated allergic contact dermatitis and IgE-mediated urticaria, rhinoconjunctivitis, asthma, and anaphylaxis.

Disease classification

- Latex refers to natural rubber latex, a product manufactured from a milky fluid derived from the tropical rubber tree *Hevea brasiliensis*. There are 14 known Hevea latex allergens: Hev b 1 through Hev b 14.

Incidence/prevalence

- Prevalence is highest in health care workers (8–17%) and patients frequently exposed to latex via multiple surgeries, such as those with spina bifida (up to 68%). Less than 1% of the general population is affected.
- In 1991, the US FDA convened an international symposium on latex allergy due to increasing prevalence, which peaked in the mid to late 1990s.
- As a result of the increased use of non-latex gloves, prevalence rates have dramatically decreased.

Economic impact

- Conversion to a latex-safe environment was associated with an initial increase in cost but has been offset by the decreased costs of diagnosis and disability incurred by latex sensitivity.

Mount Sinai Expert Guides: Allergy and Clinical Immunology, First Edition. Edited by Hugh A. Sampson.
© 2015 John Wiley & Sons, Ltd. Published 2015 by John Wiley & Sons, Ltd.
Companion website: www.mountsinaiexpertguides.com

Etiology

- Universal precautions were implemented during the 1980s AIDS crisis. In 1992, the US Occupational Safety and Health Administration (OSHA) issued the Blood-born Pathogens Standard which required protective glove use. Increased demand for natural rubber latex combined with limited supply resulted in the use of stimulant chemicals that induced higher levels of latex allergen. Rapid turnover minimized latex protein denaturation, which occurs naturally during storage.

Pathology/pathogenesis

- Latex is ammoniated to prevent microbial growth and subsequently utilized to manufacture dipped products such as medical gloves and catheters. The majority of allergic reactions to latex result from exposure to dipped rubber products. In addition, the presence of powder in gloves permits latex allergen to aerosolize, thereby potentially inducing respiratory symptoms.

Predictive/risk factors

- Use of powdered latex products.
- Frequent exposure via occupation and frequent surgeries.
- Atopy.

Section 2: Prevention

> **BOTTOM LINE/CLINICAL PEARLS**
> - Use non-latex gloves for handling non-infectious materials.
> - If latex gloves are used, use powder-free gloves.
> - Avoid oil-based creams and lotions that cause latex deterioration, thereby increasing allergen exposure.
> - Wash and dry hands after latex exposure.

Screening

- It is not recommended to screen patients for latex allergy in the absence of a suggestive history.

Primary prevention

- Avoid exposure to latex.

Secondary prevention

- Avoid contact with latex.
- Avoid areas where powder from latex gloves may be inhaled.
- Wear medical alert identification.

Section 3: Diagnosis

> **BOTTOM LINE/CLINICAL PEARLS**
> - The most reliable indicator of latex allergy is a strong clinical history.
> - Examination findings immediately after latex exposure include urticaria, rhinoconjunctivitis, asthma symptoms, and anaphylaxis.
> - Serologic testing for IgE sensitization to latex can be performed to confirm diagnosis, but negative serology does not absolutely exclude latex allergy.

Differential diagnosis

Differential diagnosis	Features
Irritant contact dermatitis	Dry, itchy, irritated skin (usually hands)

Typical presentation
- Symptoms usually begin within minutes to hours of exposure. Reactions may be more significant with mucosal exposure. Mild reactions can present with erythema, urticaria, and itching. More severe reactions may produce respiratory symptoms such as rhinorrhea, laryngeal pruritus, cough, wheeze, or shortness of breath. Rarely, shock may occur. A life-threatening reaction is seldom the first sign of allergy.

Clinical diagnosis
History
- Assess the patient's symptoms and timing of reaction to potential latex exposure. Assess potential sources of latex exposure in medical, dental, school, and household supplies. Examples include toys, balloons, cleaning gloves, condoms, swim caps, erasers, pacifiers, adhesives, and elasticized fabrics.

Physical examination
- Evaluate skin for erythema, urticaria, and pruritus within 10–15 minutes of direct contact. If the patient is being evaluated during the reaction, evaluate for signs of rhinitis, asthma, or anaphylaxis.

Useful clinical decision rules and calculators
- Patients allergic to fruits have a significantly lower risk of latex reaction whereas patients with latex allergy have a relatively higher risk of reaction to fruits implicated in the latex–fruit syndrome. Examples of cross-reactive foods include banana, avocado, kiwi, and chestnut as well as apple, carrot, celery, melon, papaya, potato, and tomato.

Disease severity classification
Not applicable for this topic.

Laboratory diagnosis
List of diagnostic tests
- Testing for type I (immediate) hypersensitivity to latex can be performed via serology or skin prick testing to assess the presence of IgE sensitization to latex proteins. Sensitization without a history of a reaction, however, is not sufficient to make a diagnosis of latex allergy given the high rate of false positive test results.
- There is no commercial skin prick test reagent available in the United States. Individually prepared extracts from latex products have been shown to vary widely in allergen content. Puncturing through a latex glove as an alternative is not encouraged because of the risk of systemic allergic reactions from a potentially high dose exposure.
- Type IV hypersensitivity (contact dermatitis) is diagnosed primarily via history. Patch testing may be performed if a reagent is available.
- Provocation testing is generally not recommended except by trained specialists.

Not applicable for this topic.

Potential pitfalls/common errors made regarding diagnosis of disease

- Contact irritant dermatitis is the most common adverse reaction to latex and may be exacerbated by sweating caused by occlusion, prolonged contact with alkaline pH (powder), frequent handwashing, and use of chemical sanitizers. This is a relatively benign and non-life-threatening condition.

Section 4: Treatment

Treatment rationale

- Implementation of latex avoidance measures is key. Topical steroids may be used to treat contact allergic dermatitis. Oral antihistamines may be used to treat pruritus, urticaria, or mild upper respiratory symptoms (i.e. rhinitis). Treatment of asthma symptoms and anaphylaxis are addressed fully in other chapters.

When to hospitalize

- Individuals experiencing severe anaphylactic reactions.

Managing the hospitalized patient

- It is recommended that patients who are latex allergic have surgical procedures performed as first cases in the morning when levels of latex aeroallergens are lowest. All medical products should be made of non-latex materials.

Table of treatment

Not applicable for this topic.

Prevention/management of complications

- Prophylaxis with H1-blockers, H2-blockers, and steroids is not recommended for patients with a documented latex allergy undergoing a surgical procedure. Complete avoidance of latex-containing materials is the treatment of choice.

CLINICAL PEARLS
- Prevention is the cornerstone in the management of latex sensitization.
- Non-latex materials should be substituted for all latex-containing items.

Section 5: Special populations

- Prevalence is highest for patients receiving multiple surgeries and for individuals having occupational exposures to latex gloves.

Section 6: Prognosis

BOTTOM LINE/CLINICAL PEARLS
- Avoidance of latex is the only way to prevent an allergic reaction.
- People at risk of anaphylaxis to latex should carry self-injectable epinephrine with them at all times.

Natural history of untreated disease

Not applicable for this topic.

Prognosis for treated patients

Not applicable for this topic.

Follow-up tests and monitoring

Not applicable for this topic.

Section 7: Reading list

Bousquet J, Flahault A, Vandenplas O, Ameille J, Duron JJ, Pecquet C, et al. Natural rubber latex allergy among health care workers: a systemic review of the evidence. J Allergy Clin Immunol 2006:118:447–54

Cabañes N, Igea JM, de la Hoz B, Agustín P, Blanco C, Domínguez J, et al. Latex allergy: Position Paper. J Investig Allergol Clin Immunol 2012;22:313–30

Hamilton RG. Latex allergy. UpToDate, updated June 20, 2012.

Hepner DL, Castells MC. Latex allergy: an update. Anesth Analg 2003:96:1219–29

Suggested websites

www.Latexallergyresources.org

https://www.osha.gov/SLTC/latexallergy/

http://www.cdc.gov/niosh/topics/latex/

Section 8: Guidelines
National society guidelines

Guideline title	Guideline source	Date
The diagnosis and management of anaphylaxis: an updated practice parameter	Joint Task Force on Practice Parameters; American Academy of Allergy, Asthma and Immunology (AAAAI); American College of Allergy, Asthma and Immunology (ACAAI); Joint Council of Allergy, Asthma and Immunology	2005 (http://www.ncbi.nlm.nih.gov/pubmed/15753926)

International society guidelines

Guideline title	Guideline source	Date
Latex allergy: Position Paper	Committee of Latex Allergy; Spanish Society of Allergology and Clinical Immunology (SEAIC)	2012 (http://www.ncbi.nlm.nih.gov/pubmed/23101306)

Section 9: Evidence

Not applicable for this topic.

Section 10: Images
Not applicable for this topic.

Additional material for this chapter can be found online at:
www.mountsinaiexpertguides.com
This includes a case study, multiple choice questions, advice for
patients, and ICD codes

CHAPTER 33

Allergy to Antibiotics

Jennifer S. Kim

NorthShore University HealthSystem, Evanston, IL, USA

OVERALL BOTTOM LINE
- Hypersensitivity reactions to antibiotics are commonly reported but often over-diagnosed.
- Penicillin is the most commonly reported drug allergy, but in large-scale studies approximately 90% of these individuals were able to tolerate penicillins.
- Skin tests have been well validated for beta-lactams (penicillins and cephalosporins) but less so for other classes of antibiotics.
- Skin testing is indicated only for type I and IV hypersensitivity reactions.

Section 1: Background

Definition of disease

- Antibiotics can act as antigens and elicit an immune response. Reactions should be defined as allergic when an immunologic mechanism is demonstrated.

Disease classification

- Drug reactions can be classified clinically as immediate (within 1 hour of drug administration) and non-immediate, as recommended by the World Allergy Organization.

Incidence/prevalence

- Antibiotic hypersensitivity reactions have an estimated prevalence of 5–10%.

Economic impact

- Over-diagnosis of drug allergy creates an increase in treatment costs because of unnecessary use of broad-spectrum antibiotics, which is a risk factor for development of multiple drug-resistant bacteria.
- Studies have shown penicillin skin testing in those patients with a history of penicillin allergy results in large decreases in use of vancomycin and quinolones. Use of expensive broad-spectrum antibiotics results in higher medical costs and compromised clinical care because of the development of multiple drug-resistant bacteria.

Etiology

- In order to cause an allergic reaction, the antibiotic must be recognized by the immune system.

Mount Sinai Expert Guides: Allergy and Clinical Immunology, First Edition. Edited by Hugh A. Sampson.
© 2015 John Wiley & Sons, Ltd. Published 2015 by John Wiley & Sons, Ltd.
Companion website: www.mountsinaiexpertguides.com

Pathology/pathogenesis

- Immunologic hypersensitivity reactions can be classified into four categories according to the Gell and Coombs system:
  - *Type I:* immediate in onset and mediated by IgE and mast cells and/or basophils;
  - *Type II:* delayed in onset and caused by antibody (usually IgG) mediated cell destruction;
  - *Type III:* delayed in onset and caused by IgG: drug immune complex deposition and complement activation; and
  - *Type IV:* delayed in onset and T-cell-mediated.
- Types I, II, and III are antibody-mediated while type IV is mediated by T cells.

Predictive/risk factors

- Female sex.
- Recurrent drug exposure.
- HIV/AIDS, particularly for sulfonamides.
- Certain HLA-B alleles may represent risk factors for reactions to a particular drug. Examples include SJS/TEN to carbamazepine in Han Chinese is strongly associated with HLA-B*15:02, drug-induced hypersensitivity syndrome (aka DRESS) and STS/TEN to allopurinol with HLA-B*58:01, and DRESS to abacavir in HLA-B*57:01 patients.

Section 2: Prevention

No interventions have been demonstrated to prevent the development of the disease.

Screening

- HLA-B typing is generally not recommended at this time. The exception is for patients being considered for therapy with abacavir as hypersensitivity occurs exclusively in HLA-B*57:01 patients.

Primary prevention

Not applicable for this topic.

Secondary prevention

- Based on limited data, 10–38% of patients selectively allergic to amoxicillin or ampicillin (tolerant of penicillin) react to the corresponding cephalosporin. Thus, patients with amoxicillin allergy should avoid cephalosporins with identical R-group side chains (cefadroxil, cefprozil, and cefatrizine). Similarly, patients with ampicillin allergy should avoid cephalexin, cefaclor, cephradine, cephaloglycin, and loracarbef.

Section 3: Diagnosis (Algorithm 33.1)

> **BOTTOM LINE/CLINICAL PEARLS**
> - Immunologic drug reactions may be divided into four categories according to the Gell and Coombs system. Types I and IV are far more common than types II and III.
> - These different types of allergic reactions each have characteristic signs and symptoms although clinically there may be significant overlap.
> - The diagnosis of type I (immediate) allergic reactions to antibiotics is based on clinical history, skin testing when available, and graded challenge if indicated. Patch testing can be used to confirm type IV reactions.

Algorithm 33.1 Diagnosis of immediate allergic reactions to beta-lactams

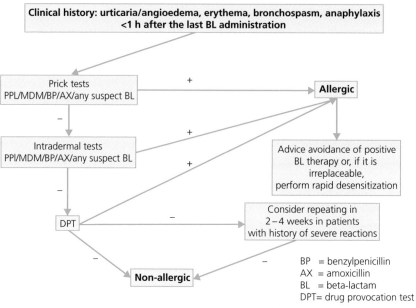

Source: Romano A, Caubet JC. Antibiotic allergies in children and adults: from clinical symptoms to skin testing diagnosis. J Allergy Clin Immunol Pract 2014;2:3–12. Reproduced with permission of Elsevier.

Differential diagnosis
- This is dependent on the clinical presentation of the individual patient as drug allergy represents a spectrum of hypersensitivity reactions with heterogeneous mechanisms and clinical presentations.

Typical presentation
Not applicable for this topic.

Clinical diagnosis
History
- Evaluation involves a meticulous history of past and present drug reactions, review of the medical record, and analysis of temporal patterns between drug administration and onset of symptoms.

Physical examination
- Perform a meticulous skin examination. Assess for lymphadenopathy or organomegaly.

Useful clinical decision rules and calculators
- Patients having a history of severe delayed-onset systemic reactions and/or exfoliating dermatoses should not receive the suspected antibiotic again under any circumstances and need not undergo diagnostic testing.

Disease severity classification
Not applicable for this topic.

Laboratory diagnosis

List of diagnostic tests
- Skin testing has been well validated for penicillins. The negative predictive value of penicillin skin testing (with PPL, penicillin G, and penicilloate and/or penilloate) for serious immediate-type reactions approaches 99%. Consider performing graded challenges in patients with a low likelihood of being allergic (e.g. those with distant (>10 years) or vague reaction histories).
- Specific IgE in vitro assays are available, although most are not adequately validated with unclear specificity and sensitivity and lack internal positive controls
- For moderate to severe allergic reactions, a complete blood count and differential and tests of liver and renal function should be obtained. This evaluation is indicated if the exanthema is substantial, bullous or pustular, confluent, involves a substantial portion of the body surface area, or if general symptoms (malaise, skin pain, lymphadenopathy) are present.
- Serum tryptase may be elevated if measured within 1–3 hours of symptom onset of anaphylaxis.

Lists of imaging techniques
Not applicable for this topic.

Potential pitfalls/common errors made regarding diagnosis of disease
- Maculopapular exanthems and delayed skin eruptions are common in children and are mainly associated with viral infections.
- Routine repeat penicillin skin testing is not indicated in patients with a history of penicillin allergy who have tolerated one or more courses of oral penicillin.

Section 4: Treatment
Treatment rationale
- There are three options for providing continued treatment in patients with confirmed drug allergy: administration of an unrelated medication, administration of a related medication, and desensitization to the culprit drug.

When to hospitalize
- Stevens–Johnson syndrome (SJS), toxic epidermal necrolysis (TEN), and acute generalized exanthematous pustulosis (AGEP) are severe reactions that may require hospitalization depending on extent of skin involvement. Consider treatment in a burn care unit.
- Patients having drug reaction or rash with eosinophilia and systemic symptom (DRESS) must be monitored for progression of skin eruption and/or development of organ failure (liver, kidney, lung).

Managing the hospitalized patient
Not applicable for this topic.

Table of treatment

Treatment	Comment
Conservative Avoid antibiotic suspected to induce reaction. If continued antimicrobial therapy necessary, utilize drug from unrelated class	This is appropriate for patients in whom the diagnosis of drug allergy has been confirmed
Medical Consult with infectious disease specialist to provide effective antibiotic alternatives. Allergist will then perform risk assessment to select antibiotic of lowest potential risk to patient	If skin test results are negative to a related drug (e.g. beta-lactams), then graded challenge to the related drug can be performed

Prevention/management of complications
- Desensitization should be considered in patients who are proven or strongly suspected to have an immediate, IgE-mediated allergy, for whom there are no acceptable alternative antibiotics. The potential benefits must outweigh the potential risks. Desensitization is temporary as sensitivity returns after the antibiotic is cleared from the body. This procedure should be performed in the hospital setting by trained clinicians and experienced staff equipped to treat and manage anaphylaxis.
- Graded challenges are contraindicated in patients demonstrating exfoliative dermatitis, end-organ involvement, or mucous membrane involvement as part of their allergic reaction.

> **CLINICAL PEARLS**
> - Immediate reactions (type I IgE-mediated) develop within 1 hour of the administered dose.
> - Delayed reactions typically begin after multiple doses and mostly consist of relatively benign rashes. However, rare delayed systemic reactions can be severe.
> - Skin testing has been validated mainly for beta-lactams. Use of graded challenges is recommended in those deemed as having low risk of reaction.

Section 5: Special populations
Pregnancy
Not applicable for this topic.

Children
- Children are more likely to present with a benign rash while taking antibiotic treatments. Immediate hypersensitivity to beta-lactams is particularly rare in children.

Elderly
Not applicable for this topic.

Others
- Patients with positive penicillin skin test responses have a slightly increased risk of reacting to cephalosporins.
- Beside penicillins, sulfonamide antibiotics are the most common cause of drug-induced allergic reactions. They most commonly cause delayed cutaneous eruptions; IgE-mediated reactions are relatively infrequent. Sulfonamides are by far the most common cause of SJS and TEN.

Section 6: Prognosis

> **BOTTOM LINE/CLINICAL PEARLS**
> - Limit antibiotic use. Obtain cultures to confirm diagnosis. Administer appropriate vaccines.
> - Consider treating through mild cutaneous reactions if alternative treatments incur greater risk of adverse events.
> - Initiate new medications at lower doses than normal when feasible.

Natural history of untreated disease

Not applicable for this topic.

Prognosis for treated patients

Not applicable for this topic.

Follow-up tests and monitoring

Not applicable for this topic.

Section 7: Reading list

Khan DA, Solensky R. Drug allergy. J Allergy Clin Immunol 2010;125(Suppl 2):S126–37
Romano A, Caubet JC. Antibiotic allergies in children and adults: from clinical symptoms to skin testing diagnosis. J Allergy Clin Immunol Pract 2014;2:3–12
Solensky R. Allergy to β-lactam antibiotics. J Allergy Clin Immunol 2012;130:1442–2.e5

Suggested website

Uptodate.com

Section 8: Guidelines
National society guidelines

Guideline title	Guideline source	Date
Executive summary of disease management of drug hypersensitivity: a practice parameter	Joint Task Force on Practice Parameters; American Academy of Allergy, Asthma and Immunology (AAAAI); American College of Allergy, Asthma and Immunology (ACAAI); Joint Council of Allergy, Asthma and Immunology	1999 (http://www.ncbi.nlm.nih.gov/pubmed/10616910)
The diagnosis and management of anaphylaxis: an updated practice parameter	Joint Task Force on Practice Parameters; American Academy of Allergy, Asthma and Immunology (AAAAI); American College of Allergy, Asthma and Immunology (ACAAI); Joint Council of Allergy, Asthma and Immunology	2005 (http://www.ncbi.nlm.nih.gov/pubmed/15753926)
Drug allergy: an updated practice parameter	Joint Task Force on Practice Parameters; American Academy of Allergy, Asthma and Immunology (AAAAI); American College of Allergy, Asthma and Immunology (ACAAI); Joint Council of Allergy, Asthma and Immunology	2010 (http://www.ncbi.nlm.nih.gov/pubmed/20934625)

Section 9: Evidence

Not applicable for this topic.

Section 10: Images

Penicillin   **Cephalosporin**

Figure 33.1 The solid arrows indicate the core four-member beta-lactam ring within both penicillins and cephalosporins. Open arrows indicate the five- and six-member side rings for penicillins and cephalosporins, respectively. R indicates additional side chain sites where substitutions of various chemical groups produce different antimicrobial spectra, pharmacokinetics, or stability to beta-lactamases.

Additional material for this chapter can be found online at:
www.mountsinaiexpertguides.com
This includes a case study, multiple choice questions, advice for patients, and ICD code

CHAPTER 34

Allergy to Non-Antibiotic Drugs

Jacob D. Kattan

Division of Allergy/Immunology, Department of Pediatrics, Icahn School of Medicine at Mount Sinai, New York, NY, USA

OVERALL BOTTOM LINE

- Drug allergy, or an immunologic drug reaction, is unpredictable, is unrelated to the pharmacologic actions of the drug, and occurs in susceptible individuals.
- An allergic drug reaction results from a specific immunologic response to a medication.
- Immunologic reactions are classified into four types according to the Gell and Coombs system:
  - *Type I:* immediate in onset and mediated by IgE and mast cells and/or basophils;
  - *Type II:* delayed in onset and caused by antibody-mediated cell destruction;
  - *Type III:* delayed in onset and caused by immune complex deposition and complement activation;
  - *Type IV:* delayed in onset and T-cell mediated.
- In addition to antibiotics, drugs that commonly cause allergic reactions include cancer chemotherapeutic agents, neuromuscular blocking agents, local anesthetics, opiates, radiocontrast media, aspirin, non-steroidal anti-inflammatory drugs, angiotensin-converting enzyme inhibitors, biologic modifying agents, and medications for patients with HIV infections and AIDS such as antiretroviral drugs.

Section 1: Background

Definition of disease

- A drug allergy is a hypersensitivity drug reaction that results from a specific immunologic mechanism (either drug-specific antibody or T cell) to a medication. It is usually unpredictable, occurs in a susceptible subgroup of patients, and has signs and symptoms that are not a result of the pharmacologic actions of the drug.

Disease classification

- The World Allergy Organization recommends dividing immunologic drug reactions into immediate reactions (typical onset within 1 hour of exposure) and non-immediate (onset after 1 hour). Examples of immediate reactions include urticaria, angioedema, and anaphylaxis. Examples of non-immediate reactions include fixed drug eruptions, Stevens–Johnson syndrome, and drug reaction with eosinophilia and systemic symptoms (DRESS).

Mount Sinai Expert Guides: Allergy and Clinical Immunology, First Edition. Edited by Hugh A. Sampson.

© 2015 John Wiley & Sons, Ltd. Published 2015 by John Wiley & Sons, Ltd.

Companion website: www.mountsinaiexpertguides.com

Incidence/prevalence
- Drug hypersensitivity reactions affect more than 7% of the general population.
- It is difficult to determine a precise prevalence as there may be under-diagnosis of drug allergy due to under-reporting or over-diagnosis due to an overuse of the term allergy.

Etiology
- A drug allergic reaction is caused by recognition of the drug by the immune system.

Pathology/pathogenesis
- Immunologic reactions are classified into four types:
  - *Type I:* immediate in onset and mediated by IgE and mast cells and/or basophils;
  - *Type II:* delayed in onset and caused by antibody (usually IgG) mediated cell destruction;
  - *Type III:* delayed in onset and caused by immune complex deposition and complement activation;
  - *Type IV:* delayed in onset and T-cell mediated.

Predictive/risk factors
- Amount and duration of drug exposure.
- Parenteral and cutaneous administration of the drug.
- Female sex.
- Prior history of allergic reaction to one or more drugs.
- HLA B 5701 in Caucasians (abacavir).
- HLA B 1502 in Han Chinese, Indian, and Thai populations (carbamazepine).
- HLA A 3101 in northern Europeans (carbamazepine).
- HLA B 5801 in Han Chinese and Caucasians (allopurinol).
- HIV/AIDS.
- Systemic lupus erythematosus.

Section 2: Prevention
There are no interventions that have been demonstrated to prevent the development of disease.

Screening
Not applicable for this topic.

Primary prevention
- Use of oral drugs when possible is likely to produce fewer drug reactions than the use of topical or parenteral medications.
- Avoid unnecessary prescribing of drugs that are often associated with adverse reactions.

Secondary prevention
- Withdrawal of the offending drug is the first step in preventing future reactions.
- Desensitization to a medication that is known to have caused an allergic reaction in the past can temporarily prevent reoccurrence if the medication is required in the future.
- Avoidance of cross-reactive drugs may prevent other drug allergic reactions.

Section 3: Diagnosis (Algorithm 34.1)

BOTTOM LINE/CLINICAL PEARLS
- The history should focus on previous and current medication use and the timing of onset of the reaction in relation to both the initiation of therapy and the precipitating dose.
- The different types of allergic reactions (see Pathology/pathogenesis section) may have different characteristic signs and symptoms, although cutaneous manifestations are the most common presentation for drug allergic reactions. The cutaneous findings include exanthems, angioedema, urticaria, erythema multiforme, bullous eruptions, purpura, and fixed drug eruptions.
- IgE-mediated drug reactions may be confirmed by skin testing, while delayed type IV reactions may be confirmed by patch testing.
- Graded challenge, involving administration of a medication in a graduated manner, can exclude an allergy, and is most appropriate for a patient who is unlikely to be allergic to that drug. These challenges are contraindicated in patients with reactions such as exfoliative dermatitis (Stevens–Johnson syndrome, toxic epidermal necrolysis), blistering or sloughing of the skin, DRESS, or erythema multiforme.

Differential diagnosis
- The differential diagnosis is dependent on the clinical presentation of the individual patient as drug allergy represents a spectrum of hypersensitivity reactions with heterogeneous mechanisms and clinical presentations.

Algorithm 34.1 Diagnosis of drug allergy

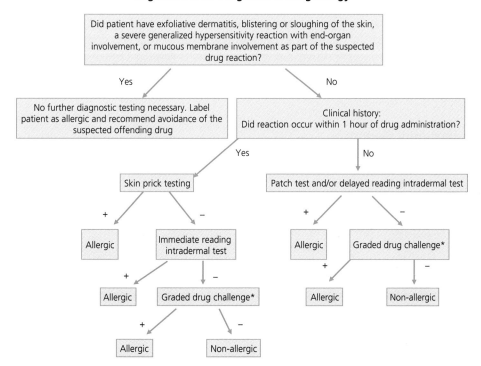

*Graded challenge is used to exclude an allergy to the drug in question, and is typically only performed in patients considered unlikely to be allergic to that drug

Typical presentation
- There are a wide variety of clinical presentations of drug allergy, as this disorder represents a spectrum of hypersensitivity reactions. Immediate drug reactions usually present with urticaria, angioedema, rhinitis, wheezing, vomiting, diarrhea, or anaphylaxis. Non-immediate reactions usually present with a variety of cutaneous symptoms, although other organ symptoms are frequently also involved.

Clinical diagnosis
History
- The history should involve a detailed determination of past and present drug reactions, previous and current medication use, and the timing of onset of the reaction in relation to both the initiation of therapy and the precipitating dose.

Physical examination
- As cutaneous manifestations are the most common presentation for drug allergic reactions, the physical examination should involve a meticulous skin examination. The characterization of cutaneous lesions can be important in determining the cause of the reaction and management decisions. On physical examination, one should also assess for symptoms of anaphylaxis, lymphadenopathy, organomegaly, and all systems that could account for the clinical presentation.

Useful clinical decision rules and calculators
- Severe exfoliative dermatitides, such as Stevens–Johnson syndrome and toxic epidermal necrolysis, are potentially life-threatening reactions characterized by fever and mucocutaneous lesions leading to necrosis and sloughing of the epidermis.
- Patients having a history of delayed-onset systemic reactions or exfoliating dermatitides should never again receive the suspected drug and do not need to undergo diagnostic testing.

Disease severity classification
Not applicable for this topic.

Laboratory diagnosis
List of diagnostic tests
- Testing for drug allergy is limited. While skin testing can be helpful to confirm an immediate hypersensitivity reaction to medication, it has only been fully validated for penicillin.
- An elevated serum tryptase level can help confirm a diagnosis of anaphylaxis, although it may only remain elevated for 2–4 hours after symptom onset because of its short half-life.
- With moderate to severe allergic reactions, a complete blood count and differential and tests of liver and renal function should be obtained.
- Laboratory abnormalities in patients with DRESS include leukocytosis with eosinophil counts >700/μL, increased serum alanine aminotransferase, increased serum creatinine, low grade proteinuria, human herpes virus 6 (HHV-6) infection, and atypical lymphocytosis.

Lists of imaging techniques
Not applicable for this topic.

Potential pitfalls/common errors made regarding diagnosis of disease

- Maculopapular exanthems and delayed skin eruptions are common in children and are mainly associated with viral infections.
- A drug allergy is different from a drug side effect. Drug allergy is a reaction to a drug that occurs as a result of a specific immunologic response in a small number of people while side effects are unwanted effects that anyone who is given enough of a drug can develop.

Section 4: Treatment

Treatment rationale

- Once a drug allergy is confirmed, there are three options for continuing treatment in a patient:
  1. Administer a different, unrelated medication. This is the most straightforward option, although a second line therapy may have its own toxicities or a higher cost.
  2. Administer a related medication. Providing a similar, but not identical medication to the offending drug is an option, although there are cross-reactive reactions that are possible depending on the drug and type of allergic reaction in question.
  3. Desensitize to the culprit drug. This option is available for patients with type I, IgE-mediated drug allergy, and is typically approached when an equally effective alternative drug is not available.

When to hospitalize

- Patients suspected to have Stevens–Johnson syndrome or toxic epidermal necrolysis should be admitted to the hospital, possibly to the intensive care unit or a burn unit depending on the extent of skin involvement and presence of comorbidities.
- Patients with DRESS must be monitored for progression of skin eruption and/or development of organ failure (liver, kidney, lung).
- For patients with anaphylaxis, observation periods must be individualized to each patient, with a minimum observation period of 4–6 hours. In general, those with severe anaphylaxis involving hypoxia, hypotension, or neurologic compromise, or those with moderate reactions that do not respond promptly to epinephrine should be admitted to a hospital.

Managing the hospitalized patient

Not applicable for this topic.

Table of treatment

Treatment	Comment
Conservative Discontinue and avoid the drug suspected to have induced the reaction. Administer a related or unrelated medication	This is appropriate for patients in whom a drug allergy has been confirmed
Medical Desensitize to the offending drug	This is an option in patients with type I IgE-mediated reactions when suitable alternatives are not available

Prevention/management of complications

- Graded challenges and future use of a drug is contraindicated in patients with a history of exfoliative dermatitis, end-organ involvement, or mucous membrane involvement as part of their drug allergy.

CLINICAL PEARLS
- Epinephrine is the treatment of choice for anaphylaxis.
- Glucocorticoids may be necessary for immune complex reactions, drug-induced hematologic diseases, early stages of erythema multiforme, and contact sensitivities.
- When an alternate non-cross-reacting medication cannot be used, induction of drug tolerance procedures can modify a patient's response to a medication and temporarily allow treatment with it safely.

Section 5: Special populations
Not applicable for this topic.

Section 6: Prognosis

BOTTOM LINE/CLINICAL PEARLS
- Avoidance measures are the most effective treatment for preventing recurrent episodes of anaphylaxis.
- Prognosis for patients with Stevens–Johnson syndrome or toxic epidermal necrolysis can be determined by applying a prognostic scoring system called SCORTEN, a system based on clinical and laboratory variables that include patient age, presence of malignancy, body surface area detached, tachycardia, serum urea, glucose, and bicarbonate.
- Most patients with DRESS recover completely in weeks to months after drug withdrawal, although there is a reported mortality rate of 5–10%.

Natural history of untreated disease
Not applicable for this topic.

Prognosis for treated patients
Not applicable for this topic.

Follow-up tests and monitoring
Not applicable for this topic.

Section 7: Reading list

Demoly P, Adkinson NF, Brockow K, Castells M, Chiriac AM, Greenberger PA, et al. International consensus on drug allergy. Allergy 2014;69:420–37

Joint Task Force on Practice Parameters; American Academy of Allergy, Asthma and Immunology; American College of Allergy, Asthma and Immunology; Joint Council of Allergy, Asthma and Immunology. Drug Allergy: an updated practice parameter. Ann Allergy Asthma Immunol 2010;105:259–73

Khan DA. Cutaneous drug reactions. J Allergy Clin Immunol 2012;130:1225

Liu A, Fanning L, Chong H, Fernandez J, Sloane D, Sancho-Serra M, et al. Desensitization regimens for drug allergy: state of the art in the 21st century. Clin Exp Allergy 2011;41:1679–89

Macy E, Ho NJ. Multiple drug intolerance syndrome: prevalence, clinical characteristics, and management. Ann Allergy Asthma Immunol 2012;108:88–93

Suggested websites

American Academy of Allergy Asthma and Immunology. www.aaaai.org

American College of Allergy, Asthma and Immunology. www.acaai.org

Uptodate.com

Section 8: Guidelines

National society guidelines

Guideline title	Guideline source	Date
Drug allergy: an updated practice parameter	Joint Task Force on Practice Parameters, representing the American Academy of Allergy, Asthma and Immunology (AAAAI), the American College of Allergy, Asthma and Immunology (ACAAI), and the Joint Council of Allergy, Asthma and Immunology (JCAAI)	2010 (https://www.aaaai.org/Aaaai/media/MediaLibrary/PDF%20Documents/Practice%20and%20Parameters/drug-allergy-updated-practice-param.pdf)

International society guidelines

Guideline title	Guideline source	Date
International consensus on drug allergy	The International Collaboration in Asthma, Allergy and Immunology (iCAALL), formed by the European Academy of Allergy and Clinical Immunology (EAACI), the AAAAI, the ACAAI, and the World Allergy Organization (WAO)	2014 (http://onlinelibrary.wiley.com/doi/10.1111/all.12350/abstract)

Section 9: Evidence

See guidelines listed in Section 8.

Section 10: Images

Not applicable for this topic.

Additional material for this chapter can be found online at:
www.mountsinaiexpertguides.com
This includes a case study, multiple choice questions, advice for patients, and ICD codes

CHAPTER 35

Drug Desensitization

Julie Wang

Department of Pediatrics, Division of Allergy/Immunology, Icahn School of Medicine at Mount Sinai, New York, NY, USA

OVERALL BOTTOM LINE

- Desensitization entails the administration of incremental increases in doses of the drug to induce temporary unresponsiveness, allowing a patient with hypersensitivity to receive a course of medication safely.
- This procedure is indicated for those who have had IgE-mediated or non-IgE-mediated reaction to a drug. It is contraindicated for those who have had more severe reactions such as Stevens–Johnson syndrome, toxic epidermal necrolysis, and serum sickness.
- Protocols have been published for many drugs including antibiotics, chemotherapeutic agents, insulin, and aspirin.
- Allergic reactions can occur during the desensitization procedure, but are often mild and do not prevent the completion of the procedure.
- Hypersensitivity to the drug returns when the medication is discontinued or treatment is interrupted.

Section 1: Background

Definition of disease

- Drug desensitization is a procedure that induces a temporary state of unresponsiveness to allow the safe administration of a drug. Drug desensitization is indicated for patients who require a drug that previously caused immediate hypersensitivity when use of alternative non-cross-reacting drugs is not possible.

Disease classification

Not applicable for this topic.

Incidence/prevalence

Not applicable for this topic.

Economic impact

Not applicable for this topic.

Mount Sinai Expert Guides: Allergy and Clinical Immunology, First Edition. Edited by Hugh A. Sampson.
© 2015 John Wiley & Sons, Ltd. Published 2015 by John Wiley & Sons, Ltd.
Companion website: www.mountsinaiexpertguides.com

Etiology
- Many drugs can cause hypersensitivity reactions, including antibiotics and chemotherapeutic agents.
- Drugs known to cause IgE-mediated reactions include penicillins, cephalosporins, and platinum-based chemotherapy agents.
- Medications such as trimethoprim-sulfamethoxazole, vancomycin, aspirin, and taxane chemotherapeutic agents cause non-IgE-mediated reactions.

Pathology/pathogenesis
- The mechanisms underlying drug desensitization are not fully understood. Proposed mechanisms include blocking IgG antibodies, sub-threshold doses of drugs causing mast cells and basophils to be unresponsive to antigen stimulation, monomeric binding to IgE receptors without cross-linking so that cell activation does not occur, and depletion of mediators or signal transduction components such as syk kinase.

Predictive/risk factors
There are no known risk factors.

Section 2: Prevention
No interventions have been demonstrated to prevent the development of the disease.

Screening
Not applicable for this topic.

Primary prevention
Not applicable for this topic.

Secondary prevention
Not applicable for this topic.

Section 3: Diagnosis

> **BOTTOM LINE/CLINICAL PEARLS**
> - Drug desensitization is contraindicated for those who have had severe non-IgE-mediated reactions including Stevens–Johnson syndrome, toxic epidermal necrolysis, erythema multiforme, serum sickness, nephritis, and hepatitis.
> - Prior to desensitization, asthma and other lung diseases should be optimally managed and medications that may impact the safety of the procedure or interfere with treatment of anaphylaxis should be discontinued (e.g. beta-blockers).
> - Informed consent should be obtained because desensitization involves the administration of a known or suspected allergen and there is a risk for allergic reaction.
> - Drug desensitization should be performed by allergy specialists trained in the procedure in a monitored setting where personnel, medications, and equipment necessary to treat anaphylaxis are readily available.

Differential diagnosis
Not applicable for this topic.

Typical presentation

- Prior reactions to the medication in question should be reviewed to ensure that desensitization is an appropriate procedure to pursue. Desensitization is contraindicated for severe, non-IgE-mediated reactions such as Stevens–Johnson syndrome, toxic epidermal necrolysis, and serum sickness. Desensitization is indicated for individuals who require the medication to which they have previously experienced a reaction and no alternative medication is available.

Clinical diagnosis

History

- The diagnosis of drug hypersensitivity should be confirmed by history and testing where indicated. History should exclude the possibility that the prior reaction was caused by a severe non-IgE-mediated process for which desensitization is contraindicated (e.g. Stevens–Johnson syndrome, toxic epidermal necrolysis, serum sickness). Desensitization is considered when the patient requires treatment with the implicated medication and alternative medications are not possible.

Physical examination

- Prior to starting the desensitization procedure, a complete physical assessment of the patient should be performed to document the baseline status, including vital signs. Asthma or other chronic lung conditions should be stable. Frequent assessments are performed throughout the procedure to assess for any changes from baseline that would suggest an allergic reaction.

Useful clinical decision rules and calculators

Not applicable for this topic.

Disease severity classification

Not applicable for this topic.

Laboratory diagnosis

List of diagnostic tests

- Identification of the triggering medication and associated symptoms should be determined prior to considering drug desensitization (see Chapters 33 and 34).

Lists of imaging techniques

No imaging studies are indicated for drug desensitization.

Potential pitfalls/common errors made regarding diagnosis of disease

- Reactions during the desensitization procedure can occur so appropriate treatments should be immediately available.

Section 4: Treatment

Treatment rationale

- Desensitization entails administering incremental doses of the drug administered via the oral, intravenous, or subcutaneous routes. Pretreatment with antihistamines and glucocorticoids is not used for IgE-mediated reactions, but is often used for non-IgE-mediated reactions or when desensitizing to chemotherapeutic or biologic agents.

- Specific protocols have been published for penicillin, cephalosporins, insulin, and other medications. Generally, the initial dose is 1/10 000 of the full dose. The dose is doubled every 15–30 minutes. The duration of the procedure depends on the drug and route of administration, but most are completed within 4–12 hours. If the intravenous route is used, a continuous infusion may be used.
- Once the desensitization procedure is completed, the drug is given normally for the duration of the treatment course. If future treatment courses are necessary, the desensitization procedure will need to be repeated.

When to hospitalize

- Drug desensitization procedures should be performed in a monitored setting with personnel, medications, and equipment necessary to treat anaphylaxis readily available.

Managing the hospitalized patient

The management of anaphylaxis is discussed elsewhere (see Chapter 29).

Table of treatment

Treatment	Comment
Conservative • Mild reactions may be treated with slowing or temporarily stopping the desensitization procedure	• This is applicable to all patients
Medical • Antihistamines are used to treat mild reactions • If a severe reaction leading to anaphylaxis occurs, intramuscular epinephrine (0.01 mg/kg) is the treatment of choice • Bronchodilators are used for respiratory symptoms, including wheezing	• Appropriate treatments for allergic reactions should be immediately available throughout the desensitization procedure

Prevention/management of complications

- Complications of drug desensitization generally involve reactions that can range from localized symptoms to systemic reactions or anaphylaxis. Approximately one-third of penicillin desensitization procedures are associated with allergic reactions, and 11% of patients undergoing desensitization to chemotherapeutic agents experience allergic reactions.
- In some cases, reactions such as serum sickness, hemolytic anemia, and nephritis have occurred following desensitization in patients who were treated with high doses or prolonged courses of medication.
- Other adverse reactions to drugs resulting from toxicity, intolerance, or idiosyncratic reactions are possible.

CLINICAL PEARLS
- The drug desensitization procedure should be performed by a physician trained in the procedure and in a monitored setting equipped to treat anaphylaxis.
- Allergic reactions during desensitization are common, but often do not prevent the completion of the procedure.
- Specific protocols for desensitization with various medications are published.
- Several sample desensitization protocols can be found in 2010 Drug allergy: an updated practice parameter (see Reading list).

Section 5: Special populations
Pregnancy
Desensitization has been safely performed in pregnant women.

Children
Drug desensitization can be performed in patients of any age.

Elderly
Drug desensitization can be performed in patients of any age.

Section 6: Prognosis

> **BOTTOM LINE/CLINICAL PEARLS**
> - Desensitization can be successfully performed without significant adverse events in most cases to allow treatment with a medication that previously caused a reaction.
> - Desensitization is a temporary state of unresponsiveness. Hypersensitivity returns within days of discontinuing the medication.
> - Repeat desensitization is necessary if a repeat course of treatment with the medication is indicated.

Natural history of untreated disease
Not applicable for this topic.

Prognosis for treated patients
Not applicable for this topic.

Follow-up tests and monitoring
Not applicable for this topic.

Section 7: Reading list

Joint Task Force on Practice Parameters; American Academy of Allergy, Asthma and Immunology; American College of Allergy, Asthma and Immunology; Joint Council of Allergy, Asthma and Immunology. Drug allergy: an updated practice parameter. Ann Allergy Asthma Immunol 2010;105:259–73

Khan DA, Solensky R. Drug allergy. J Allergy Clin Immunol 2010;125:S126–37

Liu A, Fanning L, Chong H, Fernandez J, Sloane D, Sancho-Serra M, et al. Desensitization regimens for drug allergy: state of the art in the 21st century. Clin Exp Allergy 2011;41:1679–89

Scherer K, Brockow K, Aberer W, Gooi JH, Demoly P, Romano A, et al. Desensitization in delayed drug hypersensitivity reactions: an EAACI position paper of the Drug Allergy Interest Group. Allergy 2013;68: 844–52

Suggested websites
American Academy of Allergy, Asthma and Immunology (AAAAI). www.aaaai.org
American College of Allergy, Asthma and Immunology (ACAAI). www.acaai.org

Section 8: Guidelines
National society guidelines

Guideline title	Guideline source, comment	Date
Drug allergy: an updated practice parameter	Ann Allergy Asthma Immunol. **Comment:** Includes several sample desensitization protocols for various drugs	2010 (http://www.allergyparameters.org/published-practice-parameters/alphabetical-listing/drug-allergy-download/)

International society guidelines

Guideline title	Guideline source	Date
Desensitization in delayed drug hypersensitivity reactions: an EAACI position paper of the Drug Allergy Interest Group	European Network on Drug Allergy (ENDA); European Academy of Allergy and Clinical Immunology (EAACI) Drug Allergy Interest Group	2013 (http://www.ncbi.nlm.nih.gov/pubmed/23745779)

Section 9: Evidence
Not applicable for this topic.

Section 10: Images
Not applicable for this topic.

Additional material for this chapter can be found online at:
www.mountsinaiexpertguides.com
This includes a case study, multiple choice questions, advice for patients, and ICD codes

CHAPTER 36

Immunotherapy (Procedure)

Beth E. Corn

Department of Clinical Immunology, Icahn School of Medicine at Mount Sinai, New York, NY, USA

OVERALL BOTTOM LINE

- Allergy immunotherapy: subcutaneous injections of allergen(s) causing a patient to be less sensitive to the particular offending allergen.
- Approved for the treatment of allergic rhinitis, allergic conjunctivitis, allergic asthma, and atopic dermatitis caused by aeroallergens such as cat, dog, cockroach, dust mites, pollens, and molds. It is also indicated for Hymenoptera stings resulting in systemic reactions caused by honeybees, yellow jackets, white faced hornets, and fire ants.
- Candidates for aeroallergen immunotherapy are those patients who are not controlled by avoidance and medication, and those who experience untoward effects from current treatments.
- In the United States, only subcutaneous immunotherapy (SCIT) is an FDA-approved form of immunotherapy. Recently, sublingual immunotherapy (SLIT) for grass pollen allergy was approved, but SLIT for many aeroallergens are currently approved in Europe and Canada. Many studies indicate that SLIT seems to be as efficacious as SCIT with fewer adverse effects.
- Potential adverse effects range from local erythema at the injection site to systemic reactions including rhinitis, respiratory symptoms, and even anaphylaxis. Treatment of local reactions is mainly symptomatic: ice packs, topical corticosteroids, or antihistamines. Systemic reactions can be mild or severe. Mild systemic reactions can be treated with steroids and antihistamines. Epinephrine is indicated in moderate to severe systemic reactions and in the treatment of anaphylaxis.

Section 1: Background

- The first documented use of allergy immunotherapy was to grass pollen for the treatment of hay fever in the early 1900s. For immunotherapy, the particular allergens are extracted from source materials such as animal pelt, mold cultures, and pollens. Combinations of these proteins and glycoproteins are mixed in a particular way to formulate a therapeutic immunotherapy solution. This is prepared for individual patients, serially diluted, and used in sequentially increasing incremental treatment doses. Incremental treatment is usually performed in one of two ways. Conventionally, the build-up phase involves giving an incrementally increasing weekly injection over 6 months to achieve maintenance therapy. An alternative approach is cluster immunotherapy, which involves administering several incrementally increasing doses in

---

Mount Sinai Expert Guides: Allergy and Clinical Immunology, First Edition. Edited by Hugh A. Sampson.
© 2015 John Wiley & Sons, Ltd. Published 2015 by John Wiley & Sons, Ltd.
Companion website: www.mountsinaiexpertguides.com

a single day or non-consecutive days thereby reaching the maintenance dose and symptom relief within 4–8 weeks. Of patients who achieve maintenance dose, 85% achieve some level of symptom relief. Monthly treatment is continued for 3–5 years.

Section 2: Prevention
- Allergen immunotherapy is used to prevent the progression of symptoms or the development of asthma in allergic patients and to prevent patients with allergy to one antigen from developing multiple allergies (i.e. sensitivity to many antigens).

Section 3: Diagnosis
- The initial steps involve examining and obtaining a detailed history from patients presenting with symptoms of rhinitis/conjunctivitis including rhinorrhea, congestion, post-nasal drip, allergic conjunctivitis, asthma, or systemic reactions to stinging insects.
- Following the initial history and physical examination, tests for IgE to particular environmental allergens are performed via allergy skin testing or by blood testing for specific IgE (usually allergen-specific IgE levels). While both methods of testing reveal circulating IgE, the skin test offers immediate evidence of hypersensitivity to a particular allergen. Candidates for allergen immunotherapy are those patients with demonstrable IgE via skin or blood tests and clinical symptoms of allergy.

Section 4: Treatment (Algorithm 36.1)
See Section 1.

Section 5: Special populations
- Candidates for allergy immunotherapy include those patients with allergic symptomatology as well as objective measures of hypersensitivity demonstrated by a positive skin test or allergen-specific serum IgE, regardless of age.
- Immunotherapy is approved in patients who are pregnant, have an autoimmune disorder, and in immunodeficient patients including those with early or middle stages of HIV disease with CD4 counts of 400 or more and no history of opportunistic infections.
- The only population where the standard protocol differs is pregnant women. Pregnant women can continue to receive immunotherapy but must be maintained on the dosage they were receiving prior to becoming pregnant.

Section 6: Prognosis
- Allergen immunotherapy is very effective at controlling and decreasing the symptoms of allergic rhinitis. In a large retrospective study of both children and adults with allergic rhinitis, a significant cost saving was demonstrated in those treated with allergen immunotherapy.

Algorithm 36.1 Procedure of immunotherapy

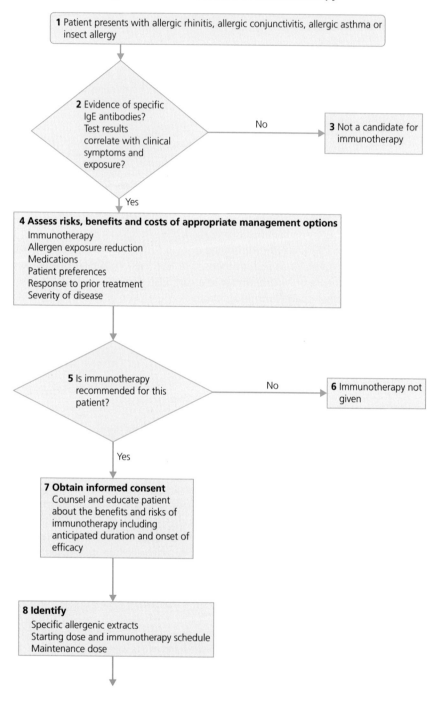

1 Patient presents with allergic rhinitis, allergic conjunctivitis, allergic asthma or insect allergy

2 Evidence of specific IgE antibodies? Test results correlate with clinical symptoms and exposure?

No → **3** Not a candidate for immunotherapy

Yes

4 Assess risks, benefits and costs of appropriate management options
Immunotherapy
Allergen exposure reduction
Medications
Patient preferences
Response to prior treatment
Severity of disease

5 Is immunotherapy recommended for this patient?

No → **6** Immunotherapy not given

Yes

7 Obtain informed consent
Counsel and educate patient about the benefits and risks of immunotherapy including anticipated duration and onset of efficacy

8 Identify
Specific allergenic extracts
Starting dose and immunotherapy schedule
Maintenance dose

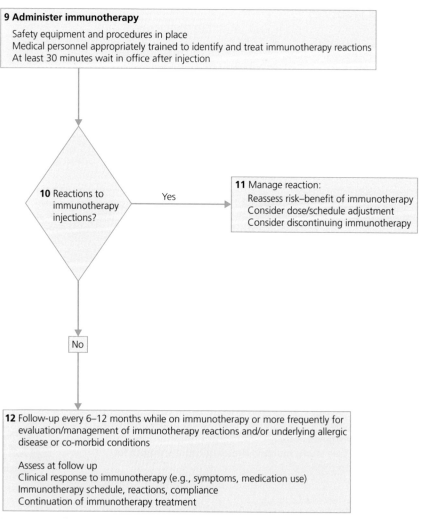

9 Administer immunotherapy

Safety equipment and procedures in place
Medical personnel appropriately trained to identify and treat immunotherapy reactions
At least 30 minutes wait in office after injection

10 Reactions to immunotherapy injections?

Yes

11 Manage reaction:

Reassess risk–benefit of immunotherapy
Consider dose/schedule adjustment
Consider discontinuing immunotherapy

No

12 Follow-up every 6–12 months while on immunotherapy or more frequently for evaluation/management of immunotherapy reactions and/or underlying allergic disease or co-morbid conditions

Assess at follow up
Clinical response to immunotherapy (e.g., symptoms, medication use)
Immunotherapy schedule, reactions, compliance
Continuation of immunotherapy treatment

Source: Cox L. Allergen immunotherapy: a practice parameter third update. J Allergy Clin Immunol 2011;127:S1–S55. Reproduced with permission of Elsevier.

Section 7: Reading list

DiBona D, Plaia A, Leto-Barone M, La Piana S, Di Lorenzo G. Efficacy of subcutaneous and sublingual immunotherapy with grass allergens for seasonal allergic rhinitis: a meta-analysis-bases comparison. J Allergy Clin Immunol 2012;130:1097–107

Dretzke J, Meadows A, Novielli N, Huissoon A, Fry-Smith A, Meads C. Subcutaneous and sublingual immunotherapy for seasonal allergic rhinitis: a systematic review and indirect comparison. J Allergy Clin Immunol 2013;131:1361–6

Hankin CS, Cox L, Bronstone A, Wang Z. Allergy immunotherapy: reduced heath care costs in adults and children with allergic rhinitis. J Allergy Clin Immunol 2013;131:1084–91

Lieberman P, Nicklas RA, Oppenheimer J, Kemp SF, Lang DM, Bernstein DI, et al. The diagnosis and management of anaphylaxis practice parameter: 2010 update. J Allergy Clin Immunol 2010;126:477–80

Nieto García A, Nevot Falcó S, Carrillo Díaz T, Cumplido Bonny JA, Izquierdo Calderón JP, Hernández-Peña J. Safety of cluster specific immunotherapy with a modified high-dose house dust mite extract. Eur Ann Allergy Clin Immunol 2013;45:78–83

Suggested websites

www.aaaai.org
www.acaai.org
www.eaaci.org

Section 8: Guidelines
National society guidelines

Guideline title	Guideline source	Date
Allergen immunotherapy: a practice parameter third update	American Academy of Allergy, Asthma and Immunology (AAAAI)	2011 (www.aaaai.org/practice-resources/statements-and-practice-parameters/ practice-parameters-and-other-guidelines-page.asp/)

Section 9: Evidence
Not applicable for this topic.

Section 10: Images
Not applicable for this topic.

**Additional material for this chapter can be found online at:www.
mountsinaiexpertguides.com
This includes a case study, multiple choice questions, advice for
patients, and ICD codes**

CHAPTER 37

Allergy Testing (Procedures: Skin Testing; Blood Tests)

Scott H. Sicherer

Department of Pediatrics, Division of Allergy/Immunology, Mount Sinai Hospital, New York, NY, USA

OVERALL BOTTOM LINE

- Allergy testing with prick or intradermal skin tests or with serum immunoassays are a means to detect allergen-specific IgE antibodies. These tests are used to confirm IgE sensitization to aeroallergens, foods, some drugs, and a few chemicals.
- The test must be selected and interpreted in context of the clinical history because positive tests (sensitization) may occur without any clinical implications.
- Patch testing is performed to identify contactant allergens that are triggers of allergic or irritant contact dermatitis.

Section 1: Skin prick testing

Indications

- To confirm clinical sensitization to aeroallergens, foods, some insect venoms, some drugs, and a few chemicals.
- Importantly, the test detects sensitization, but this may not indicate clinical reactivity upon exposure to the allergen.
- The number of skin tests and the allergens selected should be determined based on the medical history, taking into consideration factors such as age, environment and living conditions, occupation, activities, and diet. Routine use of large batteries of tests or routine annual testing without a clinical indication are not justified.

Procedure

- Patient must be off antihistaminic medications for approximately 5 half-lives of the specific agent.
- A number of sharp instruments are available for prick–puncture testing. Some comparative studies champion specific devices, but objective comparisons have not shown a clear-cut advantage of a specific device. Optimal results are expected from choosing a single device and properly training users.
- To ensure proper interpretation, positive (histamine) and negative (saline) controls should be performed at the same time as test allergens.
- The test site, which should be rash-free, is cleansed with alcohol before placement of the tests. The volar aspect of the arm is typically used, but the back is another site that may be used, especially in young children.

Mount Sinai Expert Guides: Allergy and Clinical Immunology, First Edition. Edited by Hugh A. Sampson.

© 2015 John Wiley & Sons, Ltd. Published 2015 by John Wiley & Sons, Ltd.

Companion website: www.mountsinaiexpertguides.com

- Measurement (e.g. diameter in millimeters) of wheal and erythema should be made at the peak of reactivity, approximately 15–20 minutes, and compared with controls. Results are expressed by size rather than comparison to controls (e.g. 1+, 2+ is not recommended).
- Reliability depends upon the skill of the tester, the test instrument, skin color, reactivity, patient age, and potency of extracts.

Management of complications
- Discomfort (itch) at the site of test placement is expected and transient. Antihistamines may be administered, if needed, after the tests are completed.
- Systemic allergic reactions from skin prick tests are uncommon. They are more likely if large numbers of tests are applied, or when using fresh foods rather than extracts, especially in infants. However, patients should be observed for systemic reactions and medical personnel and equipment to treat anaphylaxis should be readily available.

Follow-up
- Physicians should discuss the relevance, implications, and associated treatment instructions of positive and negative tests in the context of the medical history.

Section 2: Intradermal (intracutaneous) skin testing
Indications
- Compared with skin prick testing, intracutaneous tests are more sensitive and will identify a larger number of patients with lower skin test sensitivity. These tests are therefore indicated when increased sensitivity is the main goal of testing.
- Intracutaneous tests are *not* recommended for foods because of safety concerns and a lack of need for increased sensitivity.
- Intracutaneous tests may be useful in evaluating anaphylaxis to insect stings and penicillin.
- Pre-screening with prick–puncture tests is generally undertaken, with intracutaneous tests considered when sensitivity needs to be higher with negative skin prick tests.
- There are limited data about equivalency of intracutaneous testing to skin prick testing and relationship to end-organ responses. Clinical use is usually restricted to a single test dose (i.e. 1 : 1000 wt/vol) which may be an irritant and so predictive accuracy is often confounded by false positive results.

Procedure
- Intracutaneous tests are performed with small volumes (0.02–0.05 mL) injected intracutaneously to raise a small bleb.
- The starting dose is generally 100- to 1000-fold more dilute than that used for skin prick tests.
- See Skin prick testing section for information on patient preparation and measurement of results.

Management of complications
- Immediate systemic reactions are more common with intracutaneous tests than skin prick tests; six fatalities were reported in a retrospective survey.
- If skin prick test pre-screening is not used, preliminary intracutaneous serial threshold dilutions that begin with low concentrations should be considered, especially when evaluating anaphylactic allergies.
- Patients should be observed for systemic reactions and medical personnel and equipment to treat anaphylaxis should be readily available.

Follow-up
- Physicians should discuss the relevance, implications, and associated treatment instructions of positive and negative tests in the context of the medical history.

Section 3: Patch testing (epicutaneous patch test)
Indications
- To identify contactant allergens that are triggers of allergic (ACD) or irritant contact dermatitis.
- In the evaluation of chronic eczematous dermatitis when allergic contact dermatitis is suspected.
- Patch tests are most effective when patients are selected on the basis of a clinical suspicion and tests are performed to relevant triggers.
- Limitations include lack of a gold standard, reproducibility, lack of known irritant thresholds and minimum eliciting concentrations, and ability to correlate results with patient exposures. Negative tests may result despite proper application because other circumstances of exposure are not duplicated, for example washing hands with solvents.
- A variation, the atopy patch test (APT), uses foods or drugs. The role of these tests in diagnosis is evolving. The APT is not recommended for routine evaluation of food allergy.

Procedure
- The operator may use individual Finn Chambers. In addition, an FDA approved screening method (T.R.U.E. TEST®) is preloaded with 23 common contactants.
- The test remains in place for 48 hours and then removed with readings upon removal and again at 3–4 days or more to differentiate early irritant and later allergic responses.
- Results are read according to standard systems of evaluation developed by two major ACD research groups: the International Contact Dermatitis Research Group and the North American Contact Dermatitis Group.

Management of complications
- Approximately 6% of patients develop "angry back" where generalized erythema develops and reduces the ability to determine test results, whether irritant or allergic.
- Systemic ACD after patch testing is rare.
- Sensitization by patch testing is possible, particularly with plant contactants such as poison ivy and aniline dyes.

Follow-up
- Physicians should discuss the relevance, implications, and associated treatment instructions of positive and negative tests in the context of the medical history.

Section 4: Serum tests for detection of specific IgE
Indications
- To confirm clinical sensitization to aeroallergens, foods, and some drugs.
- Importantly, the test detects sensitization but this may not indicate clinical reactivity upon exposure to the allergen.
- The number of tests and the allergens selected should be determined based on the medical history, taking into consideration factors such as age, environment and living conditions, occupation, activities, and diet. Routine use of large batteries of tests, or routine annual testing without a clinical indication, is not justified.

- The test may be preferable to skin prick testing under conditions such as widespread rash, use of antihistamine medications, or for following responses over time.
- There are three FDA-cleared automated test systems: Thermofisher, Siemens, and Hycor. Each has excellent test characteristics (e.g. reliability, reproducibility). However, the assays either detect different populations of IgE antibody or do not measure the same antibodies with comparable efficiencies and so the results from the three assays are not interchangeable or equivalent.
- Tests that determine IgE binding to specific proteins within foods (component testing) are becoming available and may be indicated when there is clinical suspicion of sensitization without significant clinical consequence and differentiation of reactivity may impact clinical decision-making.

Procedure

- A blood or serum sample is procured and tested.

Management of complications

- Pain, infection, and vasovagal reactions may occur as for any blood test.

Follow-up

- Physicians should discuss the relevance, implications, and associated treatment instructions of positive and negative tests in the context of the medical history.

Section 5: Reading list

American Academy of Allergy, Asthma and Immunology; American College of Allergy, Asthma and Immunology. Contact dermatitis: a practice parameter. Ann Allergy Asthma Immunol 2006; 97(3 Suppl 2):S1–38

Bernstein IL, Li JT, Bernstein DI, Hamilton R, Spector SL, Tan R, et al. Allergy diagnostic testing: an updated practice parameter. Ann Allergy Asthma Immunol 2008;100(Suppl 3):S1–148

Boyce JA, Assa'ad A, Burks AW, Jones SM, Sampson HA, Wood RA, et al. Guidelines for the diagnosis and management of food allergy in the United States: report of the NIAID-sponsored expert panel. J Allergy Clin Immunol 2010;126(Suppl):S1–58

Hamilton RG, Williams PB. Human IgE antibody serology: a primer for the practicing North American allergist/immunologist. J Allergy Clin Immunol 2010;126:33–8

Sicherer SH, Wood RA. Allergy testing in childhood: using allergen-specific IgE tests. Pediatrics 2012; 129:193–7

Suggested websites

www.aaaai.org
www.acaai.org
www.contactderm.org

Section 6: Guidelines

Guideline title	Guideline source	Date
Allergy diagnostic testing: an updated practice parameter	Joint Council	2008 (http://www.aaaai.org/Aaaai/media/MediaLibrary/PDF%20Documents/Practice%20and%20Parameters/allergydiagnostictesting.pdf)

Section 7: Evidence
Not applicable for this topic.

Section 8: Images
Not applicable for this topic.

Additional material for this chapter can be found online at:
www.mountsinaiexpertguides.com
This includes a case study, multiple choice questions (provided by
Hugh Sampson), advice for patients, and ICD code

PART 2

Clinical Immunology

CHAPTER 38

Evaluating the Child with Recurrent Infections

Shradha Agarwal

Division of Allergy/Immunology, Icahn School of Medicine at Mount Sinai, New York, NY, USA

OVERALL BOTTOM LINE

- A child with a history of recurrent or unusual infections presents a diagnostic challenge to pediatricians.
- The main causes of recurrent and chronic infections in children include atopic disorders, anatomic and functional defects, and primary or secondary immunodeficiency.
- Careful attention to the medical history and physical examination will help differentiate children who are healthy from those with underlying disorders.
- Early diagnosis and treatment can help improve the quality of life for these children.
- For children suspected to have a primary immunodeficiency, prompt referral to an immunologist will provide life-saving treatment, and genetic counseling may help identify future affected individuals.

Section 1: Background

Definition of disease

- Recurrent infections are defined as infections that occur too frequently in number, are too severe, or last too long (chronic). However, sometimes even one infection with an unusual pathogen could warrant an immune evaluation. Severe infections are those that fail to respond to oral antibiotics, require hospitalization, or involve unusual pathogens. Chronic infections fail to respond to treatment and often require prophylactic antibiotics.

Disease classification

Not applicable for this topic.

Incidence/prevalence

Not applicable for this topic.

Economic impact

Not applicable for this topic.

Mount Sinai Expert Guides: Allergy and Clinical Immunology, First Edition. Edited by Hugh A. Sampson.
© 2015 John Wiley & Sons, Ltd. Published 2015 by John Wiley & Sons, Ltd.
Companion website: www.mountsinaiexpertguides.com

Etiology

- At birth the immune system is not fully developed and therefore transplacentally acquired maternal antibodies continue to protect the infant in the first 6–9 months of life. The immune system may continue to mature in some children until school age.
- Even healthy children with normally functioning immune systems can develop up to 6–8 respiratory tract infections per year in the first 5 years of life.
- Children attending day care or who have siblings attending school can have even more infections because of increased exposure.

Pathology/pathogenesis

Not applicable for this topic.

Predictive/risk factors

- Increased exposure to infections from day care or school-age siblings.
- Atopic disease.
- Anatomic or functional defects.
- Primary immunodeficiency.
- Secondary immunodeficiency.

Section 2: Prevention

No interventions have been demonstrated to prevent the development of the disease.

Screening

- Currently, the states of Wisconsin, Massachusetts, New York, California, Connecticut, Michigan, Colorado, Mississippi, Delaware, Florida, Texas, Minnesota, Iowa, Pennsylvania, and Utah include severe combined immunodeficiency (SCID) on their newborn screening panel.

Primary prevention

Not applicable for this topic.

Secondary prevention

Not applicable for this topic.

Section 3: Diagnosis (Algorithm 38.1)

> **BOTTOM LINE/CLINICAL PEARLS**
> - The age of onset, frequency, duration, and severity of infections as well as response to various treatments are important to note.
> - Those who present for medical attention have variable examination findings from a normal physical examination to eczema, post-nasal drip, or rales on chest examination. A thorough physical examination including height and weight should be performed.
> - Initial laboratory evaluation includes complete blood count with differential, quantitative immunoglobulins with specific and functional antibody responses, and complement assay. More advance testing should be performed based upon the results of the initial screening tests.

Algorithm 38.1 Evaluating the child with recurrent infections

Evidence of recurrent infections defined as too frequent in number, too severe, or lasting too long (chronic)

Evidence of infections that fail to respond to oral antibiotics, require hospitalization, or involve unusual pathogens

History of chronic infections that fail to respond to treatment and require prophylactic antibiotics

Comprehensive history (including detailed family history) and physical examination

Imaging including chest X-ray and/or CT scan

Laboratory evaluation including complete blood count, HIV, sweat chloride testing, comprehensive metabolic panel, CH50, quantitative immunoglobulins, specific antibody responses (depending on age), lymphocyte panel

Differential diagnosis

Differential diagnosis	Features
Atopy	Seasonal or year round symptoms depending on allergic sensitivities. Total IgE and eosinophil count may be elevated. Development of cough or wheezing following viral respiratory infections. Symptoms resolve with antihistamines and asthma treatments
Anatomic/functional defects	Persistent cough, wheezing, repeated infections with *Pseudomonas aeruginosa* or *Staphylococcus aureus*, and bronchiectasis are suggestive of cystic fibrosis Epigastric pain, vomiting, nausea, and aspiration indicate gastroesophageal reflux disease (GERD)
Secondary immunodeficiencies	HIV/AIDS, chronic immunosuppressive therapies (corticosteroids), malignancies, protein losing enteropathy, nephrotic syndrome
B-cell deficiencies	Recurrent sinopulmonary infections commonly due to encapsulated bacteria such as *Haemophilus influenza* or *Streptococcus pneumonia*. Chronic or recurrent gastroenteritis. Autoimmune diseases such as immune thrombocytopenic purpura
T-cell deficiencies	Lymphopenia (<1500 cells/μL) during neonatal period. Onset of recurrent bacterial and opportunistic infections in early infancy. Chronic candidiasis. Chronic diarrhea. *Mycobacterium avium-intracellulare* and *Pneumocystis carinii* are typical infections seen in patients with T-cell defects
Phagocytic defects	Delayed separation of the umbilical cord. Recurrent infections with catalase-positive pathogens. Poor wound healing. Abscesses
Complement deficiencies	Early complement component deficiency, such as C1, C2, and C4 are associated with lupus-like disorders. Late complement, C5–C9, deficiencies are associated with neisserial infections

Typical presentation
- Typical presentation is a young child with recurrent otitis media, sinusitis, and/or pneumonia. Patients often have coexisting allergic rhinitis or asthma that may be difficult to control leading to frequent sinopulmonary infections. Infections often persist or recur despite treatment with antibiotics. Cultures may reveal encapsulated bacteria such as pneumococcus or unusual organisms such as Aspergillus. Other patients may present with coexisting autoimmune disease.

Clinical diagnosis
History
- History should begin with birth, including maternal diseases (HIV) and alcohol use. Birth history should include length of gestation, birth weight, neonatal problems, or need for hospitalizations. Family history of frequent infections, early infancy deaths, or autoimmune disorders should be obtained. Immunization history should be reviewed. Infections following live vaccinations suggest primary immunodeficiency. Relevant factors of social history include exposures to smoke, animals, and whether the child attends day care or has other school-aged siblings.
- The onset of infections and the specific pathogen involved will provide clues towards the type of immune defect present. For instance, recurrent sinopulmonary infections with encapsulated organisms (pneumococcus, *Haemophilus influenza* type B) suggest B-cell defects. Chronic candidiasis may indicate T-cell defects. Children with recurrent abscesses caused by gram-negative organisms such as *Escherichia coli*, *Serratia* sp., or *Klebsiella* sp., may have abnormalities in phagocyte function. Recurrent staphylococcal skin infections, abscesses, and lung cysts are characteristic of hyper-IgE syndrome. Infections with invasive infections with *Neisseria* spp. suggest defects in the late complement components, C5–C9. Delayed detachment of the umbilical cord may be suggestive of a leukocyte adhesion defect.

Physical examination
- Physical examination should start with growth and development as documented in growth chart and milestones.
- Any facial anomalies should be noted.
- Examination of head and neck for boggy nasal turbinates, nasal discharge, sinus tenderness suggests allergic rhinitis or chronic rhinosinusitis.
- Examination of the ear for otitis media and hearing evaluation should be carried out in a child with recurrent upper respiratory tract infections.
- Oral pharynx should be examined for dentition, ulcers, and candidiasis.
- Lung examination significant for decreased breath sounds or wheezing suggests infectious process or asthma.
- Cardiac anomalies should be noted.
- Skin examination for eczema, infection, petechiae, and abscesses.
- Examination of the lymphatic system for presence or absence of adenopathy and hepatosplenomegaly is important.
- Of note, a normal physical examination does not rule out underlying immunodeficiency.

Useful clinical decision rules and calculators
Not applicable for this topic.

Disease severity classification
Not applicable for this topic.

Laboratory diagnosis

List of diagnostic tests

- Initial evaluation for all children includes complete blood count with differential, metabolic panel including protein, albumin, globulin, and HIV testing if appropriate.
- Testing for atopy includes skin prick testing or serum allergen-specific IgE testing.
- For evaluating humoral immunity, quantitative serum immunoglobulins with reference to age and antibody titers to previously administered vaccinations should be performed. In children who have not been vaccinated, these titers are not useful. In children with low antibody levels, booster immunizations can be helpful to determine capacity to make functional antibody.
- Total hemolytic complement (CH50) assay can evaluate the functional integrity of the classic complement pathway. Individual complement components are measured if the CH50 is reduced or absent.
- Lymphocyte subset analysis should be ordered when a B or T-cell defect is suspected. This can be followed by delayed hypersensitivity skin tests and lymphocyte proliferation assays for further assessment of B or T-cell function.
- More specific testing can be ordered if these screening tests are abnormal for a particular immunodeficiency, which is usually performed in a specialized laboratory.

Lists of imaging techniques

- A chest X-ray is indicated for any child with chronic cough or recurrent infections or symptoms involving the lung.
- A sinus CT for a history of recurrent sinusitis.
- A high resolution chest CT if suspicious for bronchiectasis.

Potential pitfalls/common errors made regarding diagnosis of disease

- Serum immunoglobulins should be compared with reference to the patient's age.
- Vaccination titers are not indicative of functional antibody capacity in infants who have not been vaccinated.
- A common reason for abnormal complement components is inappropriate handling of the specimen as complement is temperature labile.

Section 4: Treatment

Treatment rationale

- Treatment is according to underlying disease identified. Live attenuated vaccines such as oral polio, varicella, and MMR (measles/mumps/rubella), should be avoided in children with suspected or diagnosed T-cell deficiencies because vaccine-induced infection is a risk in these patients. Irradiated, leukocyte-poor products should be used in patients with T-cell defects who require blood transfusions to avoid graft versus host disease. Currently available treatments for primary immunodeficiency include prophylactic antibiotics, immunoglobulin replacement, enzyme-replacement, and bone marrow transplantation. Treatment for specific immunodeficiencies is discussed elsewhere in this book.

When to hospitalize

- Inability to tolerate fluids, decreased urinary output.
- Symptoms persist or worsen despite treatment with antibiotics.
- Persistent high fever, elevated heart rate, elevated respiratory rate.
- Change in mental status.

Managing the hospitalized patient

Not applicable for this topic.

Table of treatment

Treatment	Comment
Conservative	Asymptomatic patients require no treatment but should be followed at regular intervals or sooner depending on frequency of infection
Medical Antibiotics (treatment or prophylactic) Immunoglobulin (400–600 mg/kg) IV or SC	Choice and frequency of antibiotics is based on type of infection and culture/sensitivity results In a child found to have antibody deficiency who has recurrent infections despite prophylactic antibiotics
Surgical Bone marrow/stem cell transplantation	Certain cases of SCID and T-cell deficiencies
Radiological Chest X-ray or CT scan	Patient with significant upper or lower respiratory infections

Prevention/management of complications

- Infants with a history of infections found to have lymphocyte counts below 2500 cell/mm^3 or abnormal T-cell receptor excision circle (TREC) number on newborn screening require prompt referral to an immunologist to evaluate for SCID.

> **CLINICAL PEARL**
> - In patients who are considering treatment with replacement immunoglobulin, a thorough evaluation of the immune system should be performed prior to initiating immunoglobulin therapy.

Section 5: Special populations

Not applicable for this topic.

Section 6: Prognosis

> **BOTTOM LINE/CLINICAL PEARLS**
> - The signs and symptoms for a particular immunodeficiency may vary but most commonly patients with primary immunodeficiency are susceptible to infections that are often recurrent and prolonged.
> - Untreated infections or delayed diagnosis of primary immunodeficiency can be fatal.
> - Immunoglobulin replacement is used in patients who do not generate or maintain antibodies. This treatment can reduce the frequency of infections and improve their quality of life.

Natural history of untreated disease

Not applicable for this topic.

Prognosis for treated patients

Not applicable for this topic.

Follow-up tests and monitoring

- Patients with suspected immunodeficiencies should be referred to an immunologist for additional diagnostic tests and prompt treatment. Prenatal diagnosis and genetic counseling are available for some diseases.

Section 7: Reading list

Ballow M. Approach to patient with recurrent infections. Clin Rev Allergy Immunol 2008;34:129–40

Bonilla FA, Bernstein IL, Khan DA, Ballas ZK, Chinen J, Frank MM, et al. Practice parameter for the diagnosis and management of primary immunodeficiency. Ann Allergy Asthma Immunol 2005;94:S1–63

Bush A. Recurrent respiratory infections. Pediatr Clin North Am 2009;56:67

Notarangelo LD, Fischer A, Geha RS, Casanova JL, Chapel H, Conley ME, et al. Primary immunodeficiencies: 2009 update. J Allergy Clin Immunol 2009;124:1161–78

Steihm ER, Ochs HD, Winkelstein JA. Immunodeficiency disorders: general considerations. In: Stiehm ER, Ochs HD, Winkelstein JA (eds) Immunologic Disorders in Infants and Children, 5th edn. Sauders/Elsevier: 2004

Suggested websites

American Academy of Allergy Asthma and Immunology. www.aaaai.org

Clinical Immunology Society. www.clinimmsoc.org

Immune Deficiency Foundation. http://primaryimmune.org/

Jeffrey Modell Foundation. www.info4pi.org

Section 8: Guidelines
National society guidelines

Guideline title	Guideline source	Date
Practice parameter for the diagnosis and management of primary immunodeficiency	American Academy of Allergy, Asthma and Immunology (AAAAI) and American College of Allergy, Asthma and Immunology (ACAAI)	2005 (https://www.aaaai.org/Aaaai/media/MediaLibrary/PDF%20Documents/Practice%20and%20Parameters/immunodeficiency2005.pdf)

International society guidelines

Guideline title	Guideline source	Date
Primary immunodeficiency diseases: an update from the International Union of Immunological Societies Primary Immunodeficiency Diseases Classification Committee	International Union of Immunological Societies (IUIS)	2007 (http://www.ncbi.nlm.nih.gov/pubmed/17952897)

Section 9: Evidence

Not applicable for this topic.

Section 10: Images

Not applicable for this topic.

Additional material for this chapter can be found online at:
www.mountsinaiexpertguides.com
This includes a case study, multiple choice questions, and advice for patients

CHAPTER 39

Evaluating the Adult with Recurrent Infections

Charlotte Cunningham-Rundles

Departments of Medicine and Pediatrics, The Immunology Institute, Icahn School of Medicine at Mount Sinai, New York, NY, USA

OVERALL BOTTOM LINE

- Adults with chronic, recurrent, or acute infections may have a primary or secondary immune defect.
- Recurrent infections can result from many causes and these should be ruled out in the investigation.
- Other causes include untreated allergy, anatomic changes, other diseases, or medications used to treat these disorders.
- Subjects with infections caused by immune defects may be of either sex, and of any age.
- Diagnosis of the immune defect relies on the combination of clinical and laboratory data, and the exclusion of alternative diagnoses.
- The diagnostic strategies include blood tests aimed at investigating the various compartments of the immune system.
- The goal of treatment is to define the immune system deficits to provide a means to either substituting or bypassing the immune defect.

Section 1: Background

Definition of disease

- The immune system is composed of a large network of cells and organs working together. As strong immunity is so important for health, nature has provided a number of overlapping immune systems to cope with an entire range of microbes. Depending on the type and size of the immune defect, the clinical manifestations vary widely. As the immune system is also important to control infections, loss of some of these controls can result in various types of infectious diseases. However, recurrent infections can be brought about by many other causes, and these should be eliminated in any investigation so that best treatments can be instituted.

Disease classification

- To determine whether an immune defect might be present, immunologists use a classification system based on the component of the immune network at fault:
  1. *T cells:* arise in the thymus and help control viruses, and aid in antibody production;
  2. *B cells:* produce antibodies;
  3. *Combined defects:* in which both T and B cells are defective;

Mount Sinai Expert Guides: Allergy and Clinical Immunology, First Edition. Edited by Hugh A. Sampson.
© 2015 John Wiley & Sons, Ltd. Published 2015 by John Wiley & Sons, Ltd.
Companion website: www.mountsinaiexpertguides.com

4. *Phagocytic cells:* go to the site of infection and attempt to engulf and digest the bacteria;
5. *Complement:* a system of proteins that interact to aid the function of antibodies but also control immune reactions;
6. *Innate immunity:* a group of cells that do not need to be primed to work.

Incidence/prevalence
- The incidence of primary (genetic) immune defects in adults is unknown.
- Adults may also have defects that are considered "secondary" which means that a non-genetic cause can be identified: this may be a drug such as chemotherapy, another disease (such as chronic lymphocytic leukemia), or a virus (such as Epstein–Barr virus, or of course, HIV, as discussed in Chapters 51 and 52).
- In both cases, immune defects can lead to a variety of infections and also inflammatory and/or autoimmune disease.

Etiology and pathology/pathogenesis
- Immune defects result from loss or abnormality of one or more of the many components of the immune system.
- These may be due to genetic causes or may be secondary to other causes.
- Infections can also be due to untreated allergy (e.g. recurrent pneumonias), other diseases, or treatments used in these diseases.
- If a genetic cause is present, in many cases there is no family history, as complex inheritance patterns may obscure genetic contributions.
- Pathology: as the immune system contains many components and various members of this network are found in all organs, the pathology of immune defects is based on the organ itself:
  - Infections in adults commonly involve the respiratory tract (e.g. pneumonia, bronchitis, sinusitis);
  - Acute bacterial infections include skin infections, meningitis, sepsis, and solid organ abscesses;
  - Gastrointestinal infections may occur, leading to loss of absorptive surfaces, diarrhea, and malnutrition.

Section 2: Prevention
- The first step is to determine the cause of the infections, and treat these.

Screening
Not applicable for this topic.

Prevention
Not applicable for this topic.

Section 3: Diagnosis (Algorithm 39.1)
- Diagnosis of immune defects as contributors to recurrent infections relies upon laboratory tests to assess immune competence.
- These include testing the numbers of lymphocytes, granulocytes, lymphocyte subsets, immunoglobulins (IgG, IgA, and IgM, and, if pertinent, IgE) and also specific antibody production (e.g. antibodies to tetanus, diphtheria, pneumococcal serotypes after vaccination).
- More detailed tests may be needed in some cases, best ordered and interpreted by an immunologist.

Algorithm 39.1 Evaluation of recurrent infections

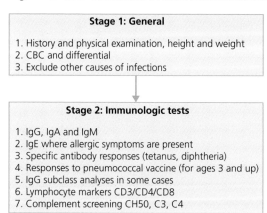

Stage 1: General

1. History and physical examination, height and weight
2. CBC and differential
3. Exclude other causes of infections

Stage 2: Immunologic tests

1. IgG, IgA and IgM
2. IgE where allergic symptoms are present
3. Specific antibody responses (tetanus, diphtheria)
4. Responses to pneumococcal vaccine (for ages 3 and up)
5. IgG subclass analyses in some cases
6. Lymphocyte markers CD3/CD4/CD8
7. Complement screening CH50, C3, C4

Differential diagnosis

- Exclusion of other causes of recurrent infections is the necessary first step: untreated allergic diseases, asthma, diabetes mellitus, HIV, cirrhosis, environmental causes, nephrotic syndrome, hemoglobinopathies, neurologic disease, inflammatory bowel disease, autoimmunity, splenectomy, malignancy, radiation therapy, and immunosuppressive agents.

Typical presentation

- The typical scenario is an adult who presents with a history of chronic infections such as sinusitis or several episodes of pneumonia. In some cases, weight loss and fatigue are other presenting signs. These lead to a suspicion of an immune defect. Physical examination may not reveal unusual features, although cervical lymphadenopathy or chest findings such as wheezing or rales may be noted. Other common presentations include adults who have an episode of giardiasis, or other gastrointestinal parasite. After exclusion of other causes, blood tests to evaluate the immune system can be carried out.

Clinical diagnosis

History

- Symptoms are heterogeneous depending on the organs and systems affected and on the nature of the immune defect. In 80% of cases, lung infections occur, specifically pneumonia or chronic bronchitis. A history of difficult to treat chronic sinusitis is very common; a history of having one or more previous sinus surgeries is often found. Gastrointestinal disease is seen in some. Details sought in the clinical history should include duration and onset of symptoms, fatigue, fever, weight loss, and shortness of breath. Weight loss is common. Obtaining a detailed family history is always important, as well as questions about smoking, drug use, and various medications tried.

Physical examination

- Physical examination should start with an evaluation for signs of systemic illness, including weight loss. Fever may be present with acute infections, otherwise chronic fever would be uncommon. Patients with lung disease may be short of breath, have a productive or non-productive cough, and may have pulmonary signs such as rhonchi or rales on examination. Lymphadenopathy is common, and enlarged spleen may be detected. Skin changes include scarring from previous herpes zoster infection; vitiligo appears to be common. Chronic conjunctivitis, iritis, or episcleritis may be observed. Joint complaints include changes due to previous joint infections, or autoimmune, chronic arthritis.

Laboratory diagnosis
- Complete blood count.
- Chemistry panel to exclude other causes.
- Rheumatologic tests if indicated.
- Serum IgG, IgA, IgM.
- Tests for functional antibody (e.g. tetanus, diphtheria, pneumococcal serotypes).
  - CRP and sedimentation rate.
  - Microbial cultures where applicable.
  - Microbiologic studies to exclude infectious etiologies.

Pathology
- Biopsies are necessary when tissue inflammation or other abnormality is present. Common areas that might be biopsied include:
  - Lymph nodes if these are chronically enlarged and the reasons are unclear;
  - Bone marrow if there are peripheral blood cell abnormalities;
  - Gastrointestinal tissues if gastrointestinal disease is found;
  - Skin biopsy for issues that need clarification.

Lists of imaging techniques
- Chest X-ray.
- Complete lung functions (spirometry and diffusion capacity).
- High-resolution CT of the chest.
- Ultrasound for splenomegaly.
- CT of the abdomen to examine organ size, lymphadenopathy.
- MRI may be preferred to minimize exposure to ionizing radiation.

Potential pitfalls/common errors made regarding diagnosis of disease
- Not diagnosing immune defects in adults leads to excess morbidity.
- Missing the correct diagnosis leads to lack of appropriate treatment.
- Over-diagnosis leads to excess medical costs as therapies can be expensive.

Section 4: Treatment
- The goals of therapy are to provide protection against infections and, where possible, to use any available therapy to enhance the immune system.
  - *Antibiotics:* when an immune deficiency has been documented, antibiotics should be started immediately for fevers and other manifestations of infection after appropriate cultures have been obtained. These cultures are important to direct further therapy if the infection does not respond to the initial antibiotic chosen. Prophylactic antibiotics can be of benefit, especially for subjects with chronic lung disease. A satisfactory combination of antibiotics includes amoxicillin-clavulanate, erythromycin, trimethoprim and sulfamethoxazole, or a cephalosporin. In adults, amoxicillin-clavulanate, trimethoprim and sulfamethoxazole, tetracyclines, or a cephalosporin are useful. Quinolones are best saved to treat acute infections.
  - *Immunoglobulin:* when significant loss of antibody production has occurred and this has been fully documented by laboratory testing, the optimum treatment is immunoglobulin replacement. The usual starting dose for the intravenous forms is 400–600 mg/kg/month; IV immunoglobulin can be given at home. Subcutaneous treatment is also quite effective; smaller doses are given once a week.

- *Specific treatment for T-cell deficiency:* there are few specific treatments for T-cell immunodeficiencies aside from bone marrow and stem cell transplants for the most severe forms (SCID). Other therapies, such as cytokines, remain investigational.
- *Specific treatment of phagocytic disorders:* there are very few treatments for the phagocytic disorders, aside from the use of antibiotics as needed, or granulocyte colony-stimulating factor (G-CFS) to raise the neutrophil count if low.
- *Specific treatment for complement deficiency:* fresh frozen plasma from healthy donors can transiently replace specific complement components in patients with isolated complement component defects and severe infections.

Table of treatment

Treatment	Comment
Medical (antibiotics)	
Prophylactic: • 60 mg trimethoprim and 800 mg sulfamethoxazole (DS) • Amoxicillin 500 mg/day • Ciprofloxacin (250 mg/day) Treatment: • Trimethoprim-sulfamethoxazole (DS) 2× day • Amoxicillin 500 mg 3× day • Ciprofloxacin (250 mg 2× day) • Azithromycin (250–500 mg/day)	Take cultures; monitor for resistance
Immunoglobulin: • Intravenous (400–600 mg/kg/month) • Subcutaneous (400–600 mg/kg/month but given weekly SC)	Only when antibody deficiency is fully documented

Section 5: Special populations
Pregnancy
- The evaluation of the pregnant patient is not different from other individuals; antibiotics used are those chosen to be acceptable at this time. All immunoglobulin products may be used.

Elderly
- Elderly subjects receive the same treatments as other subjects.

Section 6: Prognosis

> **BOTTOM LINE/CLINICAL PEARLS**
> - Adults with frequent infections may require evaluation for immune defects
> - These may be primary or secondary.
> - However, there are other causes of recurrent infections that should be excluded before immune functions are examined.
> - With appropriate treatment the prognosis is good.

Natural history of untreated disease
• This depends on the nature of the immune defect, and whether organ damage has occurred.

Follow-up tests and monitoring
• The follow-up will depend on the causes of the frequent infections. Follow-up will be dictated by these issues.

Section 7: Reading list

Boyle JM, Buckley RH. Population prevalence of diagnosed primary immunodeficiency diseases in the United States. J Clin Immunol 2007;27:497–502

Srinivasa BT, Alizadehfar R, Desrosiers M, Shuster J, Pai NP, Tsoukas CM. Adult primary immune deficiency: what are we missing? Am J Med 2012;125:779–86

Yarmohammadi H, Estrella L, Doucette J, Cunningham-Rundles C. Recognizing primary immune deficiency in clinical practice. Clin Vaccine Immunol 2006;13:329–32

Suggested websites
http://primaryimmune.org/about-primary-immunodeficiencies/relevant-info/laboratory-tests/

http://www.uptodate.com/contents/laboratory-evaluation-of-the-immune-system

http://www.worldallergy.org/professional/allergic_diseases_center/suspected_immune_deficiency/

Section 8: Guidelines
National society guidelines

Guideline title	Guideline source	Date
Practice parameter for the diagnosis and management of primary immunodeficiency	American Academy of Allergy, Asthma and Immunology (AAAAI)	2005 (https://www.aaaai.org/Aaaai/media/MediaLibrary/PDF%20 Documents/Practice%20 and%20Parameters/ immunodeficiency2005.pdf)

Section 9: Evidence
Not applicable for this topic.

Section 10: Images
Not applicable for this topic.

Additional material for this chapter can be found online at:
www.mountsinaiexpertguides.com
This includes multiple choice questions, advice for patients, and ICD codes

CHAPTER 40

Antibody Deficiencies

Charlotte Cunningham-Rundles

Departments of Medicine and Pediatrics, The Immunology Institute, Icahn School of Medicine at Mount Sinai, New York, NY, USA

OVERALL BOTTOM LINE

- Adults with chronic, recurrent, or acute infections may lack antibodies or antibody function.
- These may be due to genetic causes, or secondary to another illness or medication.
- Subjects with antibody defects may be either sex and of any age.
- The diagnosis relies on a combination of clinical, laboratory tests, and exclusion of alternative diagnoses.
- The diagnostic strategy includes blood tests to examine the levels of serum immunoglobulins, and also the functions of these immunoglobulins.
- The goal of treatment is to determine if there is a significant lack of antibody function and determine the origin.

Section 1: Background

Definition of disease

- Antibody protection is important to prevent disease. Loss of production of either immunoglobulins or the ability to create a functioning IgG antibody can lead to recurrent infections. As the immune system is also important to control inflammation, in some cases loss of some normal controls can be associated with autoimmunity.

Disease classification

- Antibody defects result from impaired production of IgG, IgG subclasses, IgA, or IgM.
- When IgG, IgA, and/or IgM are deficient and loss of antibody is documented, the diagnosis of common variable immunodeficiency is made, if no other cause is elucidated.
- When IgG or IgG subclasses are subnormal in amount (compared with age-matched criteria), this would be another diagnosis. These subjects have variable defects in antibody production.
- When IgA or IgM alone are absent, the diagnosis is selective IgA or IgM deficiency.
- These may be due to either primary (genetic) causes, or B-cell defects can be due to other diseases, the most common being malignancy (i.e. chronic lymphocytic leukemia, CLL) or, in rare cases, drug reactions (e.g. antiepileptics, chemotherapy, rituximab).

Mount Sinai Expert Guides: Allergy and Clinical Immunology, First Edition. Edited by Hugh A. Sampson.
© 2015 John Wiley & Sons, Ltd. Published 2015 by John Wiley & Sons, Ltd.
Companion website: www.mountsinaiexpertguides.com

Incidence/prevalence
- The incidence of primary or secondary antibody immune defects, taken as a whole, is unknown.
- For IgA deficiency, the incidence varies in different ethnic groups, from 1 in 500 in Finland, to a considerably less common incidence in Asian populations.
- Subjects on chemotherapy, including rituximab, may have a loss of antibody function.

Economic impact
- Unrecognized immune defects that lead to a significant loss of antibody production may lead to increased morbidity and mortality.

Etiology
- In most cases, the mechanisms for primary antibody defects are unknown.
- Medical causes of antibody deficiency include B-cell diseases such as leukemias, chemotherapy, some antiepileptic medications (e.g. Phenytoin (Dilantin)®, Carbamazepine (Tegretol)®).

Pathology/pathogenesis
- As above, antibody defects may be either primary or secondary to other causes.
- The role of genetics in some cases is clear from family studies, but complex inheritance patterns usually obscure the actual genetic contributions.
- Pathology: lack of immunoglobulin or antibody can lead to the following:
  - Acute bacterial infections of the lungs, blood, brain, joints, or solid organs;
  - Autoimmunity, in particular immune thrombocytopenia or hemolytic anemia;
  - Chronic gastrointestinal inflammation with loss of absorptive surfaces leading to diarrhea, malnutrition, iron deficiency anemia, hypoalbuminemia, and so on.
  - IgA deficiency may be common in subjects with celiac disease;
  - IgA deficiency with IgG2 deficiency can be found in association with lung disease.

Predictive/risk factors
- A family history of an immune defect suggests that an immune defect should be considered.

Section 2: Prevention
Screening
- Patients with medical histories suggestive of antibody defects (recurrent infections, auto-immunity, lymphadenopathy, etc.) can be tested to determine if serum immunoglobulins are normal. To test antibody function, selected vaccines are given to determine the production of antibodies. If the serum IgG, IgA, and IgM are very low, the number of circulating B cells can also be assessed.

Primary prevention
There are no primary preventative measures.

Secondary prevention
There are no secondary preventative measures.

Section 3: Diagnosis
- Antibody defects, from whatever cause, generally lead to acute or recurrent bacterial infections, infections with unusual organisms, or infections that prove difficult to eliminate.

- In some cases, significant infections have not occurred but various forms of inflammatory or autoimmune disease have occurred instead (e.g. interstitial lung disease, arthritis, gastrointestinal disease, hematologic cytopenias, gastrointestinal infections, or inflammation).
- The clinical examination can be normal or show non-specific signs such as lung abnormalities (rales, rhonchi) or lymphadenopathy, splenomegaly, pallor, or evidence of malnutrition of gastrointestinal disease.

Differential diagnosis

Differential diagnosis	Features
Allergy/asthma	Recurrent infections; pneumonias
Chronic viral/parasitic infection	Infections, weight loss
Malignancy/lymphoma	Weight loss, fever
Medications	Rash, fever

Typical presentation
- The typical scenario for a patient with a very significant loss of antibody is a history of the sudden onset of an acute bacterial infection such as pneumococcal pneumonia leading to an empyema. This person may or may not have a previous history of sinusitis or other more minor infections before this time.
- A second presentation is a patient who has an episode of acute immune thrombocytopenic purpura (ITP) or hemolytic anemia. The patient with autoimmunity may have had a previous episode as well, treated successfully with steroids, but who now presents with a recurrence.
- Other common presentations include an episode of giardiasis, or other gastrointestinal parasites, or an otherwise unexplained enteropathy.
- Subjects with celiac disease or allergies are also more likely to have IgA deficiency.

Clinical diagnosis
History
- Symptoms are heterogeneous as the organs and systems affected vary; depends on the nature of the immune defect. In 80% of cases, lung infections occur, specifically pneumonia or chronic bronchitis. A history of "difficult to treat" chronic sinusitis or previous sinus surgery is often found. Gastrointestinal disease is seen in some. Details sought in the clinical history should include duration and onset of symptoms, fatigue, fever, weight loss, shortness of breath. Weight loss is common. Obtaining a detailed family history is always important, as well as questions about smoking, drug use, the medications used and results obtained.

Physical examination
- Physical examination should start with evaluation for signs of systemic illness, including weight loss. However, patients with IgA or IgG deficiency may also look entirely healthy and have a normal physical examination. Fever may be present with acute infections, otherwise chronic fever would be uncommon. Patients with lung disease may be short of breath, have a productive or non-productive cough, and may have pulmonary signs such as rhonchi or rales on examinination. Lymphadenopathy is common, and enlarged spleen may be detected. Skin changes may include scarring from previous herpes zoster; vitiligo appears to be common.

Chronic conjunctivitis, iritis, or episcleritis may be observed. Joint complaints include changes resulting from previous joint infections, or autoimmune and chronic arthritis.

Laboratory diagnosis

List of diagnostic tests

- Complete blood count (anemia, leukopenia, thrombocytopenia).
- Serum IgG, IgA, IgM (based on appropriate age ranges).
- Unless the level of serum IgG is very low (perhaps less than 300 mg/dL), tests for functional antibody (tetanus, diphtheria, etc.) should be carried out to prove loss of function.
- For subjects with some retained serum IgG, immunization with pneumococcal or other vaccines and testing for antibody titers in about 1 month is useful to prove loss of antibody function.
- Microbial cultures where applicable.
- Microbiologic studies to define infectious etiologies.

Lists of imaging techniques

- Chest X-ray.
- Complete lung functions (spirometry and diffusion capacity).
- High-resolution CT of the chest.
- Ultrasound for question of splenomegaly.
- CT of the abdomen to examine organ size, lymphadenopathy.
- MRI may preferred to minimize exposure to ionizing radiation.

Potential pitfalls/common errors made regarding diagnosis of disease

- Not diagnosing significant antibody defects leads to excess morbidity.
- Over-diagnosis can lead to excess medical costs as therapies to correct these can be expensive.

Section 4: Treatment

Treatment rationale

- The goal of therapy is to provide protection against infections.
  - *Antibiotics:* when an antibody deficiency has been documented, antibiotics should be started immediately for fevers or other manifestations of acute infection after appropriate cultures have been obtained. These cultures are important to direct further therapy if the infection does not respond to the initial antibiotic chosen. Prophylactic antibiotics can be of benefit, especially for subjects with chronic lung disease. A satisfactory combination of antibiotics includes amoxicillin-clavulanate, erythromycin, trimethoprim and sulfamethoxazole, or a cephalosporin. In adults, amoxicillin-clavulanate, trimethoprim and sulfamethoxazole, tetracyclines, or a cephalosporin are useful. Quinolones are best saved to treat acute infections.
  - *Immunoglobulin:* when significant loss of antibody production has occurred and this has been fully documented, the optimum treatment is immunoglobulin replacement. The usual starting dose for the intravenous forms (IVIg) is 400–600 mg/kg/month; IVIg can be given at home. Subcutaneous treatment is also quite effective; smaller doses are given once a week. The latter is useful for persons with busy schedules, who want more independence for choosing times of treatment and poor venous access, amongst other reasons.

Table of treatment

Treatment	Comment
Conservative	Antibiotics for acute care as needed Prophylactic antibiotics for some
Medical	Immunoglobulin replacement when loss of antibody is documented; 400–600 mg/kg, IV or given subcutaneously Antibiotics as above
Surgical	Biopsies if pathology suspected
Radiological	To examine lungs or other organs as needed
Complementary	Vitamins and nutrients as needed
Other	Encourage normal activities, schooling, work, etc.

Prevention/management of complications
- For a patient on immunoglobulin replacement therapy, testing the trough values (levels in the blood just before the next treatment) is important to assure satisfactory dosing.

> **CLINICAL PEARLS**
> - Smoking is a risk factor for progressive lung disease.
> - Steroids and other immunosuppressants are to be avoided when the immune system is impaired.
> - Do not start immunoglobulin therapy unless a very complete evaluation of antibody production has been carried out.

Section 5: Special populations
Pregnancy
- Treatment is as usual but with medications approved in pregnancy. For those with loss of antibody, the immunoglobulin replacement is given, but in a dosage that is in accordance with increased body weight.

Children
- Treatment is as usual but with medications and immunoglobulin given based on weight.

Elderly
- Treatment is as usual.

Section 6: Prognosis

> **BOTTOM LINE/CLINICAL PEARLS**
> - Patients with antibody defects will do well if the correct therapy is initiated.
> - Careful evaluation of any new clinical findings that develop over time is important.
> - Use of antibiotics: choices are based on the literature which outlines the most common organisms. When new infections arise, cultures are carried out where possible.

Natural history of untreated disease
• Continued infections are likely and other complications may occur. These may lead to lung or other organ damage.

Prognosis for treated patients
• Prognosis varies with the degree of the antibody defect and with complications that may have developed but, with treatment, the prognosis is clearly improved.

Follow-up tests and monitoring
• Careful follow-up for signs of new infections.
• For patients on immunoglobulin therapy, attention to trough values (the IgG at the lowest points before retreatment) is essential.

Section 7: Reading list

Primary immunodeficiency disease. In Goldman L, Schafer, AI (eds) Cecil Textbook of Medicine, 24th edition. Philadelphia, PA: Elsevier Saunders; 2012.

Suggested websites
American Associate of Asthma Allergy and Immune Deficiency (AAAAI). http://www.aaaai.org/conditions-and-treatments/primary-immunodeficiency-disease.aspx
Immune Deficiency Foundation. www.primaryimmune.org
The Jeffrey Modell Foundation. http://www.info4pi.org/jmf
NIH. http://www.niaid.nih.gov/topics/immunedeficiency

Section 8: Guidelines

Guideline title	Guideline source	Date
Practice parameter for the diagnosis and management of primary immunodeficiency	American Academy of Allergy, Asthma and Immunology (AAAAI)	2005 (https://www.aaaai.org/Aaaai/media/MediaLibrary/PDF%20Documents/Practice%20and%20Parameters/immunodeficiency2005.pdf)

Section 9: Evidence
Not applicable for this topic.

Section 10: Images

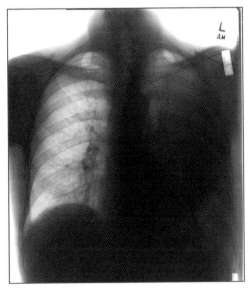

Figure 40.1 A 42-year-old healthy man developed pneumonia which led to an empyema. The culture grew *Streptococcus pneumoniae*.

Additional material for this chapter can be found online at:
www.mountsinaiexpertguides.com
This includes a case study, multiple choice questions,
and ICD codes

CHAPTER 41

Selective IgA Deficiency

Shradha Agarwal

Division of Allergy/Immunology, Icahn School of Medicine at Mount Sinai, New York, NY, USA

OVERALL BOTTOM LINE
- Selective IgA deficiency is the most common primary immunodeficiency.
- The majority of patients with IgA deficiency are asymptomatic and require routine follow-up and education regarding their disease.
- Symptomatic patients typically present with recurrent sinopulmonary infections, autoimmune disease, or gastrointestinal disorders (e.g. celiac disease, inflammatory bowel disease, nodular lymphoid hyperplasia).
- Symptomatic patients with recurrent sinopulmonary disease should be aggressively treated according to the underlying condition (e.g. allergy, asthma, chronic rhinosinusitis).
- Patient with severe symptoms or coexisting antibody deficiency may require treatment with antibiotics and/or immunoglobulin replacement.

Section 1: Background
Definition of disease
- Selective IgA deficiency is a primary antibody immunodeficiency characterized by significantly decreased (<7 mg/dL) or lack of serum IgA in the absence of any other immunodeficiency disorder in an individual older than 4 years of age. Serum levels of IgG and IgM are normal in patients with selective IgA deficiency.

Disease classification
Not applicable for this topic.

Incidence/prevalence
- The incidence varies depending on the ethnic background; however, in the United States the frequency is estimated to be 1 in 223–1000 in studies and 1 in 333–3000 in healthy blood donors.
- True incidence may be higher because most individuals with IgA deficiency are asymptomatic.

Economic impact
Not applicable for this topic.

Etiology
- The exact molecular basis for IgA deficiency is not known but is likely heterogeneous arising through several pathogenic mechanisms.

Mount Sinai Expert Guides: Allergy and Clinical Immunology, First Edition. Edited by Hugh A. Sampson.
© 2015 John Wiley & Sons, Ltd. Published 2015 by John Wiley & Sons, Ltd.
Companion website: www.mountsinaiexpertguides.com

Pathology/pathogenesis
• B cells from IgA deficient patients demonstrate defective terminal B-cell differentiation and subsequently do not mature into IgA secreting plasma cells.

Predictive/risk factors

Risk factor	Odds ratio
Family history of IgA deficiency or common variable immunodeficiency (CVID)	50-fold relative risk for first degree relatives

Section 2: Prevention
No interventions have been demonstrated to prevent the development of the disease.

Screening
Currently no populations are being screened for IgA deficiency.

Primary prevention
Not applicable for this topic.

Secondary prevention
Not applicable for this topic.

Section 3: Diagnosis (Algorithm 41.1)

Algorithm 41.1 Diagnosis of selective IgA deficiency

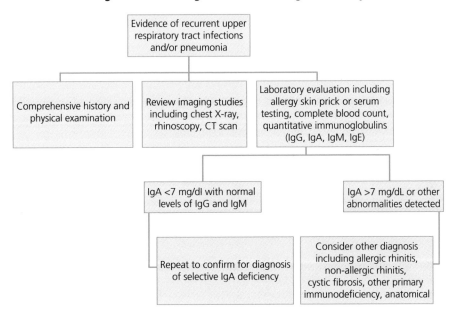

> **BOTTOM LINE/CLINICAL PEARLS**
> - The majority of patients with IgA deficiency are asymptomatic.
> - Those who present for medical attention may have variable symptoms: recurrent sinopulmonary infections, allergic disease, autoimmunity, anaphylactic transfusion reactions, and gastrointestinal infections and diseases.
> - The diagnosis should be considered in any patient who is symptomatic with unusual presentations of the diseases listed above or is difficult to manage with standard therapies.
> - The diagnosis of IgA deficiency is confirmed by isolated deficiency of serum IgA (<7 mg/dL) with normal IgG and IgM levels. Testing should be repeated for confirmation.
> - Laboratory examination is driven by the patient's history and symptoms (e.g. IgE level in an allergic patient).
> - Patients with a history of recurrent upper or lower respiratory tract infections should have IgG subclasses evaluated as IgG subclass deficiency can accompany IgA deficiency.

Differential diagnosis

Differential diagnosis	Features
Transient hypogammaglobulinemia of infancy	Physiologic hypogammaglobulinemia of infancy presenting beyond 6 months of age. Usually have reduced IgG but may have isolated IgA deficiency with spontaneous recovery of immunoglobulin levels by 2–4 years of age
Evolving common variable immunodeficiency (CVID)	Reduced serum IgG, IgA, and/or IgM with impaired antibody response. History of recurrent upper/lower respiratory tract infections; autoimmunity
Medication induced IgA deficiency	Reduction in serum immunoglobulins are reversible when medications are withdrawn. Anti-seizure medications, captopril, D-penicillamine, fenclofenac, gold, sulfasalazine, thyroxine

Typical presentation
- Typical presentation is a young patient with recurrent otitis media, sinusitis, and/or pneumonia. Patients often have coexisting allergic rhinitis or asthma that may be difficult to manage leading to frequent sinopulmonary infections. Patients with coexisting gastrointestinal symptoms may have symptoms of malabsorption, diarrhea, weight loss, or infection with *Giardia lamblia*. Other patients may present with unexplained autoimmune disease. A few patients present with a history of an anaphylactic reaction to blood products.

Clinical diagnosis
History
- Symptoms are heterogeneous. Details in the history to note include the onset and duration of infectious symptoms particularly sinopulmonary and/or gastrointestinal disorders.
- Physicians should enquire about symptoms of allergic disease such as nasal congestion, rhinorrhea, cough, and wheezing.
- Those with gastrointestinal disease may report abdominal pain, weight loss, malabsorption, and diarrhea.
- Patients with autoimmune symptoms may report joint pain, fatigue, and weight loss.

- Patients with a history of reaction to blood products may report symptoms of anaphylaxis including pruritus, flushing, shortness of breath, and wheezing.

Physical examination

- Physical examination should begin with examination of head and neck for boggy nasal turbinates, nasal discharge, and sinus tenderness which suggest allergic rhinitis or chronic rhinosinusitis.
- Lung examination significant for decreased breath sounds or wheezing suggests infectious process or asthma.
- Patients with gastrointestinal symptoms may have abdominal tenderness indicating an inflammatory disorder.
- Physical examination should include a search for autoimmune manifestations, such as joint pain/tenderness, enlarged thyroid, and petechiae.

Useful clinical decision rules and calculators

Not applicable for this topic.

Disease severity classification

Not applicable for this topic.

Laboratory diagnosis

List of diagnostic tests

- Measurement of serum immunoglobulins with reference to age. A repeat test to confirm diagnosis is necessary.

Lists of imaging techniques

Not applicable for this topic.

Potential pitfalls/common errors made regarding diagnosis of disease

- Serum immunoglobulins should be drawn with reference to the patient's age. Those younger than 4 years of age should be monitored for normalization of IgA levels over time.

Section 4: Treatment (Algorithm 41.2)

Treatment rationale

- Asymptomatic patients require no specific treatment for IgA deficiency.
- Patients should be educated that blood products can be screened for IgA antibodies to prevent infusion reactions.
- Symptomatic patients are treated according to their coexisting disease.
- Prophylactic antibiotics may be used in patients with recurrent infections. A trial of immunoglobulin (Ig) may be given, particularly in patients with coexisting IgG subclass and antibody deficiency and recurrent infections.

When to hospitalize

Not applicable for this topic.

Managing the hospitalized patient

Not applicable for this topic.

Algorithm 41.2 Treatment for selective IgA deficiency

Education	• For all patients • Asymptomatic patients do not require specific treatment and may be monitored periodically
Antihistamines, allergy immunotherapy	• For those with underlying allergic rhinitis
Antibiotics	• Choice of antibiotic may be according to past culture and sensitivity results and type of infection (bronchitis, otitis, pneumonia, sinusitis) • Trial of prophylactic antibiotics for patients with continued infections
Immunoglobulin (IgG) therapy	• A trial of immunoglobulin replacement therapy may be considered in patients with recurrent infections despite prophylactic antibiotics, particularly if there is an associated antibody deficiency and/or subclass deficiency

Table of treatment

Treatment	Comment
Conservative	Asymptomatic patients require no treatment but should be followed at regular intervals or sooner depending on frequency of infection
Medical Antibiotics (treatment or prophylactic)	Choice and frequency of antibiotics is based on type of infection and culture/sensitivity results
Immunoglobulin (400–600 mg/kg) IV or SC	In patients who have recurrent infections despite prophylactic antibiotics, particularly patients with antibody deficiency and/or IgG subclass deficiency
Radiological Chest X-ray or CT scan	Patients with significant upper or lower respiratory infections
Other IgA washed blood products	For patients who have anti-IgA antibodies

Prevention/management of complications
- Patients who require blood transfusions should consult with a hematologist to advise how blood products can be washed to remove IgA.
- Patients who require immunoglobulin should receive products that are low in IgA content or subcutaneous preparations.

CLINICAL PEARLS
- In patients with IgA deficiency, management of coexisting allergic, gastrointestinal, or autoimmune disorders should be according to standard treatment guidelines.
- A thorough evaluation of the immune system should be performed prior to initiating treatment with immunoglobulin replacement therapy.

Section 5: Special populations

Pregnancy
Not applicable for this topic.

Children
- Serum immunoglobulins in infants are comprised of maternal IgG which typically decline beginning at 6 months of age. Therefore, reduced immunoglobulins in an infant or child should be monitored for normalization until the immune system has matured.

Elderly
Not applicable for this topic.

Others
Not applicable for this topic.

Section 6: Prognosis

BOTTOM LINE/CLINICAL PEARLS
- The prognosis for patients with IgA deficiency who have no significant disease is good.
- In others, the prognosis depends on the severity of associated disorders (i.e. allergy, autoimmune).
- Some patients with IgA deficiency may progress to CVID.

Natural history of untreated disease
Not applicable for this topic.

Prognosis for treated patients
Not applicable for this topic.

Follow-up tests and monitoring
- Patient with IgA deficiency should have routine follow-up of clinical history and laboratory evaluation of serum IgG, IgA, and IgM, as some cases may evolve to CVID.

Section 7: Reading list

Hammarström L, Smith CIE. Genetic approach to common variable immunodeficiency and IgA deficiency. In: Ochs HD, Smith CIE, Puck JM (eds) Primary Immunodeficiency Diseases: A Molecular and Genetic Approach, 2nd edition. Oxford University Press, 2007: 313–25

Notarangelo LD, Fischer A, Geha RS, Casanova JL, Chapel H, Conley ME, et al. Primary immunodeficiencies: 2009 update. J Allergy Clin Immunol 2009;124:1161–78

Pan-Hammarström Q, Hammarström L. Antibody deficiency diseases. Eur J Immunol 2008;38:327–33

Wang N, Hammarström L. IgA deficiency: what is new? Curr Opin Allergy Clin Immunol 2012;12:602–8

Yel L. Selective IgA deficiency. J Clin Immunol 2010;30:10–6

Suggested websites

American Academy of Allergy Asthma and Immunology. www.aaaai.org/home.aspx

Clinical Immunology Society. www.clinimmsoc.org

Immune Deficiency Foundation. http://primaryimmune.org/

Jeffrey Modell Foundation. www.info4pi.org

Section 8: Guidelines
National society guidelines

Guideline title	Guideline source	Date
Practice parameter for the diagnosis and management of primary immunodeficiency	American Academy of Allergy, Asthma and Immunology (AAAAI); American College of Allergy, Asthma and Immunology (ACAAI)	2005 (https://www.aaaai.org/Aaaai/media/MediaLibrary/PDF%20Documents/Practice%20and%20Parameters/immunodeficiency2005.pdf)

International society guidelines

Guideline title	Guideline source	Date
Primary immunodeficiency diseases: an update from the International Union of Immunological Societies Primary Immunodeficiency Diseases Classification Committee	International Union of Immunological Societies (IUIS)	2007 (http://www.ncbi.nlm.nih.gov/pubmed/17952897)

Section 9: Evidence
Not applicable for this topic.

Section 10: Images
Not applicable for this topic.

Additional material for this chapter can be found online at:
www.mountsinaiexpertguides.com
This includes a case study, multiple choice questions, advice for patients, and ICD code

CHAPTER 42

Severe Combined Immunodeficiency

Kate Welch and Elena S. Resnick
Icahn School of Medicine at Mount Sinai, New York, NY, USA

OVERALL BOTTOM LINE
- Severe combined immunodeficiency syndrome (SCID) is a rare genetic syndrome characterized by profound deficiencies of T- and B-cell function and, in some cases, NK cell function.
- The classic symptoms of SCID manifest in the first few months of life and include recurrent infections, diarrhea, and failure to thrive.
- In infants with SCID, lymphopenia is present, serum immunoglobulins and antibodies are diminished to absent, and the thymus is very small (usually <1 g).
- SCID is a pediatric emergency. The most common widely available curative therapy for most forms of the disease is hematopoietic cell transplantation.
- Without treatment, the disease is uniformly fatal.

Section 1: Background
Definition of disease
- SCID is a rare fatal syndrome of diverse genetic origin characterized by profound defects in the development and function of T- and B-cells and leading to overwhelming infection in affected infants. There is high variability in the phenotype of circulating lymphocytes in patients with SCID, which is a result of the diverse genetic causes. Death in infancy is a universal result unless immune reconstitution can be achieved.

Disease classification
- Until a genetic diagnosis is established, SCID syndromes can be classified based upon molecular defects affecting T cells and the presence or absence of defects affecting B and/or NK cells as T–, B+ and NK+; T–, B+ and NK–; T–, B– and NK+; or T–, B– and NK–. In some cases, only T-cell function is affected. However, because B cells rely on T-cell signaling for antibody production, T-cell dysfunction precludes effective humoral immunity. These lymphocyte phenotypes are the result of at least 12 different gene mutations, which include defects in cytokine receptor genes, antigen receptor genes, and genes leading to deficiencies of adenosine deaminase and CD45.

Incidence/prevalence
- The incidence of SCID is estimated to be 1 in 40 000–50 000 live births.
- X-linked SCID, related to a defect in a cytokine receptor gene (*IL2RG*), is the most common form and accounts for roughly 45% of cases in the United States.

Mount Sinai Expert Guides: Allergy and Clinical Immunology, First Edition. Edited by Hugh A. Sampson.
© 2015 John Wiley & Sons, Ltd. Published 2015 by John Wiley & Sons, Ltd.
Companion website: www.mountsinaiexpertguides.com

Economic impact

Not applicable for this topic.

Etiology

- Mutations in 12 genes have been found to cause SCID.
- An absence of the enzyme adenosine deaminase (ADA) was the first causal gene identified (in 1972) and accounts for approximately 17% of SCID cases. ADA deficiency results in toxic accumulation of metabolites that cause T cell apoptosis.
- A defect in three cytokine receptor genes IL2RG, JAK3, and IL7Rα, lead to different T–B+ phenotypes.
- The products of other genes (e.g. RAG 1 and 2, Artemis, Ligase 4, and 3 CD3 subs) are essential for effecting antigen receptor gene rearrangement.
- A mutation in the gene that encodes the common leukocyte antigen, CD45, a phosphatase critical for regulating signaling thresholds in immune cells, also causes SCID.

Pathology/pathogenesis

- Infants with SCID are lymphopenic and have an absence of lymphocytic response to mitogens, antigens, and allogeneic cells in vitro. Serum immunoglobulin concentrations are diminished to absent, and there is no antibody formation after immunization. NK cells are present in approximately 50% of patients with SCID and may provide some degree of protection against bacterial and viral infections. Affected infants look normal outwardly, and maternally derived antibodies provide some protection during early infancy. However, in the absence of both specific cellular and humoral immunity, infants with SCID have a profound susceptibility to infection that manifests in the first few months of life.

Predictive/risk factors

Not applicable for this topic.

Section 2: Prevention

No interventions have been demonstrated to prevent the development of the disease.

Screening

- Because early diagnosis of SCID improves outcomes, a screening method for SCID was added to the recommended uniform newborn screening panel in the United States in 2010. This method for screening for T-cell lymphopenia uses dried blood spots, usually from a heel stick or cord blood, to measure T-cell receptor excision circles (TRECs) as a marker of naïve T cells. SCID babies diagnosed at birth have a decreased number of infections and overall improved survival. US states that currently screen all newborns for SCID include Wisconsin, Massachusetts, New York, California, Connecticut, Michigan, Colorado, Mississippi, Delaware, Florida, Texas, Minnesota, Iowa, Pennsylvania, Utah, and Ohio.

Primary prevention

Not applicable for this topic.

Secondary prevention

Not applicable for this topic.

Section 3: Diagnosis

Differential diagnosis

Differential diagnosis	Features
Wiskott–Aldrich syndrome	X-linked disorder Thrombocytopenia and eczema are often present
Complete DiGeorge syndrome	22q11.2 deletion Hypocalcemia, palatal abnormalities, cardiac anomalies
Omenn's syndrome	SCID-related disorder but will have other findings of exudative skin rash, lymphadenopathy, and hepatosplenomegaly
HIV/AIDS	Presence of a thymic shadow on chest radiograph Normal lymphocyte count Normal lymphocyte proliferation Elevated serum immunoglobulin levels
Extreme malnutrition	Normal lymphocyte count Clinical history of poor feeding

Typical presentation
- In the absence of effective newborn screening, the mean age at diagnosis of SCID is 6 months. Affected infants present within the first few months of life with recurrent fevers, chronic diarrhea, and failure to thrive. Recurrent infections with common and opportunistic organisms occur and can lead to death. These organisms include *Candida albicans, Pneumocystis jiroveci*, respiratory syncytial virus, varicella zoster virus, adenovirus, parainfluenza 3, herpesviruses, cytomegalovirus, Epstein–Barr virus, and influenza, among others. Patients also experience infections in response to live vaccines. They are susceptible to graft versus host disease from maternal T cells crossing into circulation in utero or from T lymphocytes in non-irradiated blood products.

Clinical diagnosis
History
- In addition to a history of infections or failure to thrive, the clinician should enquire about a family history of SCID or infants in the family who died of unexplained causes.

Physical examination

- Infants with SCID appear normal outwardly, but may become cachectic and appear malnourished with the onset of recurrent infections and diarrhea.

Useful clinical decision rules and calculators

Not applicable for this topic.

Disease severity classification

- There is no standard classification of disease severity, although different lymphocytic phenotypes (T−, B+ and NK+; T−, B+ and NK−; T−, B− and NK+; or T−, B− and NK−) exist and are linked to the various known genetic defects.
  - Adenosine deaminase deficiency (approximately 16% of patients):
    - ➤ T−, B− and NK−;
    - ➤ More profound lymphopenia than other types of SCID;
    - ➤ Mean absolute lymphocyte counts of <500/mm³ and a deficiency of all three types of immune cells;
    - ➤ Characterized by multiple skeletal abnormalities related to chondro-osseous dysplasia.
  - Common gamma chain deficiency (approximately 46% of patients):
    - ➤ T−, B+ and NK−;
    - ➤ Seen in X-linked recessive SCID;
    - ➤ B cells are present in the circulation but do not undergo class switch recombination.
  - Jak3 deficiency (approximately 6% of patients):
    - ➤ T−, B+ and NK−;
    - ➤ Autosomal recessive inheritance;
    - ➤ Lymphocyte characteristics closely resemble those of patients with X-linked SCID, with an elevated percentage of B cells.
  - IL-7 receptor alpha chain deficiency (approximately 11% of patients):
    - ➤ T−, B+ and NK+;
    - ➤ Profoundly deficient in T- and B-cell function;
    - ➤ Normal NK cell function.
  - Recombinase-activating gene deficiencies (RAG1/RAG2) (approximately 4% of patients):
    - ➤ T−, B− and NK+;
    - ➤ Mutations result in functional inability to form antigen receptors through genetic recombination;
    - ➤ More common in Europe than the United States.
  - CD3δ, ε, ζ chain deficiencies (approximately 2% of patients):
    - ➤ T−, B+ and NK+;
    - ➤ Mutations in in the genes encoding CD3ε and CD3ζ chains result in only a partial arrest of T-cell maturation and therefore only moderate immunodeficiency;
    - ➤ Nearly normal-sized thymus on chest X-ray.
  - CD45 deficiency (0.5% of patients):
    - ➤ T−, B+ and NK+;
    - ➤ Normal protein functions to regulate Src kinases required for T- and B-cell antigen receptor signal transduction.
  - Artemis deficiency (1% of patients):
    - ➤ T−, B− and NK+;
    - ➤ Inability to repair DNA after cuts have been made by RAG1 or RAG2 gene products;
    - ➤ Increased radiation sensitivity of skin fibroblasts.

Laboratory diagnosis
List of diagnostic tests
- Laboratory diagnosis of SCID requires evaluation of humoral and cellular immunity.
- Studies include the absolute numbers and percentages of lymphocyte subsets (T, B, and NK), measurement of immunoglobulin levels, and assessment of T-cell function.
- At the age of 6–7 months when most infants with SCID are diagnosed, the normal absolute lymphocyte count is high, and any count <4000 cells/mm^3 is lymphopenic. Flow cytometry and T-cell function studies should be performed to further evaluate lymphopenia.
- T-cell function is usually determined by measurement of responses to mitogens such as phytohemagglutinin and concanavalin A.
- A diagnosis of SCID is made if the absolute lymphocyte count is <2500 cells/mm^3, T cells make up less than 20% of the total lymphocytes, and the response to mitogens is less than 10% of the control.

Lists of imaging techniques
- Chest radiograph of infants with SCID is notable for the absence of the thymic shadow.
- Patients with the ADA deficiency variant of SCID will have other skeletal abnormalities on radiographic examination, including chondro-osseous dysplasia, with flaring of the costochondral junctions and a bone-in-bone anomaly in the vertebral bodies.

Potential pitfalls/common errors made regarding diagnosis of disease
Not applicable for this topic.

Section 4: Treatment
Treatment rationale
- SCID is a pediatric emergency. The most common curative therapy for all forms of SCID is bone marrow transplantation from HLA-identical or haploidentical donors. Without this, death usually occurs by 1 year of age and invariably before the patient's second birthday. No chemotherapeutic conditioning is required to achieve engraftment because the recipient is devoid of T cells at the time of transplantation.
- Some patients with ADA deficiency may be treated with enzyme replacement therapy (PEG-ADA); however, most receive transplant.
- Gene therapy has been on the horizon as a promising treatment for SCID. However, serious adverse events, including development of leukemic-like processes in treated infants, have halted its progress.

When to hospitalize
Not applicable for this topic.

Managing the hospitalized patient
Not applicable for this topic.

Table of treatment
Not applicable for this topic.

Prevention/management of complications
Not applicable for this topic.

Section 5: Special populations

Not applicable for this topic.

Section 6: Prognosis

> **BOTTOM LINE/CLINICAL PEARLS**
> * Immune reconstitution after transplant is due to thymic education of the transplanted allogeneic stem cells.
> * Thymic output appears sooner and to a greater degree in those infants transplanted in the neonatal period, thus making early diagnosis the key to survival.

Natural history of untreated disease
* If untreated, the disease is invariably fatal.

Prognosis for treated patients
* Transplantation in the first 3.5 months of life confers a >96% chance of survival.
* Death after transplant usually occurs from infectious complications.

Follow-up tests and monitoring
Not applicable for this topic.

Section 7: Reading list

Brown L, Xu-Bayford J, Allwood Z, Slatter M, Cant A, Davies EG, et al. Neonatal diagnosis of severe combined immunodeficiency leads to significantly improved survival outcome: the case for newborn screening. Blood 2011;117:3243–6

Buckley RH. Advances in the understanding and treatment of human severe combined immunodeficiency. Immunol Res 2000;22:237–51

Buckley RH. Molecular defects in human severe combined immunodeficiency and approaches to immune reconstitution. Annu Rev Immunol 2004;22:625–55

Buckley RH, Schiff RI, Schiff SE, Markert ML, Williams LW, Harville TO, et al. Human severe combined immunodeficiency: genetic, phenotypic and functional diversity in one hundred eight infants. J Pediatr 1997;130:378–87

Lipstein EA, Vorono S, Browning MF, Green NS, Kemper AR, Knapp AA, et al. Systematic evidence review of newborn screening and treatment of severe combined immunodeficiency. Pediatrics 2010;125: e1226–35

Roifman CM, Somech R, Kavadas F, Pires L, Nahum A, Dalal I, et al. Defining combined immunodeficiency. J Allergy Clin Immunol 2012;130:177–83

Suggested websites
National Human Genome Research Institute. http://www.genome.gov/13014325
Immune Deficiency Foundation. http://primaryimmune.org/
http://www.scid.net/

Section 8: Guidelines
National society guidelines

Guideline title	Guideline source	Date
Practice parameter for the diagnosis and management of primary immunodeficiency	The American Academy of Allergy, Asthma, and Immunology	2005 (http://www.aaaai.org/Aaaai/ media/MediaLibrary/PDF%20 Documents/Practice%20 and%20Parameters/ immunodeficiency2005.pdf)

Section 9: Evidence
Not applicable for this topic.

Section 10: Images
Not applicable for this topic.

Additional material for this chapter can be found online at:
www.mountsinaiexpertguides.com
This includes a case study, multiple choice questions,
and ICD code

CHAPTER 43

Wiskott–Aldrich Syndrome

Elena S. Resnick

Icahn School of Medicine at Mount Sinai, New York, NY, USA

OVERALL BOTTOM LINE
- Wiskott–Aldrich syndrome (WAS) is a rare, X-linked disease caused by a mutation in the gene for the Wiskott–Aldrich syndrome protein (WASp).
- Mutations in WASp cause classic WAS, X-linked thrombocytopenia, or X-linked neutropenia.
- Clinical features are variable, and include immune deficiency, microthrombocytopenia, eczematous dermatitis, autoimmunity, and malignancy.

Section 1: Background

Definition of disease
- Wiskott–Aldrich syndrome (WAS) is a rare, X-linked disease caused by a mutation in the gene for the Wiskott-Aldrich syndrome protein (WASp). Clinical features are variable, and include immune deficiency, thrombocytopenia, eczematous dermatitis, autoimmunity, and malignancy.

Disease classification
- Specific WASp gene mutations may cause diverse clinical manifestations, usually including immune deficiency, thrombocytopenia, and eczema. Classic WAS can be severe and include symptoms of autoimmunity and malignancy. X-linked thrombocytopenia (XLT) is a less severe phenotype consisting of isolated thrombocytopenia. X-linked neutropenia (XLN) is caused by yet another WASp mutation.

Incidence/prevalence
- The incidence of WAS is estimated at 1 in 250 000 live male births.
- The XLT phenotype accounts for approximately 50% of WASp mutations.
- The XLN phenotype is extremely rare, with <12 patients in four families having been reported in the literature.

Economic impact
Not applicable for this topic.

Mount Sinai Expert Guides: Allergy and Clinical Immunology, First Edition. Edited by Hugh A. Sampson.
© 2015 John Wiley & Sons, Ltd. Published 2015 by John Wiley & Sons, Ltd.
Companion website: www.mountsinaiexpertguides.com

Etiology

- WAS is a genetic disease caused by a mutation in the gene for the WASp on the X-chromosome.
- Many unique WAS gene mutations account for the disease phenotype, with missense mutations most common.
- A WAS-like phenotype is also seen with mutations in the gene for WIPF1, encoding the WASp-interacting protein (WIP) necessary to stabilize WASp.

Pathology/pathogenesis

- WASp is required for remodeling of the cellular actin cytoskeleton and cell chemotaxis as well as the appropriate formation of the immunologic synapse. The absence of a functional WASp leads to the WAS phenotype, which can be severe and lead to death if not recognized and treated. Mutations in WASp cause defective T-cell and NK cell function as well as decreased B-cell numbers, accounting for the immune deficiency phenotype observed in WAS patients. WASp defects also lead to a decrease in regulatory T-cell (Treg) function, which along with B-cell dysfunction and impaired cellular apoptosis can lead to increased autoimmune phenomena. Thrombocytopenia observed in WAS patients may be autoimmune in nature or due to impaired platelet formation or survival.

Predictive/risk factors

Not applicable for this topic.

Section 2: Prevention

No interventions have been demonstrated to prevent the development of the disease.

Screening

No screening is currently routinely performed.

Primary prevention

Not applicable for this topic.

Secondary prevention

Not applicable for this topic.

Section 3: Diagnosis

> **BOTTOM LINE/CLINICAL PEARLS**
> - Classic WAS typically presents in a young male presenting with recurrent infections (immunodeficiency), eczematous dermatitis, and bleeding diathesis (microthrombocytopenia).
> - Malignancy and/or autoimmunity may develop later in life.
> - T- and B-cells numbers may be reduced and/or function may be impaired.
> - Definitive diagnosis is made with the identification of a mutation in the WAS gene and/or the WASp is found to be deficient or non-functional.

Differential diagnosis

Differential diagnosis	Features
X-linked thrombocytopenia	Mild clinical phenotype including thrombocytopenia and mild eczema
X-linked neutropenia	Frequent infections due to neutropenia
WIPF1 mutation	Clinical features similar to WAS, *WIPF1* sequencing necessary to confirm diagnosis
Severe combined immunodeficiency (SCID)	Frequent severe infections from infancy
Immune dysregulation, polyendocrinopathy, X-linked (IPEX)	Immunodeficiency, autoimmune disease, severe gastrointestinal disease

Typical presentation
- WAS is most often seen in a young male presenting with immune deficiency, eczematous dermatitis, and microthrombocytopenia. Thrombocytopenia may manifest as bleeding, petechiae, purpura, gastrointestinal bleeding, epistaxis, hematuria, and/or life-threatening hemorrhage. Immune deficiency may manifest as recurrent infections due to impaired T- and B-cell numbers and function. Severe infections with encapsulated bacteria may occur, and splenectomy performed for thrombocytopenia will worsen this propensity to infection. Opportunistic infections can also be seen; fungal infections are more rare. Eczematous dermatitis is common and may be severe. Autoimmunity is present in as many as 70% of patients. Malignancy is also observed, most commonly B-cell lymphomas associated with Epstein–Barr virus.

Clinical diagnosis
History
- The history will likely be remarkable for a young male with manifestations of thrombocytopenia, sometimes present since birth. All male infants with thrombocytopenia should be investigated for WAS. Other manifestations include a history of eczema and/or frequent infections. Other autoimmune diseases such as vasculitis, autoimmune renal disease, inflammatory bowel disease, neutropenia, and autoimmune hemolytic anemia may occur. A history of malignancy, most often lymphoma, may also be present.

Physical examination
- The physical examination may reveal a young male with eczematous dermatitis, ranging from mild to severe. Physical manifestations of thrombocytopenia may include bleeding, petechiae, purpura, gastrointestinal bleeding, epistaxis, or hematuria. Evidence of infection due to immune deficiency may include fever, lethargy, or other localizing symptoms.

Useful clinical decision rules and calculators
Not applicable for this topic.

Disease severity classification

Disease severity scoring system for disorders associated with WAS mutations

Disease	XLN	iXLT	XLT			Classic WAS	
Score	0	<1	1	2	3	4	5
Thrombocytopenia	–	–/+	+	+	+	+	+
Small platelets	–	+	+	+	+	+	+
Eczema	–	–	–	(+)	+	++	–/(+)/+/++
Immunodeficiency	–/(+)	–	–/(+)	(+)	+	+	(+)/+
Infections	–/(+)	–	–	(+)	+	+/++	–/(+)/+/++
Autoimmunity and/or malignancy	–	–	–	–	–	–	+
Congenital neutropenia	+	–	–	–	–	–	–
Myelodysplasia	–/+	–	–	–	–	–	–

Scoring system:
– Absent.
–/(+) Absent or mild.
–/+ Intermittent thrombocytopenia, possible myelodysplasia.
(+) Mild, transient eczema or mild, infrequent infections not resulting in sequelae.
+ Thrombocytopenia, persistent but therapy-responsive eczema, and recurrent infections requiring antibiotics and often intravenous immunoglobulin prophylaxis.
++ Eczema that is difficult to control and severe, life-threatening infections.
iXLT: intermittent X-linked thrombocytopenia; WAS, Wiskott–Aldrich syndrome; XLN: X-linked neutropenia; XLT: X-linked thrombocytopenia.
Adapted from Stiehm ER, Ochs HD, Winkelstein JA, Rich E (Eds). Immunologic disorders in infants and children, 5th edn. Philadelphia: Saunders, 2004.

Laboratory diagnosis
List of diagnostic tests
- CBC with differential.
- T-cell number and functional studies.
- B-cell number and functional studies.
- NK cell number and functional studies.
- Immunoglobulin levels.
- Sequence of WAS gene necessary to confirm diagnosis.

Lists of imaging techniques
Not applicable for this topic.

Potential pitfalls/common errors made regarding diagnosis of disease
- As this is a relatively rare disease, it must be considered in the differential of any young male presenting with thrombocytopenia.

Section 4: Treatment
Treatment rationale
- Patients diagnosed with WAS should receive prophylactic treatment for frequent infections. This may include intravenous immunoglobulin (IVIg) therapy for patients found to be antibody deficient. Prophylactic antibiotic therapy with trimethoprim-sulfamethoxazole and acyclovir should

also be used. Platelet transfusions may be necessary for bleeding manifestations. Splenectomy has been recommended in the past for thrombocytopenia but is no longer recommended because of the increased risk of infection with encapsulated bacteria. Immunosuppressive therapies such as rituximab may be used for autoimmune disease; however, the risk of infection must be carefully considered. Hematopoitic stem cell transplant is the only definitive treatment for WAS. Gene therapy for WAS is currently under investigation and is not yet used in clinical practice.

When to hospitalize

- Patients with WAS often present with thrombocytopenia and/or severe infections and associated complications that require immediate hospitalization.
- Hospitalization should occur in a tertiary care institution with access to physicians familiar with the disease as well as immunologists, pediatric intensivists, and other pediatric specialists.

Managing the hospitalized patient

See When to hospitalize section.

Table of treatment

Treatment	Comment
Medical IVIG Prophylactic antibiotics (Bactrim®, acyclovir) Immunosuppressive medications	400–600 mg/kg/month Dosage based on weight As necessary for autoimmune disease
Other HSCT	Only curative therapy

Prevention/management of complications

See Treatment rationale section.

Section 5: Special populations

> **CLINICAL PEARLS**
> - In order to make the diagnosis, WAS must first be considered in the differential diagnosis.

Pregnancy

Not applicable for this topic.

Children

See Treatment rationale section.

Elderly

Not applicable for this topic.

Others

Not applicable for this topic.

Section 6: Prognosis

BOTTOM LINE/CLINICAL PEARLS

- Life expectancy in WAS is reduced.
- Causes of death include infection, bleeding complications, autoimmunity, and malignancy.
- Patients with platelet counts below 10 000/mm^3 are at greater risk for bleeding complications.
- Patients with autoimmunity are at greater risk of malignancy.

Section 7: Reading list

Aldrich RA, Steinberg AG, Campbell DC. Pedigree demonstrating a sex-linked recessive condition characterized by draining ears, eczematoid dermatitis and bloody diarrhea. Pediatrics 1954;13:133

Griffith LM, Cowan MJ, Kohn DB, Notarangelo LD, Puck JM, Schultz KR, et al. Allogeneic hematopoietic cell transplantation for primary immune deficiency diseases: current status and critical needs. J Allergy Clin Immunol 2008;122:1087–96

Kim AS, Kakalis LT, Abdul-Manan N, Liu GA, Rosen MK. Autoinhibition and activation mechanisms of the Wiskott–Aldrich syndrome protein. Nature 2000;404:151

Massaad MJ, Ramesh N, Geha RS. Wiskott–Aldrich syndrome: a comprehensive review. Ann N Y Acad Sci 2013;1285:26–43

Ozsahin H, Cavazzana-Calvo M, Notarangelo LD, Schulz A, Thrasher AJ, Mazzolari E, et al. Long-term outcome following hematopoietic stem-cell transplantation in Wiskott–Aldrich syndrome: collaborative study of the European Society for Immunodeficiencies and European Group for Blood and Marrow Transplantation. Blood 2008;111:439

Sullivan KE, Mullen CA, Blaese RM, Winkelstein JA. A multiinstitutional survey of the Wiskott–Aldrich syndrome. J Pediatr 1994;125:876

Wolff JA. Wiskott–Aldrich syndrome: clinical, immunologic, and pathologic observations. J Pediatr 1967;70:221

Section 8: Guidelines
Not applicable for this topic.

Section 9: Evidence
Not applicable for this topic.

Section 10: Images
Not applicable for this topic.

Additional material for this chapter can be found online at:
www.mountsinaiexpertguides.com
This includes a case study, multiple choice questions,
and ICD code

CHAPTER 44

DiGeorge Syndrome

Kate Welch and Elena S. Resnick
Icahn School of Medicine at Mount Sinai, New York, NY, USA

OVERALL BOTTOM LINE

- DiGeorge syndrome encompasses a constellation of symptoms due to defective development of mesenchyme affecting the embryologic pharyngeal pouches.
- It typically occurs in association with a heterozygous chromosomal deletion of chromosome 22q11.2. Chromosome 22q11.2 deletion syndrome includes DiGeorge and similar syndromes, such as velocardiofacial syndrome.
- The classic features include hypoplastic thymus, as well as cardiac anomalies and hypocalcemia, as a result of parathyroid hypoplasia.
- The hypoplastic thymus results in a range of T-cell deficits and varying degrees of immune deficiency. Most patients have only mild defects and few clinical manifestations. Other patients, with a complete absence of the thymus known as "complete DiGeorge syndrome," manifest similarly to severe combined immunodeficiency and need immediate treatment with immune reconstitution.

Section 1: Background

Definition of disease

- DiGeorge syndrome most often occurs as a result of a heterozygous deletion of chromosome 22q11.2 and classically encompasses the triad of hypoplastic thymus, cardiac anomalies, and hypocalcemia as a result of parathyroid hypoplasia. The immune system is affected in approximately 75% of cases, and the phenotype can range from absent thymus with no circulating T cells to completely normal T-cell counts.

Disease classification

- Most cases of DiGeorge syndrome occur as a result of hemizygous deletion of chromosome 22q11.2. However, 5–10% of patients with the clinical manifestations of the syndrome do not have the deletion. Most patients have a mild to moderate immune deficiency, and the majority have a cardiac abnormality. Additional features vary in presentation and include renal anomalies, hypoparathyroidism, skeletal defects, and developmental delay. In an effort to eliminate confusion, there has been an effort toward labeling patients with the classic chromosome deletion as having "22q11.2 deletion syndrome" and those with a distinct or no known cause as having "DiGeorge syndrome." For the sake of simplicity, they will be used interchangeably here.

Mount Sinai Expert Guides: Allergy and Clinical Immunology, First Edition. Edited by Hugh A. Sampson.
© 2015 John Wiley & Sons, Ltd. Published 2015 by John Wiley & Sons, Ltd.
Companion website: www.mountsinaiexpertguides.com

Incidence/prevalence

- The incidence of chromosome 22q11.2 deletions has been estimated as 1 in 3000–6000 births. The deletion may in fact be under-reported because the phenotypic findings can be very mild.
- The incidence is thought to be increasing because the detection and treatment of cardiac and immune anomalies has led to affected parents bearing affected offspring.

Economic impact

Not applicable for this topic.

Etiology

- Approximately 90–95% of infants with the classic constellation of cardiac anomaly, diminished T cells, and hypocalcemia have the deletion of chromosome 22q11.2. The deletion usually arises via unequal meiotic exchange of discrete blocks of four low copy number repeats. These blocks are thought to be inherently unstable because the deletion is roughly 10 times more common than the next most frequent human deletion syndrome. There are over 35 genes within the commonly deleted region of chromosome 22.

Pathology/pathogenesis

- The development of a TBX1 knockout mouse has demonstrated the importance of this gene in cardiac development. Its absence leads to impaired formation of the fourth branchial arch artery, a precursor to the right ventricle and outflow tract. In mice, TBX1 is expressed in the pharyngeal mesenchyme and endodermal pouch. The pharyngeal pouches give rise to the face and upper thorax. In humans, compromised development of the third and fourth pharyngeal pouches also affects the thymus and parathyroid glands. The phenotype is extraordinarily variable, but the following defects can be seen as a result of various gene deletions:
  - *Cardiac anomalies:* cardiac defects include tetralogy of Fallot, ventriculoseptal defect, interrupted aortic arch, truncus arteriosus, and vascular rings.
  - *Thymic hypoplasia and immunodeficiency:* the thymus is absent in patients with complete DiGeorge syndrome and hypoplastic in patients with partial DiGeorge syndrome. As a result, patients with the partial form will have varying degrees of T-cell lymphopenia. The majority of these patients will be only modestly immunocompromised and will not develop opportunistic infections. Abnormal palatal anatomy may affect sinus drainage and lead to an increase in sinopulmonary infections. Some patients will have humoral immune deficiencies and functional antibody defects. Complete DiGeorge syndrome, found in less than 1% of patients with 22q deletion syndrome, results in a severe combined immunodeficiency (SCID)-like presentation and infant fatality without prompt recognition and treatment. Other consequences of immune deficiency include autoimmune disease, seen in roughly 10% of patients, and an increase in allergic disease.
  - *Hypocalcemia:* underdevelopment of the parathyroid glands develops in up to 60% of patients with DiGeorge syndrome. This may present with tetany, low serum calcium, elevated serum phosphorus, and very low parathyroid hormone levels.
  - *Craniofacial abnormalities:* possible defects include low set and posteriorly rotated ears, ocular hypertelorism, and nasal dysmorphism.
  - *Palatal and related problems:* the most common defect is a muscular weakness that affects the ability to close off the nasopharynx when swallowing and speaking. Feeding difficulties, nasal regurgitation, and hypernasal speech may result. More significant defects such as submucous clefts and frank anatomic clefts may be seen.

- *Developmental and behavioral problems:* developmental delay is common and highly variable, with mean IQ ranging from normal to moderately disabled. Speech delay is especially common.

Predictive/risk factors

Not applicable for this topic.

Section 2: Prevention

Not applicable for this topic.

Screening

Not applicable for this topic.

Primary prevention

Not applicable for this topic.

Secondary prevention

Not applicable for this topic.

Section 3: Diagnosis

> **BOTTOM LINE/CLINICAL PEARLS**
> - The diagnosis of DiGeorge syndrome varies by age and the severity of the phenotypic variant. The emphasis of an examination in infancy should focus on high impact areas of cardiac anomaly, profound hypocalcemia, or severe immunodeficiency.
> - Cardiac defects may manifest as cyanosis; hypocalcemia with tetany or seizure; and palatal abnormalities with feeding difficulty in early infancy.
> - Immunodeficiency can be identified in infancy with T-cell lymphopenia or later in life with a history of recurrent infection.
> - Cardiac anomalies, some of which present with cyanosis, may be the first issue discovered after birth, and absence of a thymus seen in surgery or on preoperative X-ray is a clue to the diagnosis.

Differential diagnosis

Differential diagnosis	Features
CHARGE syndrome	Patients will have coloboma, choanal atresia and genital abnormalities
Zellweger's syndrome	Hepatomegaly that may be associated with cirrhosis and biliary dysgenesis
Opitz G/BBB syndrome	Asymmetry of the skull and hypospadias
SCID	Profound deficiencies of T- and B-cell function
Teratogen exposure	Phenotypic similarities may be seen with isotretinoin or ethanol exposure in utero, though genetic abnormalities are not identified

Typical presentation

- The presentation of disease varies based on age at diagnosis, which in turn depends on the severity of phenotypic abnormalities. From a cardiac standpoint, cyanosis is seen in infancy and occurs as a result of interrupted aortic arch, truncus arteriosus, or tetralogy of Fallot. Children with large septal defects may present with failure to thrive or heart failure. Vascular rings can cause feeding difficulties or varying degrees of airway obstruction. Profound hypocalcemia is a life-threatening complication in the newborn period, whereas complications of hypocalcemia are unusual later in life due to compensatory hyperplasia of existing parathyroid tissue. Immunodeficiency, if severe, as in the complete form of DiGeorge syndrome, can be detected on newborn screening. Later in life, a history of recurrent sinopulmonary infections may be the clue to diagnosis.

Clinical diagnosis

History

- If the syndrome is not detected in early infancy based on such emergencies as cyanosis, hypocalcemic tetany, or complete immunodeficiency, other clues to diagnosis may manifest as the patient ages. Evaluation should be considered in any newborn infant with a cleft palate or persistent feeding difficulties. In older children and adults, a history of recurrent infection or developmental delay, in conjunction with typical physical examination findings, can lead to diagnosis.

Physical examination

- Craniofacial and palate abnormalities may be the first abnormalities detected on physical examination. Other findings that may be seen include ocular hypertelorism, low-set posteriorly rotated ears, micrognathia, short philtrum, upslanting palpebral fissures, and hooded eyelids.

Useful clinical decision rules and calculators

Not applicable for this topic.

Disease severity classification

Not applicable for this topic.

Laboratory diagnosis

List of diagnostic tests

- Complete blood count with differential to evaluate for lymphopenia.
- Complete lymphocyte screen and immunoglobulin levels.
- Serum calcium and phosphorus levels, as well as parathyroid hormone and thyroid stimulating hormone (TSH).
- Fluorescence in situ hybridization (FISH) for 22q11.2 deletion; if negative, gene sequencing of TBS1 can be performed.
- Psychiatric and cognitive assessment for children and older adults.

Lists of imaging techniques

- Cardiac evaluation and echocardiogram is urgent for any infant with suspected anomalies.
- Chest radiograph to evaluate for thymic shadow.
- Renal ultrasound.

Potential pitfalls/common errors made regarding diagnosis of disease

• As this is a rare disease, it must be considered in the differential diagnosis in order for the appropriate diagnosis to be made.

Section 4: Treatment

Treatment rationale

• Management of the syndrome depends on phenotype and age at diagnosis. Most patients are identified shortly after birth due to a cardiac anomaly and should undergo prompt cardiac evaluation and surgical correction, if indicated. Neonatal hypocalcemia is treated with intravenous calcium supplementation. Oral supplementation can then be used, but it is important to monitor levels, because patients may outgrow the need for supplementation as existing parathyroid tissue hypertrophies. During times of stress, these patients may require transient supplementation.
• For patients with partial DiGeorge syndrome and only mild to moderate immune deficiency, no immunologic treatment is needed, and targeted antimicrobial therapy can be used as infections arise.
• For patients with complete DiGeorge syndrome and thymic aplasia, immune reconstitution is a pediatric emergency, and treatment may involve thymus transplant or a fully matched T-cell transplant.
• Palatal abnormalities are addressed on an individual basis with functional testing done to assess if surgical repair is indicated.
• As patients enter early childhood, individualized assessments of the need for speech or behavioral therapy are warranted.

When to hospitalize

Not applicable for this topic.

Managing the hospitalized patient

Not applicable for this topic.

Table of treatment

Not applicable for this topic.

Prevention/management of complications

Not applicable for this topic.

CLINICAL PEARLS
• Assessment for neonatal emergencies includes cardiac anomalies, profound hypocalcemia, and evaluation for immunodeficiency and athymia.
• Further treatment is patient-specific and focused at addressing the phenotypic abnormalities.
• Emphasis on language development and educational needs of growing children should not be underestimated.

Section 5: Special populations
Not applicable for this topic.

Section 6: Prognosis

> **BOTTOM LINE/CLINICAL PEARLS**
> • For patients with complete DiGeorge syndrome who do not undergo transplantation, life expectancy is less than 1 year.
> • For patients with partial DiGeorge syndrome or those who survive transplant, prognosis depends on the severity of cardiac defects, degree of hypocalcemia, and level of intellectual development.
> • A thorough individualized treatment plan will necessitate a multidisciplinary approach for affected patients.

Natural history of untreated disease
Not applicable for this topic.

Prognosis for treated patients
Not applicable for this topic.

Follow-up tests and monitoring
• Children with DiGeorge syndrome should be monitored for hearing difficulties, speech problems, delayed growth, as well as learning and behavioral disabilities. Schizophrenia and major depression can be seen in adolescents and adults.

Section 7: Reading list

Bassett AS, Chow EW, Husted J, Weksberg R, Caluseriu O, Webb GD, et al. Clinical features of 78 adults with 22q11 Deletion Syndrome. Am J Med Genet 2005;138:307–13

Botto LD, May K, Fernhoff PM. A population-based study of the 22q11.2 deletion: phenotype, incidence and contribution to major birth defects in the population. Pediatrics 2003;112:101–7

Conley M, Notarangelo L, Etzioni A. Diagnostic criteria for primary immunodeficiencies. Clin Immunol 1999;93:190–7

McDonald-McGinn D, Sullivan K. Chromosome 22q11.2 Deletion Syndrome. Medicine 2011;90:1–18

Sullivan K. The clinical, immunological, and molecular spectrum of chromosome 22q11.2 deletion syndrome and DiGeorge syndrome. Curr Opin Allergy Clin Immunol 2004;4:505–12

Suggested websites
Immune Deficiency Foundation. http://primaryimmune.org/
Genetics Home Reference. http://ghr.nlm.nih.gov/condition/22q112-deletion-syndrome

Section 8: Guidelines

Guideline title	Guideline source	Date
Practice parameter for the diagnosis and management of primary immunodeficiency	The American Academy of Allergy, Asthma, and Immunology	2005 (http://www.aaaai.org/Aaaai/media/MediaLibrary/PDF%20 Documents/Practice%20 and%20Parameters/ immunodeficiency2005.pdf)

Section 9: Evidence

Not applicable for this topic.

Section 10: Images

Not applicable for this topic.

> **Additional material for this chapter can be found online at:**
> **www.mountsinaiexpertguides.com**
> **This includes a case study, multiple choice questions,**
> **and ICD code**

CHAPTER 45

Chronic Mucocutaneous Candidiasis

Shradha Agarwal

Division of Allergy/Immunology, Icahn School of Medicine at Mount Sinai, New York, NY, USA

OVERALL BOTTOM LINE

- Chronic mucocutaneous candidiasis (CMC) is characterized by persistent or recurrent mucocutaneous infections caused by the *Candida* sp. affecting the nails, skin, and mucosa.
- CMC can be an isolated phenomenon or seen in patients with severe acquired or primary T-cell immunodeficiency and/or in patients on immunosuppressive, antibiotic, or steroid therapies.
- In addition to the chronic candidiasis, patients may have associated endocrinopathies, autoimmune manifestations, or thymoma.
- CMC secondary to primary immunodeficiency has been associated with defects in STAT3, IL-17, AIRE, DOCK8, CARD9, and dectin-1.
- Patients with CMC are managed with antifungal medications and treatment of the associated primary immunodeficiency, endocrinopathy, or autoimmune disorder.

Section 1: Background
Definition of disease

- CMC refers to susceptibility to recurrent or chronic candidiasis of the skin, nails, and mucous membranes occurring within a spectrum of immunologic, endocrine, and autoimmune disorders. The infection is rarely invasive and unlikely to cause sepsis. The clinical manifestation, severity, and genetic features can vary according to the underlying defect.

Disease classification

- CMC can be classified according to its association with other conditions such as endocrinopathy, autoimmunity, and immune dysregulation.

Incidence/prevalence

- There is no racial preference for CMC.
- The male : female ratio for CMC is equal.

Economic impact

Not applicable for this topic.

Mount Sinai Expert Guides: Allergy and Clinical Immunology, First Edition. Edited by Hugh A. Sampson.
© 2015 John Wiley & Sons, Ltd. Published 2015 by John Wiley & Sons, Ltd.
Companion website: www.mountsinaiexpertguides.com

Etiology

- *Candida albicans* is an opportunistic yeast that is part of the normal flora. Defects in immune regulation, specifically cell-mediated immunity, are responsible for infection by *Candida* organisms.

Pathology/pathogenesis

- The molecular basis of CMC varies according to the associated immunodeficiency, although in some cases the exact etiology is unknown.

Predictive/risk factors

Not applicable for this topic.

Section 2: Prevention

No interventions have been demonstrated to prevent the development of the disease.

Screening

Currently no populations are being screened for CMC.

Primary prevention

Not applicable for this topic.

Secondary prevention

Not applicable for this topic.

Section 3: Diagnosis (Algorithm 45.1)

> **BOTTOM LINE/CLINICAL PEARLS**
> - Patients present with recurrent or chronic superficial *Candida* infections of the oral cavity, intertriginous or peri-orificial areas.
> - Examination of the oral cavity may reveal white plaques of thrush. Nails may be thickened, split, and discolored. Skin may be erythematous with hyperkeratotic plaques which may involve the scalp.
> - Scraping from the infected area in 10–20% KOH examined microscopically for the presence of yeast cells and pseudohyphae can confirm a cutaneous diagnosis.
> - Screening tests for associated endocrinopathy include glucose levels, thyroid function, comprehensive metabolic panel, and cortisol levels. Complete blood count and lymphocyte panel screening for leukopenia and HIV testing should be performed. Lymphocyte proliferation to *Candida* antigen is typically reduced.
> - Advanced immune testing including quantitative immunoglobulins should be considered in patients with a history of recurrent infections.

Differential diagnosis

Differential diagnosis	Features
Overgrowth of *Candida*	Responsive to treatment. Can occur in setting of chronic antibiotic or inhaled/oral corticosteroid therapy; in persons with hyperglycemia, diabetes mellitus, iron deficiency. In infants, oral thrush is common in the first 3 months of life; however, this is self-limited and resolves within a few days
Persistent oral thrush	T-cell immunodeficiencies such as DiGeorge syndrome, SCID, and HIV
Autosomal dominant hyper IgE syndrome	Elevated IgE, recurrent staphylococcal skin abscesses, recurrent bacterial pneumonias, eczematous dermatitis, connective tissue defects
Autoimmune polyendocrinopathy, candidiasis, and ectodermal dystrophy (APECED)	CMC associated with autoimmune polyendocrinopathy, commonly hypoparathyroidism and adrenal insufficiency, skin dystrophy

Typical presentation
* Typical clinical presentation varies according to the underlying cause but features include chronic non-invasive candidiasis of the nail, skin, and oral mucous membranes resistant to topical therapies.

Clinical diagnosis
History
* Associated symptoms vary according to the underlying cause, for example symptoms of endo-crinopathy are particular to the organ involved. Hypoparathyroidism and adrenal insufficiency are the most common endocrinopathies seen in patients with APECED. Autoimmune phenomena may occur such as vitiligo, alopecia, hepatitis, and pernicious anemia.

Physical examination
* Cutaneous examination may be characterized by erythematous, pustular, crusted, and thickened plaques resembling psoriasis. Oropharyngeal candidiasis causes white plaques on buccal mucosa, tongue, and lips that may cause bleeding when scraped. The corners of the mouth may show cracks and fissures infected with *Candida*. The intertriginous and peri-anal areas will reveal erythematous patches and are pruritic. Vulvovaginal candidiasis can also cause pruritus and discharge. Distal separation of fingernails with white or yellow discoloration of the subungual area can be seen in cases of chronic paronychia.

Useful clinical decision rules and calculators
Not applicable for this topic.

Disease severity classification
Not applicable for this topic.

Algorithm 45.1 Diagnosis of chronic mucocutaneous candidiasis

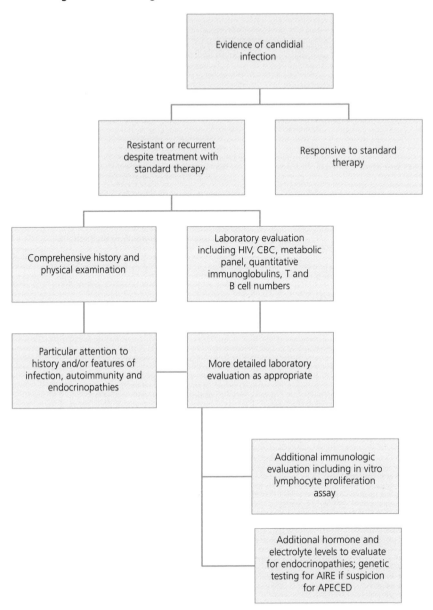

Laboratory diagnosis

List of diagnostic tests

- Scraping from the infected site in 10–20% KOH examined under a microscope will reveal the presence of yeast cells and pseudohyphae. Additional staining with chlorazol black E stain or Parker blue–black ink may be used to highlight the organism.
- Laboratory tests including glucose levels, thyroid function, blood chemistries, liver function, and cortisol levels should be performed as screening for associated endocrine dysfunction.
- Complete blood count and lymphocyte panel screening for leukopenia and HIV testing should be performed.

- Quantitative immunoglobulins (IgG, IgA, IgM, IgE) should be considered in patients with a history of recurrent infections.
- In vivo and in vitro T-cell responses to *Candida* antigens are poor or absent.
- More advanced immune testing in cases of CMC associated with primary immunodeficiency examining the associated gene or molecular defect is available in specialized laboratories.

Lists of imaging techniques
Not applicable for this topic.

Potential pitfalls/common errors made regarding diagnosis of disease
- Invasive candidiasis is rare and other diagnoses should be considered.

Section 4: Treatment (Algorithm 45.2)
Treatment rationale
- Topical therapies such as clotrimazole troches or oral nystatin solution can be given as a therapeutic trial; however, these drugs are generally not effective in cases of CMC.
- Systemic antifungal therapy with azoles is the treatment of choice and can be use alone or in combination with an immunomodulatory agent. Patients on systemic antifungal therapy must be monitored for toxicity, recurrence following completion of therapy, and resistance.
- Endocrine dysfunction should be treated according to the abnormalities found with hormone and/or electrolyte replacement.
- Primary immunodeficiency with antibody deficiency should be treated with immunoglobulin replacement.

Algorithm 45.2 Treatment of chronic mucocutaneous candidiasis

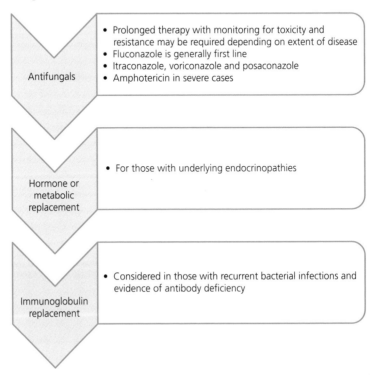

Antifungals
- Prolonged therapy with monitoring for toxicity and resistance may be required depending on extent of disease
- Fluconazole is generally first line
- Itraconazole, voriconazole and posaconazole
- Amphotericin in severe cases

Hormone or metabolic replacement
- For those with underlying endocrinopathies

Immunoglobulin replacement
- Considered in those with recurrent bacterial infections and evidence of antibody deficiency

When to hospitalize
Not applicable for this topic.

Managing the hospitalized patient
Not applicable for this topic.

Table of treatment

Treatment	Comment
Medical Azole family antifungal therapy	Long-term therapy may be used with monitoring for liver toxicity at regular intervals

Prevention/management of complications
- Long-term systemic antifungal therapy may cause liver toxicity requiring reduction or discontinuation of therapy.

CLINICAL PEARLS
- Avoid use of proton pump inhibitors, which may increase the risk of esophageal candidiasis.
- Treatment can be challenging in patients with a history of recurrent bacterial infections requiring chronic antibiotics, which exacerbate the candidiasis.

Section 5: Special populations
Not applicable for this topic.

Section 6: Prognosis

BOTTOM LINE/CLINICAL PEARLS
- The prognosis is good in patients with CMC without associated endocrine or autoimmune disorders although persistent infections with *Candida* organisms should be expected.
- The lesions, while not life-threatening, can be disfiguring and debilitating and impact the patient's quality of life.

Natural history of untreated disease
Not applicable for this topic.

Prognosis for treated patients
Not applicable for this topic.

Follow-up tests and monitoring
- Patient with CMC and associated endocrinopathies, autoimmunity, or immune dysregulation should have routine follow-up with a specialist.

Section 7: Reading list

Engelhardt KR, Grimbacher B. Mendelian traits causing susceptibility to mucocutaneous fungal infections in human subjects. J Allergy Clin Immunol 2012;129:294–305; quiz 306–7

Eyerich K, Eyerich S, Hiller J, Behrendt H, Traidl-Hoffmann C. Chronic mucocutaneous candidiasis, from bench to bedside. Eur J Dermatol 2010;20:260–5

Glocker E, Grimbacher B. Chronic mucocutaneous candidiasis and congenital susceptibility to Candida. Curr Opin Allergy Clin Immunol 2010;10:542–50

Hanna S, Etzioni A. New host defense mechanisms against Candida species clarify the basis of clinical phenotypes. J Allergy Clin Immunol 2011;127:1433–7

Puel A, Cypowyj S, Maródi L, Abel L, Picard C, Casanova JL. Inborn errors of human IL-17 immunity underlie chronic mucocutaneous candidiasis. Curr Opin Allergy Clin Immunol 2012;12:616–22

Suggested websites

American Academy of Allergy Asthma and Immunology. http://www.aaaai.org/home.aspx

Clinical Immunology Society. www.clinimmsoc.org

Immune Deficiency Foundation. http://primaryimmune.org/

Jeffrey Modell Foundation. www.info4pi.org

Section 8: Guidelines
National society guidelines

Guideline title	Guideline source	Date
Practice parameter for the diagnosis and management of primary immunodeficiency	American Academy of Allergy, Asthma and Immunology (AAAAI); American College of Allergy, Asthma and Immunology (ACAAI)	2005 (https://www.aaaai.org/Aaaai/media/MediaLibrary/PDF%20Documents/Practice%20and%20Parameters/immunodeficiency2005.pdf)

International society guidelines

Guideline title	Guideline source	Date
Primary immunodeficiency diseases: an update from the International Union of Immunological Societies Primary Immunodeficiency Diseases Classification Committee	International Union of Immunological Societies (IUIS)	2007 (http://www.ncbi.nlm.nih.gov/pubmed/17952897)

Section 9: Evidence

Not applicable for this topic.

Section 10: Images

Not applicable for this topic.

Additional material for this chapter can be found online at:
www.mountsinaiexpertguides.com
This includes a case study, multiple choice questions,
and ICD code

CHAPTER 46

X-linked Immune Dysregulation with Polyendocrinopathy (IPEX) Syndrome

Elena S. Resnick

Icahn School of Medicine at Mount Sinai, New York, NY, USA

OVERALL BOTTOM LINE

- Immunodysregulation, polyendocrinopathy, enteropathy, X-linked (IPEX) is a rare, X-linked disease caused by a mutation in the gene for FOXP3.
- FOXP3 is essential for the immunosuppressive function of T-regulatory cells; absence or dysfunction of FOXP3 leads to autoimmune and atopic manifestations.
- Cardinal signs and symptoms include severe chronic diarrhea due to autoimmune enteropathy, neonatal type 1 diabetes and/or thyroiditis due to autoimmune endocrinopathy, and eczematous dermatitis.
- Treatment includes referral to a tertiary care center and active management of disease complications until definitive treatment with hematopoietic stem cell transplantation can be performed.

Section 1: Background

Definition of disease

- Immunodysregulation, polyendocrinopathy, enteropathy, X-linked (IPEX) is a rare disease caused by an X-linked mutation in the gene for the transcription factor Foxp3 (FOXP3). Patients with IPEX present with gastrointestinal enteropathy, autoimmune endocrinopathy, and dermatitis.

Disease classification

- Patients presenting with the triad of symptoms listed above are diagnosed with "IPEX" if a mutation is detected in FOXP3. Patients with similar symptoms but without identified mutations are designated "IPEX-like."

Incidence/prevalence

- IPEX is extremely rare, likely under-diagnosed and epidemiologic data are scarce.
- One Australian study identified one case of IPEX in 10 cases of neonatal diabetes in a national registry 1989–2007, thus estimating incidence at 1 in 1 609 490.

Etiology

- IPEX is caused by a mutation in FOXP3, a member of the forkhead box P family of transcription factors, located on chromosome Xp11.23.

Mount Sinai Expert Guides: Allergy and Clinical Immunology, First Edition. Edited by Hugh A. Sampson.
© 2015 John Wiley & Sons, Ltd. Published 2015 by John Wiley & Sons, Ltd.
Companion website: www.mountsinaiexpertguides.com

- The etiology of IPEX-like syndromes (IPEX triad of symptoms without identified FOXP3 mutation) is unknown. New evidence suggests that gain-of-function mutations in STAT1 can cause an IPEX-like phenotype with normal frequency and function of T-regulatory cells (Tregs).

Pathology/pathogenesis

- As described above, IPEX is caused by a mutation in FOXP3, a transcription factor essential to the function of CD4$^+$ Treg cells. Tregs act as natural suppressors of autoimmune and atopic immune responses. Tregs are dependent on the cytokine IL-2 to perform their suppressive function, and FOXP3 interacts with the IL-2 promoter. Adequate levels of FOXP3 are necessary, but not sufficient, for Tregs to suppress immune responses. IPEX-causing mutations are usually loss-of-function mutations in FOXP3 that may be inherited or sporadic. Mutations in FOXP3 result in decreased numbers or impaired function of Tregs, thus increased autoimmune and atopic manifestations including the classic triad of chronic diarrhea due to autoimmune enteropathy, neonatal type 1 diabetes and/or thyroiditis due to autoimmune endocrinopathy, and eczematous dermatitis.

Predictive/risk factors

Not applicable for this topic.

Section 2: Prevention

No interventions have been demonstrated to prevent the development of the disease.

Screening

No routine screening methods are currently utilized to identify cases of this disease.

Primary prevention

Not applicable for this topic.

Secondary prevention

Not applicable for this topic.

Section 3: Diagnosis (Algorithm 46.1)

> **BOTTOM LINE/CLINICAL PEARLS**
> - IPEX is most often seen in a male infant with autoimmune and atopic diseases, including but not limited to diarrhea, type 1 diabetes, thyroiditis, cytopenias, hepatitis, interstitial nephritis, severe food allergies, eczematous dermatitis, and exaggerated response to infections.
> - Examination findings including failure to thrive, developmental delay, as well as the specific manifestations of the complications listed above.
> - Pathology from affected tissues (e.g. gut) may show lymphocytic infiltrates and/or associated autoantibodies.
> - Investigations include CBC, serum glucose, anti-islet antibodies, thyroid function studies, antithyroid antibodies, anti-enterocyte antibodies, immunoglobulin levels, IgE-mediated food allergy testing, lymphocyte subset and proliferation assays, endoscopy with biopsy, skin biopsy, and Treg quantitative and functional studies.
> - Confirmation of the disease is through genetic testing for mutations in FOXP3.

Algorithm 46.1 Diagnosis of IPEX syndrome

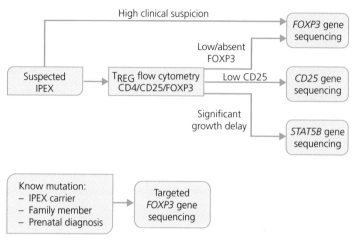

Source: http://www.seattlechildrens.org/research/immunity-and-immunotherapies/ipex/
Last accessed November 2014. Reproduced with permission of Troy R. Torgerson,
MD, PhD, Seattle Children's Hospital.

Differential diagnosis

Differential diagnosis	Features
IPEX-like syndrome	Clinical findings similar to IPEX without identifiable FOXP3 mutation. Can occur in females
CD25 or IL2RA deficiency	Infectious complications, antigen-specific responses impaired, profound cytomegalovirus (CMV) infection, early onset enteropathy
STAT5b deficiency	Growth failure, chronic mucocutaneous candidiasis, CMV infection, lung disease
STAT1 deficiency	Polyendocrinopathy, enteropathy, dermatitis, chronic mucocutaneous candidiasis, disseminated fungal infections, arterial aneurysms, thyroid disease, short stature, squamous cell carcinomas, normal Treg function
Enteropathy of infancy	Includes food allergy, eosinophilic enteropathy, infectious enteropathy, celiac disease, microvillus inclusion disease, enteroendocrine cell dysgenesis, inflammatory bowel disease
Neonatal diabetes	Diabetes due to any cause (not only autoimmune)
Other immune deficiency: severe combined immune deficiency (SCID), neonatal onset multisystemic inflammatory disease (NOMID), autoimmune lymphoproliferative disorder (ALPS), autoimmune polyendocrinopathy, candidiasis, ectodermal dysplasia (APECED)	Severe immune deficiencies associated with infections, autoimmunity, and inflammation

Typical presentation
- IPEX presents in an acutely ill newborn male infant with failure to thrive and developmental delay. Cardinal features include severe diarrhea, neonatal type 1 diabetes, thyroiditis, and severe eczematous dermatitis. Other autoimmune and atopic manifestations may include cytopenias, hepatitis, interstitial nephritis, severe food allergies, and exaggerated response to infections.

Clinical diagnosis
History
- Clinical history will reveal a male infant who has likely been ill since birth with severe diarrhea and metabolic derangements. Failure to thrive and developmental delay are common. A family history of other severely ill male infants or male infants who died of unexplained causes may be present.

Physical examination
- Physical examination findings may include an acutely ill male infant with failure to thrive and developmental delay. Severe diarrhea, metabolic derangements from endocrinopathies, and severe eczematous dermatitis may be present on examination.

Useful clinical decision rules and calculators
Not applicable for this topic.

Disease severity classification
Not applicable for this topic.

Laboratory diagnosis
List of diagnostic tests
- CBC.
- Serum glucose.
- Anti-islet antibodies.
- Thyroid function studies.
- Antithyroid antibodies.
- Anti-enterocyte antibodies.
- Immunoglobulin levels.
- IgE-mediated food allergy testing.
- Lymphocyte subset and proliferation assays.
- Endoscopy with biopsy.
- Skin biopsy.
- Treg quantitative and functional studies.

Lists of imaging techniques
Not applicable for this topic.

Potential pitfalls/common errors made regarding diagnosis of disease
- As this disease is quite rare, it is often not included in the differential diagnosis of acutely ill infants.
- Any infant with autoimmune and atopic disease should be investigated for IPEX as described above.

Section 4: Treatment

Treatment rationale

- IPEX patients are often acutely ill at baseline; however, they may also have disease "flares" as a result of infections, immunizations, or unknown triggers. Treatment requires hospitalization, preferably at a tertiary care institution with access to clinical immunologists and other pediatric specialists. Patients should be treated as severely immune compromised and placed in isolation; blood products should be irradiated and CMV-negative. Vaccines should be strictly avoided. Immunosuppression with high dose steroids (1–2 mg/kg/day) may be necessary but the risks of active infection must be weighed carefully against the benefits of immunosuppressive therapy. Steroid-sparing agents such as calcineurin inhibitors and sirolimus should be used when possible. Enteropathy may require gut rest and total parenteral nutrition, as well as the use of extensively hydrolyzed formula to minimize exposure to food antigens. Hematopoietic stem cell transplantation (HSCT) is the only definitive treatment available; however, complications due to end-organ damage often persist even after HSCT.

When to hospitalize

- Infants with IPEX are often acutely ill and must be managed in the hospital setting.

Managing the hospitalized patient

- Patients with IPEX should be treated as severely immunocompromised.
- Patients should be kept in isolation; blood products should be irradiated and CMV-negative; vaccinations should be strictly avoided.
- Transfer to a tertiary care institution with access to a clinical immunologist familiar with the disease as well as pediatric intensivists and specialists is necessary.
- Treatment involves immunosuppression and active management of the complications listed.
- Definitive treatment can be accomplished only with HSCT.

Table of treatment

No standardized or proven treatment exists.

Prevention/management of complications

- Immunosuppression with high dose steroids may be necessary to manage disease complications; however, the risks of active infection must be weighed carefully against the benefits of immunosuppressive therapy.

> **CLINICAL PEARLS**
> - IPEX patients are often acutely ill and should be managed by a team in a tertiary care center including a clinical immunologist and pediatric intensivists and specialists.

Section 5: Special populations

Not applicable for this topic.

Section 6: Prognosis

> **BOTTOM LINE/CLINICAL PEARLS**
> - Prognosis for IPEX patients is generally quite poor.
> - Even with HSCT, many cases are fatal.

Natural history of untreated disease
Untreated disease is likely to be uniformly fatal.

Prognosis for treated patients
Not applicable for this topic.

Follow-up tests and monitoring
As determined by clinical course and disease complications.

Section 7: Reading list

d'Hennezel E, Bin Dhuban K, Torgerson T, Piccirillo CA. The immunogenetics of immune dysregulation, polyendocrinopathy, enteropathy, X linked (IPEX) syndrome. J Med Genet 2012;49:291–302

Katoh H, Zheng P, Liu Y. FOXP3: genetic and epigenetic implications for autoimmunity. J Autoimmun 2013;41:72–8

Ochs HD, Torgerson TR. Immune dysregulation, polyendocrinopathy, enteropathy, X-linked inheritance: model for autoaggression. Adv Exp Med Biol 2007; 601:27

Powell BR, Buist NR, Stenzel P. An X-linked syndrome of diarrhea, polyendocrinopathy, and fatal infection in infancy. J Pediatr 1982;100:731

Uzel G, Sampaio EP, Lawrence MG, Hsu AP, Hackett M, Dorsey MJ, et al. Dominant gain-of-function STAT1 mutations in FOXP3 wild-type immune dysregulation-polyendocrinopathy-enteropathy-X-linked-like syndrome. J Allergy Clin Immunol 2013;131:1611–23

Wiedemann B, Schober E, Waldhoer T, Koehle J, Flanagan SE, Mackay DJ, et al. Incidence of neonatal diabetes in Austria–calculation based on the Austrian Diabetes Register. Pediatr Diabetes 2010;11:18–23

Wildin RS, Smyk-Pearson S, Filipovich AH. Clinical and molecular features of the immunodysregulation, polyendocrinopathy, enteropathy, X linked (IPEX) syndrome. J Med Genet 2002;39:537

Section 8: Guidelines
Not applicable for this topic.

Section 9: Evidence
Not applicable for this topic.

Section 10: Images
Not applicable for this topic.

Additional material for this chapter can be found online at:
www.mountsinaiexpertguides.com
This includes a case study, multiple choice questions, and ICD codes

CHAPTER 47

Autoimmune Lymphoproliferative Syndrome

Charlotte Cunningham-Rundles

Departments of Medicine and Pediatrics, The Immunology Institute, Icahn School of Medicine at Mount Sinai, New York, NY, USA

OVERALL BOTTOM LINE

- Autoimmune lymphoproliferative syndrome (ALPS) is an inherited disorder of the immune system that affects both children and adults caused by a group of genetic defects.
- Genetic mutations responsible for ALPS can be passed on from generation to generation or can occur spontaneously.
- In this disorder, unusually high numbers of lymphocytes accumulate in the lymph nodes, liver, and spleen.
- These organs may be enlarged.
- The syndrome leads to anemia, thrombocytopenia, and sometimes neutropenia.
- Lymphoma is more common in ALPS.

Section 1: Background

- Autoimmune lymphoproliferative syndrome (ALPS), a lymphoproliferative syndrome with autoimmunity, results from genetic defects of programmed cell death, or apoptosis, which leads to abnormal lymphocyte homeostasis. Patients with ALPS have an enlarged spleen and lymph nodes, and various manifestations of autoimmunity. One of the cardinal features is the presence of a circulating population of "double negative T-cells," T lymphocytes bearing αβ T-cell receptors but neither CD4 nor CD8 surface antigens. When lymphocytes from ALPS patients are cultured in vitro, they are more resistant to programmed cell death than cells from healthy controls. The incidence of lymphoma is increased in ALPS.

Disease classification

- ALPS is a syndrome caused by genetic defects of cell death.
- The inheritance of the most common forms are in a dominant pattern but family members may have very mild disease, which can only be detected in laboratory studies.
- The main features are enlarged spleen and lymph nodes.
- Patients have autoimmunity – hemolytic anemia, thrombocytopenia, and sometimes auto-immune neutropenia.

Incidence/prevalence

The incidence of ALPS is unknown.

Mount Sinai Expert Guides: Allergy and Clinical Immunology, First Edition. Edited by Hugh A. Sampson.

Economic impact
Unrecognized immune defects may lead to morbidity and mortality.

Etiology
- The causes are a group of genetic defects, which lead to delayed programmed cell death.

Pathology/pathogenesis
- *Genetics:* ALPS is generally inherited from a parent but spontaneous mutations also occur. Depending on the mutation, in some cases other family members may not display the syndrome, even though they carry the affected gene.
- *Pathology:* defects of the death (apoptotic) pathways can lead to the following:
  - Enlarged spleen, lymph nodes, or both;
  - Autoimmune blood cytopenias are common;
  - Glomerulonephritis, Guillain–Barré syndrome, autoimmune hepatitis, uveitis, and vasculitis have also been observed.

Predictive/risk factors
- A family history of a similar clinical syndrome might suggest that an immune defect should be considered.

Section 2: Prevention
Screening
- Patients with medical histories suggestive of ALPS can be screened by determining if there is a gap between the sum of percentages of CD4 plus CD8 bearing cells as compared to the total T-cell percentage as measured by CD3.

Primary prevention
There are no primary preventive measures.

Secondary prevention
There are no secondary preventive measures.

Section 3: Diagnosis
- Childhood onset of acute or recurrent immune thrombocytopenia (ITP).
- Hemolytic anemia.
- Lymphadenopathy.
- Splenomegaly.
- Skin rashes.
- Suggestive family history.

Differential diagnosis

Differential diagnosis	Features
Liver disease	Enlarged spleen with thrombocytopenia but with signs of liver disease
Hemophagocytic syndrome	Biopsy: signs of hemophagocytosis
Collagen vascular disease	Cytopenias
Lymphoma	Enlarged lymph nodes and spleen
Other immune defects	Features of Wiskott–Aldrich syndrome, common variable immunodeficiency

Typical presentation
- A typical scenario of a child with ALPS includes acute or recurrent ITP or hemolytic anemia. The physical examination may reveal lymphadenopathy and splenomegaly. The family history may include a first degree relative who has had autoimmunity, or possibly a previous splenectomy, or, in some cases, a lymphoma or Hodgkin's disease.

Clinical diagnosis
History
- Symptoms are heterogeneous as the organs and systems affected depend on the nature of the immune defect. In 80% of cases, lung infections occur, specifically pneumonia or chronic bronchitis. A history of difficult-to-treat chronic sinusitis or previous sinus surgery is often found. Gastrointestinal disease is seen in some. Details sought in the clinical history should include duration and onset of symptoms, fatigue, fever, weight loss, and shortness of breath. Weight loss is common. Obtaining a detailed family history is always important, as well as questions about smoking, drug use, the medications used, and results obtained.

Physical examination
- Physical examination should start with evaluation for signs of systemic illness, including weight loss. However, patients with IgA or IgG deficiency may also look healthy and have a normal physical examination.
- Fever may be present with acute infections, otherwise chronic fever would be uncommon.
- Patients with lung disease may be short of breath, have a productive or non-productive cough, and may have pulmonary signs such as rhonchi or rales on examination.
- Lymphadenopathy is common, and enlarged spleen may be detected.
- Skin changes may include scarring from previous herpes zoster; vitiligo appears to be common.
- Chronic conjunctivitis, iritis, or episcleritis, may be observed.
- Joint complaints include changes due to previous joint infections, or autoimmune, chronic arthritis.

Laboratory diagnosis
List of diagnostic tests
- Elevated numbers of double-negative T cells.
- Elevations of B- and T-cell numbers.
- Significant titers of autoantibodies.
- Serum IL-10 levels are commonly elevated.
- Serum vitamin B_{12} levels are commonly elevated.
- Soluble Fas ligand.
- In vitro defective lymphocyte apoptosis (a research test).
- Genetic mutational studies.

Lists of imaging techniques
- Chest X-ray.
- Ultrasound for splenomegaly.
- CT of the abdomen to examine organ size, lymphadenopathy.
- MRI may be preferred to minimize exposure to ionizing radiation.

Potential pitfalls/common errors made regarding diagnosis of disease
- Not diagnosing immune defects leads to excess morbidity.

Section 4: Treatment

Treatment rationale

- The goal of therapy is to provide amelioration of the cytopenias:
  - Episodes of autoimmune hemolytic anemia and thrombocytopenia are generally responsive to short courses of high dose glucocorticosteroids;
  - Splenectomy has been required in some, but is to be avoided as post-splenectomy sepsis has occurred.

Table of treatment

Treatment	Comment
Conservative Medical	Short-term steroids for thrombocytopenia or hemolytic anemia Recombinant granulocyte colony-stimulating factor for neutropenia IVIg for cytopenias with steroids Rituximab in standard 375 mg/m^2 for 4 weeks Mycophenylate mofetil (MMF) 600 mg/m^2 Rapamycin loading dose 3 mg/m^2 and then tapered
Surgical	Node biopsies if indicated Avoid splenectomy
Radiological	To examine organs as needed
Other Hematopoietic stem cell transplant	Encourage normal activities, schooling, work, etc. Reserved for severe cases

Prevention/management of complications

- Steroids or other immunosuppressants used for only short periods as needed. Splenectomy is to be avoided.

> **CLINICAL PEARLS**
> - ALPS is a genetic disease that leads to lymphadenopathy and cytopenias.
> - It usually presents in childhood.
> - Treatment is dictated by the medical need but immunosuppression is to be minimized.
> - There is an increased risk of lymphoma.

Section 5: Special populations

Pregnancy

- Treatment is as usual but with medications approved in pregnancy.

Children

- Treatment is as usual but with medications given based on weight.

Elderly

- Treatment is as usual.

Section 6: Prognosis

> **BOTTOM LINE/CLINICAL PEARLS**
> - Patients with ALPS may do well with conservative treatment.
> - Careful evaluation of any new clinical findings that develop over time is important.
> - Some subjects, depending on the mutation, will require other medical treatments or possibly splenectomy.
> - There is an increased risk of lymphoma.

Natural history of untreated disease
- Continued bouts of autoimmunity are likely.
- Increased splenomegaly and lymphadenopathy are likely.

Prognosis for treated patients
- Varying with the degree of the genetic defect.

Follow-up tests and monitoring
- Careful follow-up for signs of autoimmunity.

Section 7: Reading list

Oliveira JB, Bleesing JJ, Dianzani U, Fleisher TA, Jaffe ES, Lenardo MJ, et al. Revised diagnostic criteria and classification for the autoimmune lymphoproliferative syndrome (ALPS): report from the 2009 NIH International Workshop. Blood 2010;116:e35–40
Rao VK, Oliveira JB. How I treat autoimmune lymphoproliferative syndrome. Blood 2011;118:5741–51
Teachey DT. New advances in the diagnosis and treatment of autoimmune lymphoproliferative syndrome. Curr Opin Pediatr 2012;24:1–8

Suggested websites
National Institute of Allergy and Infectious Diseases. http://www.niaid.nih.gov/topics/ALPS/research/Pages/description.aspx

Section 8: Guidelines
Not applicable for this topic.

Section 9: Evidence
Not applicable for this topic.

Section 10: Images
Not applicable for this topic.

Additional material for this chapter can be found online at:
www.mountsinaiexpertguides.com
This includes a case study, multiple choice questions, advice for patients, and ICD codes

CHAPTER 48

Hyper IgE Syndrome

Shradha Agarwal

Division of Allergy/Immunology, Icahn School of Medicine at Mount Sinai, New York, NY, USA

OVERALL BOTTOM LINE

- Hyper IgE syndrome (HIES) was first described as Job's syndrome in 1966 in two girls with recurrent staphylococcal abscesses, sinopulmonary infections, and severe eczema.
- The disorder was later expanded to include an associated increase in serum levels of IgE, coarse facial features, and skeletal abnormalities, which can be seen in both males and females.
- Laboratory levels of IgE typically range from 2000 to >50 000 IU/mL and variable eosinophilia.
- Mutations in the STAT3 signaling protein have been identified in both the sporadic and familial forms of HIES.
- Management focuses on skin care and prevention of infection, often with prophylactic administration of trimethoprim-sulfamethoxazole. IFN-γ has been used in the setting of life-threatening infections.

Section 1: Background

Definition of disease

- Hyper IgE syndrome (HIES) is a primary antibody immunodeficiency characterized by recurrent "cold" staphylococcal infections, severe eczema, pneumonia that can result in pneumatoceles, and elevated concentrations of serum IgE. Affected patients often have coarse facial features, skeletal, vascular, and connective tissue abnormalities.

Disease classification

Not applicable for this topic.

Incidence/prevalence

- The prevalence of HIES is unknown but the condition is rare.
- There is no reported gender or racial preference.

Economic impact

Not applicable for this topic.

Etiology

- Dominant negative mutations in STAT3 were identified as the cause of autosomal dominant HIES (AD-HIES). An autosomal recessive pattern of inheritance, commonly associated with mutations in DOCK8, is rarer and represents a separate entity.

Mount Sinai Expert Guides: Allergy and Clinical Immunology, First Edition. Edited by Hugh A. Sampson.
© 2015 John Wiley & Sons, Ltd. Published 2015 by John Wiley & Sons, Ltd.
Companion website: www.mountsinaiexpertguides.com

Pathology/pathogenesis

- HIES is caused by defects in the Janus activated kinase/signal transduced and activator of transcription (JAK-STAT) mediated cytokine signals such as IL-6 and IL-23. Defects in STAT3 lead to impaired TH17 function, which has been suggested to be the cause of susceptibility to infection.

Predictive/risk factors

- Those with a parent affected with AD-HIES have a 50% chance of inheriting the mutation.

Section 2: Prevention

No interventions have been demonstrated to prevent the development of the disease.

Screening

Currently no populations are being screened for HIES.

Primary prevention

Not applicable for this topic.

Secondary prevention

Not applicable for this topic.

Section 3: Diagnosis (Algorithm 48.1)

> **BOTTOM LINE/CLINICAL PEARLS**
> - Patients with HIES often report a history of papulopustular rash within the newborn period. The rash is often on the face and scalp and later spreads to the trunk and progresses to an eczematous pruritic rash similar to atopic dermatitis. Skin lesions can lead to recurrent cellulitis, abscesses, or lymphadenitis often secondary to *Staphylococcus aureus* or *Candida albicans*.
> - Patients present with recurrent upper respiratory infections and pneumonias complicated by bronchiectasis, fistulae, and pneumatoceles, which can become infected with *Aspergillus* or *Pseudomonas*.
> - Non-immunologic characteristics include characteristic features of facial asymmetry, broad nasal bridge, wide outer canthal distances, and deep-set eyes. Patients often retain primary teeth which may require extraction. Osteopenia, minimal trauma fractures, and scoliosis are noted. Vascular abnormalities including aneurysms can be seen.
> - Laboratory examination is driven by IgE levels; serum IgE levels in affected patients range from 2000 to >50 000 IU/mL, but normal levels have also been noted. IgE levels do not correlate with the severity of disease. Eosinophilia >700/μL is present in most patients.
> - A clinical scoring system reflecting the heterogeneous manifestations has been developed by the National Institutes of Health (NIH) (see Table 48.1: A clinical scoring system). The scoring system includes 20 clinical features including total IgE level; for each clinical feature a point value 0–10 is assigned. A score >40 is suggestive of HIES and <20 makes it unlikely.

Algorithm 48.1 Diagnosis of hyper-IgE syndrome

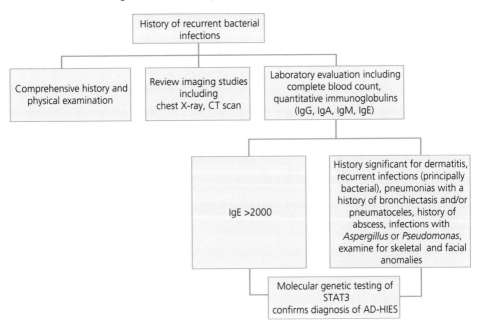

Differential diagnosis

Differential diagnosis	Features
Atopic dermatitis	Superficial skin infections can occur, but it is not common to have abscesses or pneumonia. Patients with atopic dermatitis do not have the bone abnormalities or the coarse facial features of HIES. Patients with atopic dermatitis often have food and/or environmental allergies, which is not common in HIES
Wiskott–Aldrich syndrome	Elevated total IgE presents with triad of recurrent infections, thrombocytopenia, and eczema
Omenn's syndrome	Can present with a rash in the newborn period and elevated IgE similar to HIES. Affected individuals are typically sicker at a young age with associated lymphadenopathy, hepatosplenomegaly, and opportunistic infections

Typical presentation
- Typical presentation includes recurrent staphylococcal skin infections or abscesses, recurrent respiratory infections leading to pneumatoceles, and increased concentrations of serum IgE.

Clinical diagnosis
History
- Symptoms are heterogeneous. Typical presentation begins with a rash in the newborn infant that develops into eczematoid dermatitis. Patients usually develop recurrent staphylococcal skin abscess and bacterial pneumonias after the first year of life. Complications of pneumatoceles

and bronchiectasis may develop. During adolescence, abnormal facies and coarse facial features are apparent.
- Opportunistic infections may be seen in patients with significant immunodeficiency. Skeletal deformities including scoliosis, delayed shedding of primary teeth, minimal trauma fractures, and osteopenia are common. Vascular abnormalities including aneurysms may develop. Symptoms of reflux, dysmotility, and fungal infections of the gastrointestinal tract can occur.

Physical examination
- Physical examination should start with the skin, looking for a papulopustular or eczematous rash similar to atopic dermatitis. Skin may be infected and abscesses may be present, especially on the face, neck, and scalp. Skeletal examination may reveal retained primary teeth, scoliosis, osteopenia. Facial features of prominence of the forehead or chin, wide set eyes, coarse skin, high arched palate, and broad nasal bridge.

Useful clinical decision rules and calculators
- A clinical scoring system (Table 48.1) to include manifestations of HIES developed by the NIH is available.

Disease severity classification
Not applicable for this topic.

Laboratory diagnosis
List of diagnostic tests
- Measurement of serum IgE with reference to age. A repeat test to confirm diagnosis is necessary.
- Complete blood count with differential.
- Molecular genetic testing of STAT3 polymorphisms confirms diagnosis of AD-HIES.

List of imaging techniques
- CT scan of the lungs should be performed in patients with recurrent lung infections to evaluate for bronchiectasis or pneumatoceles.
- Spine images examining scoliosis and bone density for osteopenia.

Potential pitfalls/common errors made regarding diagnosis of disease
- Serum immunoglobulins should be drawn with reference to the patient's age.

Section 4: Treatment (Algorithm 48.2)
Treatment rationale
- Treatment is aimed at early recognition of the syndrome and resulting infections with aggressive management when actively infected. Prophylactic trimethoprim-sulfamethoxazole is used for prevention of *Staphylococcus aureus* and may also be helpful in preventing bacterial infections such as abscesses, sinusitis, otitis media, and possibly pneumonia. Skin care consists of adequate hydration, use of emollients, and antihistamines to control pruritus.

When to hospitalize
- Deep infections may require surgical drainage and intravenous antibiotics.

Managing the hospitalized patient
Not applicable for this topic.

Table 48.1 A clinical scoring system to include manifestations of hyper-IgE syndrome (HIES) developed by the Natonal Institutes of Health (NIH) is available. A score >40 is suggestive of AD-HIES

Clinical Findings	Points[a]									
	0	1	2	3	4	5	6	7	8	10
Highest serum-IgE level (IU/ml)[b]	<200	200–500			501–1000				1001–2000	>2000
Skin abscesses	None		1–2		3–4				>4	
Pneumonia (episodes over lifetime)	None		1		2		3		>3	
Parenchymal lung anomalies	Absent						Bronchiectasis		Pneumatocele	
Retained primary teeth	None	1	2		3					
Scoliosis maximum curvature	<10°		10–14°		15°–20°				>20°	
Fractures with minor trauma	None				1–2				>2	
Highest eosinophil count (cells/µl)[c]	<700			700–800			>800			
Characteristic face	Absent		Mildly present			Present				
Midline anomaly[d]	Absent					Present				
Newborn rash	Absent				Present					
Eczema (worst stage)	Absent	Mild	Moderate		Severe					
Upper respiratory infections per year	1–2	3	4–6		>6					
Candidiasis	None	Oral	Fingernails		Systemic					
Other serious infections	None				Present					
Fatal infection	Absent				Present					
Hyperextensibility	Absent				Present					
Lymphoma	Absent				Present					
Increased nasal width[e]	<1 SD	1–2 SD		>2 SD						
High palate	Absent		Present							
Young-age correction	>5 years			2–5 years		1–2 years		≤1 year		

[a] The entry in the furthest-right column is assigned the maximum points allowed for each finding.

[b] Normal <130IU/ml.

[c] 700/µl =1 SD, 800/µl =2 SD above the mean value for normal individuals.

[d] For example, cleft palate, cleft tongue, hemivertebrae, other vertebral anomaly, etc. (see Grimbacher et al. 1999a).

[e] Compared with age- and sex-matched controls.

Source: Grimbacher B, et al. Genetic linkage of hyper-IgE syndrome to chromosome 4. Am J Hum Genet 1999b;65:735–44. Reproduced with permission of Elsevier.

Algorithm 48.2 Treatment of hyper-IgE syndrome

Skin care, antihistamines, topical emollients, topical steroids

- To control pruritus and eczematous dermatitis in order to prevent occurrence of systemic infection

Prophylactic antibiotics

- Prophylactic trimethoprim- sulfamethoxazole used in the prevention of cutaneous staphylococcal infections

Antifungals, antibiotics, antivirals

- Choice of therapy is according to culture and sensitivity results and type of infection (bronchitis, otitis, pneumonia, sinusitis)
- Deep infections may require surgical drainage and intravenous antibiotics.

IFN-γ

- A trial of IFN-γ therapy is reserved/considered in patients with serious infections

Table of treatment

Treatment	Comment
Medical Antibiotics (treatment or prophylactic)	Choice and frequency of antibiotics is based on type of infection and culture/sensitivity results In patients with recurrent staphylococcal infections, prophylactic administration of trimethoprim-sulfamethoxazole is recommended Antifungal therapies to control mucocutaneous candidiasis may be necessary
Surgical	Patients with deep infections may require surgical drainage. Patients with recurrent lung infections leading to pneumatoceles may require segmental removal of the lung or lobectomy
Radiological Chest X-ray or CT scan	Patients with significant upper or lower respiratory infections should have CT scan for bronchiectasis and pneumatoceles

Treatment	Comment
Complementary	Bleach baths and swimming in chlorinated pools may be used to control superficial skin infections Vitamin D and calcium supplementation in patients with significant bone involvement should be considered
Other	IFN-γ therapy can be considered in patients with serious infections such as pulmonary aspergillosis

Prevention/management of complications
- Patients with HIES are at increased risk for lymphoma and require chemotherapy and/or transplantation.

CLINICAL PEARLS
- Treatment of HIES is focused on skin care and prevention of systemic infection.
- Prophylactic trimethoprim-sulfamethoxazole is recommended for the prevention of cutaneous infections.
- Antibiotic coverage may be extended if pulmonary complications develop with secondary infections commonly involving *Pseudomonas* or *Aspergillus*.

Section 5: Special populations
Pregnancy
- Termination of prophylactic antibiotics may be advised during pregnancy; however, the risk of infection should be considered.
- Female patients with significant pulmonary and skeletal disease such as scoliosis should discuss these complications with their physician, as they can affect pregnancy.

Children
- Children should be monitored for scoliosis. Bone fractures may occur following minor trauma and can be recurrent. Therefore additional precautions should be taken for children participating in sports.

Elderly
Not applicable for this topic.

Others
Not applicable for this topic.

Section 6: Prognosis

BOTTOM LINE/CLINICAL PEARLS
- Patients survive into adulthood but lifespan may be shortened secondary to complications.
- Pulmonary complications including pneumatoceles and bronchiectasis contribute to the majority of mortality in patients with HIES.
- Infected pneumatoceles can lead to recurrent pneumonia, sepsis, or pulmonary hemorrhage.
- Patients who develop lymphoma have a poor prognosis.

Natural history of untreated disease

Not applicable for this topic.

Prognosis for treated patients

Not applicable for this topic.

Follow-up tests and monitoring

- Patients with HIES should have regular follow-ups with an immunologist. Patients with HIES sometimes lack signs of systemic infection and a high index of suspicion for infection by an immunologist to initiate treatment to prevent complications is needed. Therapy should be culture directed whenever possible. Patients with significant pulmonary involvement may require periodic imaging.

Section 7: Reading list

Freeman AF, Holland SM. The hyper-IgE syndromes. Immunol Allergy Clin North Am 2008;28:277–91

Grimbacher B, Puck JM, Holland SM. Hyper-IgE syndrome. In: Ochs H, Smith HIE, Puck JM (eds) Primary Immunodeficiency Diseases: A Molecular and Genetic Approach, 2nd edn. New York, NY: Oxford University Press, 2007: 496–504

Grimbacher B, Schäffer AA, Holland SM, Davis J, Gallin JI, Malech HL, et al. Genetic linkage of hyper-IgE syndrome to chromosome 4. Am J Hum Genet 1999;65:735–44

Holland SM, DeLeo FR, Elloumi HZ, Hsu AP, Uzel G, Brodsky N, et al. STAT3 mutations in the hyper-IgE syndrome. N Engl J Med 2007;357:1608–19

Notarangelo LD, Fischer A, Geha RS, Casanova JL, Chapel H, Conley ME, et al. Primary immunodeficiencies: 2009 update. J Allergy Clin Immunol 2009;124:1161–78

Woellner C, Gertz EM, Schäffer AA, Lagos M, Perro M, Glocker EO, et al. Mutations in STAT3 and diagnostic guidelines for hyper-IgE syndrome. J Allergy Clin Immunol 2010;125:424–32

Suggested websites

American Academy of Allergy, Asthma and Immunology. http://www.aaaai.org/home.aspx

Clinical Immunology Society. www.clinimmsoc.org

Immune Deficiency Foundation. http://primaryimmune.org/

Jeffrey Modell Foundation. www.info4pi.org

Section 8: Guidelines
National society guidelines

Guideline title	Guideline source	Date
Practice parameter for the diagnosis and management of primary immunodeficiency	American Academy of Allergy, Asthma and Immunology (AAAAI); American College of Allergy, Asthma and Immunology (ACAAI)	2005 (https://www.aaaai.org/Aaaai/media/MediaLibrary/PDF%20Documents/Practice%20and%20Parameters/immunodeficiency2005.pdf)

International society guidelines

Guideline title	Guideline source	Date
Primary immunodeficiency diseases: an update from the International Union of Immunological Societies Primary Immunodeficiency Diseases Classification Committee	International Union of Immunological Societies (IUIS)	2007 (http://www.ncbi.nlm.nih.gov/pubmed/17952897)

Section 9: Evidence
Not applicable for this topic.

Section 10: Images
Not applicable for this topic.

Additional material for this chapter can be found online at:
www.mountsinaiexpertguides.com
This includes a case study, multiple choice questions, advice for patients, and ICD codes

CHAPTER 49

Deficiencies of Complement

Paula J. Busse

Department of Medicine, Division of Clinical Immunology, Mount Sinai School of Medicine, New York, NY, USA

OVERALL BOTTOM LINE

- Deficiencies in early components of the classic complement pathway (e.g. C1, C4, C2) may predispose patients to autoimmune diseases such as systemic lupus erythematosus (SLE) or recurrent infections.
- Deficiencies in later components of the classic pathway may put patients at risk for recurrent infections with encapsulated organisms (e.g. pneumococcus and *Haemophilus influenzae*, with C3 deficiency) and neisserial infections (with C5–C9 deficiency).
- Properdin deficiency is the most common deficiency in the alternative pathway and results in increased risk of neisserial infections in males.
- Patients with complement deficiencies should be educated to seek medical attention with early signs of infection.
- Patients with complement deficiencies, which can predispose to increased risk of infection, should receive vaccination against pneumococcus, *H. influenzae*, and meningococcal disease.

Section 1: Background
Definition of disease

- The complement system is part of the innate immune system and is an important defense against pyogenic organisms and promotes the inflammatory response. Depending upon the specific complement deficiency, patients may develop recurrent sinopulmonary infections, sepsis and meningitis, or autoimmune disease.

Disease classification

- Complement deficiencies can be classified based upon whether it affects the classical, alternative or lectin pathway or an inhibitor of these pathways (see Table: Inherited complement deficiencies and clinical associations).

Incidence/prevalence

- Complement deficiencies are rare.

Etiology

- Most inherited disorders of the classic pathway are transmitted as autosomal co-dominant (recessive) traits (Table 49.1).

Mount Sinai Expert Guides: Allergy and Clinical Immunology, First Edition. Edited by Hugh A. Sampson.
© 2015 John Wiley & Sons, Ltd. Published 2015 by John Wiley & Sons, Ltd.
Companion website: www.mountsinaiexpertguides.com

Table 49.1 Inherited complement deficiencies and clinical associations.

Presenting syndrome	Component	Pathway	Inheritance	Major clinical correlates
Infection	C1q, C1r, C1s, C4, C2	CP	Autosomal	Most commonly autoimmune conditions, particularly SLE. Also higher than normal incidence of encapsulated bacterial infections.
	C3	Common to CP, AP, LP	Autosomal	Severe, recurrent pyogenic infections early in life. Also might have glomerulonephritis.
	C5, C6, C6, C8, or C9	MAC	Autosomal	Recurrent *Neisseria* infections, less common with C9.
	Factor H, factor I	AP inhibitors	Autosomal	Recurrent pyogenic infections as a result of C3 deficiency. Factor H deficiency is also associated with glomerulonephritis and HUS.
	Properdin	AP stabilizer	X-linked	Recurrent *Neisseria* infections
	MBL	LP	Autosomal	Pyogenic infections and sepsis in children and neonates; also an association with SLE
	CR3	Receptor	Autosomal	Leukocyte adhesion defect: leukocytosis, pyogenic infections, delayed umbilical cord separation
Rheumatic disorders	C1, C2, C4	CP	Autosomal	As above; mainly SLE
	MBL	LP	Autosomal	As above; SLE is associated as well.
HAE	C1-Inh	CP inhibitor	Autosomal	HAE
Kidney damage	C3	Common to CP, AP, LP	Autosomal	Membranoproliferative glomerulonephritis and overwhelming infections
	Factor H	AP inhibitor	Autosomal	Atypical HUS, glomerulonephritis
	CD46	AP inhibitor	Autosomal	Atypical HUS
PNH	Decay accelerating factor, CD59	AP and MAC inhibitors	Somatic mutation on X chromosome	Hemolysis and thrombosis

AP, alternative pathway; CP, classic pathway; HAE, hereditary angioma; LP, lectin pathway.
Source: Wen L, Atkinson JP, Giclas PC. Clinical and laboratory evaluation of complement deficiency. J Allergy Clin Immunol 2004; 113: 585–93. Reproduced with permission of Elsevier.

Pathology/pathogenesis

- There are three major pathways of the complement cascade that converge at component C3 (Figure 49.1). Activation of C3 then produces C3b, which attaches to antigens and targets them for ingestion by phagocytic cells (opsonization). Production of C5b by activated C3b generates the membrane attack complex (MAC). The three pathways are the following:
  - *Classic pathway:* activated when IgM or IgG antibodies bind to antigens (e.g. virus, bacteria).
  - *Lectin pathway:* similar activation as the classic pathway except that instead of an antibody binding to the antigen, a lectin (such as mannose-binding protein, MBP) binds to the antigen.
  - *Alternative pathway:* does not require antigen binding for activation. Activated by activated C3 binding to a target.

Section 2: Prevention

No interventions have been demonstrated to prevent the development of the disease.

Screening

- Indications for screening include the following:
  - Recurrent, unexplained pyogenic infections in patients with normal immunoglobulin and white blood cell counts (classic pathway, CH50);
  - Recurrent neisserial infections and families with multiple members with a history of neisserial infection;
  - Any patient with SLE.

Primary prevention

Not applicable for this topic.

Secondary prevention

- Patients should be instructed to seek medical attention with high fevers and/or a stiff neck, which may suggest meningitis.
- Vaccination against pneumococcus, *H. influenzae,* and meningococcus.

Section 3: Diagnosis

BOTTOM LINE/CLINICAL PEARLS
- A history of SLE may suggest a deficiency in early components of the classic complement pathway.
- A history of recurrent infections with pneumococcus and *H. influenzae* may indicate a defect in later components of the classic complement pathway.
- Males with a familial predisposition to neisserial infections (in particular meningitis) may have properdin deficiency.

Differential diagnosis

Differential diagnosis	Features
Decreased C4	Low C4 may be secondary to consumption in patients with SLE and may not indicate C4 specific deficiency. Decreased C2 and C3 suggest consumption
Specific antibody deficiency	Complement deficiencies will have normal immunoglobulin levels and antibody responses (see Chapter 40)

Typical presentation

- The typical presentation depends upon the component of the complement cascade that is involved:
  - *C1 deficiencies (C1q, C1r, C1s):* deficiencies of C1 can develop SLE and have recurrent infections. Patients with deficiencies of C1r or C1s are at increased risk of renal and cutaneous sequelae.
  - *C4 deficiency:* partial C4 deficiency predisposes a patient to develop SLE; total deficiency of C4 is rare. Deficiency of C4A or C4B can be associated with scleroderma, IgA nephropathy, Henoch–Schönlein purpura, childhood diabetes.
  - *C2 deficiency:* patients with complete C2 deficiency can present with SLE-like illness; children can present with recurrent pyogenic infections from encapsulated bacteria; associated with IgG subclass deficiency. Partial C2 deficiency is asymptomatic.
  - *C3 deficiency:* complete C3 deficiency results in severe, recurrent infections with encapsulated bacteria that begin shortly after birth. Partial C3 deficiency has no clinical significance.
  - *C5–C9 deficiency:* associated with infection by *Neisseria* species (meningococcus and gonococcus) which are recurrent and clinically mild to moderate.
  - *Properdin deficiency:* affects males (gene on X chromosome). Unusual subtypes of *Neisseria* meningitis.
  - *Mannose-binding lectin (MBL) deficiency:* neonates and infants presenting with infections from encapsulated bacteria.
  - *Mannan-binding lectin-associated protease 2 (MASP-2):* severe pneumococcal pneumonia.
  - *C1-inhibitor deficiency:* (see Chapter 28).
  - *Factor H or I:* a complete deficiency may produce recurrent infections and glomerulonephritis. Heterozygous mutations have been associated with atypical hemolytic uremic syndrome (HUS).
  - *Complement receptor 3 (CR3):* also known as leukocyte adhesion deficiency syndrome (see Chapter XX).
  - *Decay accelerating factor (DAF) and CD59:* deficiencies predispose red blood cells to lysis and subsequent hemolytic anemia and paroxysmal nocturnal hemoglobinuria (PNH).

Clinical diagnosis

History

- History should be focused on infection history, both in early childhood and later in life; episodes of meningitis; joint pains (suggesting SLE).

Physical examination

No specific physical examination findings for complement deficiency.

Laboratory diagnosis

List of diagnostic tests
- *CH50:* a complete deficiency caused by a homozygous mutation in the classic pathway gives an undetectable CH50 (with the exception of homozygous C9 deficiency which can give a low, but detectable value). Heterozygous deficiencies will have a normal CH50.
- *Specific complement proteins (e.g. C2, C4, C1q):* performed if the CH50 is low.
- *AH50:* a low value suggests deficiency of C3, C5, C6, C7, C8 or C9, properdin, or factor D.

Lists of imaging techniques
Not applicable for this topic.

Section 4: Treatment
Treatment rationale
- The present goal of therapy of patients with complement deficiencies is to treat infection and autoimmunity. At present, there are no commercially available replacement complement components available. The use of plasma or blood transfusions to replace missing complements is not standard of care. Inhibition of complement (with a monoclonal antibody to C5) for treatment of PNH has been approved for clinical use. Depending on the complement deficiency, patients at increased risk of infection should be educated to seek medical attention quickly for symptoms of fever, stiff neck, purpuric rash, and so on. In addition, patients should be vaccinated against meningococcus, pneumococcus, and *H. influenzae*.

Section 5: Special populations
Not applicable for this topic.

Section 6: Prognosis
- Deficiencies of C3 result in recurrent pyogenic infections with encapsulated bacteria and high rates of morbidity and mortality.
- Deficiencies of the early classic pathway (C1, C4, C2) are not usually associated with an increased risk of infection.
- Defects in the MAC (later complement pathway) do not have as high rates of morbidity and mortality as deficiencies of C3.

Section 7: Reading list

Botto M, Kirschfink M, Macor P, Pickering MC, Wurzner R, Tedesco F. Complement in human diseases: lessons from complement deficiencies. Mol Immunol 2009;46:2774–83

Frank MM. Complement deficiencies. Pediatr Clin North Am 2000;47:1339–54

Nilsson B, Ekdahl KN. Complement diagnostics: concepts, indications, and practical guidelines. Clin Dev Immunol 2012;2012:962702

O'Neil KM. Complement deficiency. Clin Rev Allergy Immunol 2000;19:83–108

Walport MJ. Complement. First of two parts. N Engl J Med 2001;344:1058–66

Walport MJ. Complement. Second of two parts. N Engl J Med 2001;344:1140–4

Wen L, Atkinson JP, Giclas PC. Clinical and laboratory evaluation of complement deficiency. J Allergy Clin Immunol 2004;113:585–93; quiz 94

Section 8: Guidelines
Not applicable for this topic.

Section 9: Evidence

Not applicable for this topic.

Section 10: Images

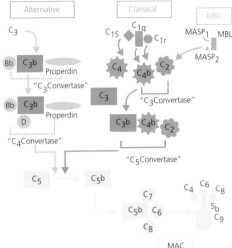

Classical (C1 q,r,s C4 and C2) deficiencies: are associated with an increased predisposition for develpoing immune complex diseases such as SLE.

MBL deficiencies: are associated with an increased risk of infection with the yeast saccharomyces cerevisiae and with encapsulated bacteria.

Alternative pathway (factor D, B, Properdin and C3): are associated with decreased opsonization ability and a subsequent increased risk of infection, especially with encapsulated bacteria.

C3 deficiencies: are associated with defective opsonization, deficient leukocyte chemotaxis, and decreased bactericidal killing activity (because of decreased MAC formation). These deficiencies are associated with overwhelming infections with encapsulated bacteria. There is also a 79% association with the development of immune complex disease.

MAC deficiencies: are associated with an increased risk of infection, especially with the bacteria *N. meningitidis*, but have decreased morbidity and mortality rates than C3 deficiencies.

Figure 49.1 Complement pathways and deficiencies. Deficiencies in complement increase susceptibility for infection by decreasing the ability for opsonization, which is particularly important for encapsulated bacteria. Additionally, a defect in the MAC decreases the ability of the immune system to generate lytic activity, which also increases the risk of infection with encapsulated bacteria. Source: http://emedicine. medscape.com/article/135478-overview. Last accessed November 2014. Reproduced with permission of Medscape Reference.

Additional material for this chapter can be found online at:
www.mountsinaiexpertguides.com
This includes a case study, multiple choice questions, advice for patients, and ICD code

CHAPTER 50

Phagocytic Cell Disorders

Charlotte Cunningham-Rundles
Departments of Medicine and Pediatrics, The Immunology Institute, Icahn School of Medicine at Mount Sinai, New York, NY, USA

OVERALL BOTTOM LINE
- Phagocytic disorders can be the result of inherited defects of the immune system.
- However, exclusion of other medical causes may be important.
- The genetic disorders affect both children and adults.
- Genetic mutations responsible for these can be passed on from generation to generation in various inheritance patterns, or can occur spontaneously.
- Because of these defects, infections occur because there are too few neutrophils or there is impaired neutrophil function.
- Infections may be acute or recurrent.

Section 1: Background
Definition of disease
- Genetic phagocytic disorders can be divided into several groups:
  - Defects of neutrophil differentiation (neutropenia);
  - Defects of motility; and
  - Defects of respiratory burst.
- The results in each case lead to recurrent and/or severe infections with fungi (e.g. *Candida* and *Aspergillus* spp.) and/or bacteria (e.g. *Staphylococcus aureus, Pseudomonas* sp. and *Nocardia* sp.). While those discussed here are genetic defects, impaired phagocytic functions can also occur secondary to drug reactions, diabetes mellitus, metabolic storage diseases, malnutrition, immaturity, or burns, among others. In addition, loss of neutrophils may be associated with autoimmunity, or other immune deficiency diseases.

Disease classification
- *Defects of neutrophil differentiation:* circulating neutrophils are deficient (<1000 cells/mm). This may be due to different forms of agranulocytosis (Kostmann's syndrome), cyclic neutropenia, glycogen storage disease type Ib, or failure of release of neutrophils from bone marrow, one version of which is WHIM syndrome (warts, hypogammaglobulinemia, infections, and myelokathexis). This is a rare, dominantly inherited, congenital, immunodeficiency disorder characterized by chronic neutropenia and cutaneous warts. Neutropenia may also be caused by other immune defects (e.g. X-linked hyper IgM, X-linked agammaglobulinemia) or secondary to autoimmunity that accompanies Wiskott–Aldrich syndrome, common variable immune deficiency, or conditions such as hypersplenism.

Mount Sinai Expert Guides: Allergy and Clinical Immunology, First Edition. Edited by Hugh A. Sampson.
© 2015 John Wiley & Sons, Ltd. Published 2015 by John Wiley & Sons, Ltd.
Companion website: www.mountsinaiexpertguides.com

- *Defects of motility:* leukocyte adhesion deficiency (LAD) type I results from mutations in the adhesion molecules on neutrophils, leading to an inability of these cells to leave the circulation. This leads to high peripheral blood leukocyte counts, recurrent bacterial sinopulmonary and skin infections, and poor wound healing. Delayed separation of the umbilical cord may be identified in the clinical history. LAD type II results from a defect of a fucose transporter needed to glycosylate selected leukocyte adhesion molecules. LAD-3, caused by mutations in *Kindlin* gene, is associated with infections but also a bleeding disorder. Shwachman–Diamond syndrome leads to neutrophil dysfunction, amongst other syndromic features. The Shwachman–Diamond protein co-localizes with the mitotic spindle; this binds to and stabilizes purified microtubules. Defects in this protein lead to poor neutrophil chemotaxis. Less well understood are the chemotactic syndromes, which lead to severe, early onset periodontitis.
- *Defects of respiratory burst:* chronic granulomatous disease (CGD) is caused by defects in genes contributing to phagocyte NADPH oxidase. These lead to recurrent life-threatening bacterial and fungal infections, with the formation of granulomatous changes in tissues. The majority of patients with CGD are males with defects in the X-linked gene encoding the gp91phox subunit of flavocytochrome b_{558}, a membrane-bound protein forming a main unit of the oxidase. More rarely, CGD is caused by autosomal mutations in genes encoding p47phox, p67phox, or p22phox. When neutrophils are exposed to inflammatory stimuli, these components assemble, become activated, and induce superoxide formation leading to killing of microbes.
- *Other neutrophil defects:* these include myeloperoxidase deficiency, which is quite common. In this autosomal recessive disease, myeloperoxidase, an enzyme found in the azurophilic granules of neutrophils and monocytes, is absent. While it can be involved in killing microbes, loss of this enzyme is not normally associated with any illnesses. A second defect, neutrophil-specific granule deficiency, is quite rare but is associated with severe bacterial infections. Chediak–Higashi syndrome is a very rare autosomal recessive disorder with severe congenital neutropenia. The main features include recurrent pyogenic infections, partial oculocutaneous albinism, progressive neurologic abnormalities, mild coagulation defects, and a lymphoma-like accelerated phase in some.

Incidence/prevalence
- The overall incidence of phagocytic defects is unknown. Most of these are rare; the estimated incidence of CGD is 1 in 250 000 persons. Myeloperoxidase deficiency is more common, perhaps 1 in 2727 persons in one estimate.

Economic impact
- Phagocytic defects can lead to severe and recurrent infections. As patients often present in childhood and are not readily cured, over time the economic impact of these diseases is quite great. Treatments to raise the neutrophil count can be used (G-CSF) but are similarly expensive and may be lifelong. In some cases, hematopoietic stem cell transplantation is needed, leading to an additional economic burden. Patients with unrecognized defects will have severe infections, surgical interventions, and increased morbidity and mortality.

Etiology
- The causes of the primary phagocytic defects are mutations in genes that are required for normal neutrophil numbers and functions. It is important to remember that secondary phagocytic defects may be observed in subjects with diabetes mellitus, metabolic diseases, or in those with medication-induced neutropenia.

Pathology/pathogenesis
- *Genetics:* a number of genes can lead to phagocytic disorders. These are categorized according to whether genes are involved in phagocyte cell development, cell motility, or respiratory burst.

Pathology

- Defects of the phagocytic pathways can lead to the following:
  - Recurrent bacterial and fungal infections;
  - Organ damage, fistulae;
  - Skin abscesses, inflammatory bowel disease, oral ulcers, stomatitis, gingivitis, and periodontitis leading to loss of teeth.

Predictive/risk factors

- A family history of a similar clinical history might suggest that an immune defect should be considered.

Section 2: Prevention

Screening

- Patients with medical histories suggestive of phagocytic disorders can be screened by evaluating neutrophil numbers, morphology, and function.

Primary prevention

There are no primary preventative measures.

Secondary prevention

There are no secondary preventative measures.

Section 3: Diagnosis

- Childhood onset of acute or recurrent bacterial or fungal infections.
- Oral ulcers; gingivitis.
- Rectal fistulae.
- Unexplained inflammatory bowel disease.
- Organ abscesses.
- Suggestive family history.
- Isolation of unusual organisms.

Differential diagnosis

Differential diagnosis	Features
Neutropenia, chronic	Drug reaction, autoimmunity and congenital causes (gene mutations: *ELANE; GFI1; HAX1; G6PC3; G6PT1; ROBLD3; TAZ*)
Neutropenia, cyclic	Congenital causes *(ELANE)*
Persistent neutrophilia	Chronic infection, leukocyte adhesion defects, *LAD1, LAD2, LAD3*
Staphylococcus aureus liver or organ abscess	Chronic granulomatous disease *(CYBB; CYBA; NCF1; NCF2; NCF4)*
Burkholderia cepacia pneumonia or other unusual infection such as *Aspergillus* or *Nocardia*	Chronic granulomatous disease *(CYBB; CYBA; NCF1; NCF2; NCF4)*
Severe early periodontitis	Localized juvenile periodontitis *(FPR1)*

Typical presentation

- A typical scenario for CGD is a 5-year-old male child, with a newly diagnosed liver abscess. His whole blood count is elevated to 18 000 with 80% neutrophils. On abscess drainage and culture, *Staphylococcus aureus* is isolated. On history, the mother recalls that at age 2, the child had a rectal abscess that was successfully treated with oral antibiotics. The child recovers well with intravenous antibiotics. There is no family history of an immune defect as far as the parents know.

Clinical diagnosis

History

- Symptoms are heterogeneous as the organs and systems affected, and depend on the phagocytic defect. For cases of neutropenia, severe and early onset bacterial infections are prominent. For subjects with CGD, lymphadenitis, organ abscesses, or pneumonias with typical organisms are common. In CGD, early onset gastrointestinal disease is not uncommon. Details sought in the clinical history should include the microbiology of any previous cultures. Obtaining a detailed family history is always important.

Physical examination

- Physical examination should start with evaluation for signs of systemic illness. Fever may be present with acute infections, otherwise chronic fever would be uncommon. Patients with acute lung infections may be short of breath, have a productive or non-productive cough, and may have pulmonary signs such as rhonchi or rales on examination. Lymphadenitis is common. Gingivitis, oral ulcers, canker sores, and/or swollen gums are common findings in subjects with phagocytic defects.

Laboratory diagnosis

List of diagnostic tests

- CBC with differential.
- Neutrophil oxidative burst.
- Genetic mutational studies as indicated.

Lists of imaging techniques

- Chest X-ray and/or CT if lung findings are suspected.
- Ultrasound for organ abscesses.
- CT of the abdomen to examine organ size, lymphadenopathy.
- MRI may be preferred to minimize exposure to ionizing radiation.

Potential pitfalls/common errors made regarding diagnosis of disease

- Failing to diagnose phagocytic defects leads to excess morbidity.

Section 4: Treatment
Treatment rationale

- The goal of therapy is to provide amelioration of the phagocytic defect.

Table of treatment

Treatment	Comments
Conservative (Medical)	Recombinant G-CSF given at sufficient intervals to raise the neutrophil counts into the normal or near-normal range, 3–5 μg/kg SC/IV every day, as needed
	For neutopenic patients: chronic antibiotics are used, potentially trimethoprim-sulfamethoxazole (5 mg/kg twice daily), and perhaps itraconazole 100 or 200 mg/day
	If neutropenia is due to autoimmunity, short courses of steroids can be tried. If persistent, rituximab in standard 375 mg/m^2 for 4 weeks may be of use
	For CGD: standard of care includes trimethoprim-sulfamethoxazole (5 mg/kg twice daily), and itraconazole 100 or 200 mg/day
	IFN-γ in some cases: patients with a body surface area of ~0.5 m^2, 0.05 mg/m^2; for those with a body surface area of ~0.5 m^2, 0.0015 mg/kg; administered SC 3 times weekly
	For new infections, a first choice is often ciprofloxacin
Surgical	Drainage of abscesses
Radiological	To examine organs as needed
Other	Encourage normal activities, schooling, work, etc.
Hematopoetic stem cell transplantation	Required for cases of severe congenital neutropenia; reserved for selected cases of CGD

Prevention/management of complications
- Steroids or other immunosuppressants are used for only short periods as needed.

CLINICAL PEARLS
- Phagocytic disorders may lead to severe bacterial and fungal infections.
- These usually present in childhood.
- Inheritance may be X-linked, autosomal dominant or recessive.
- Treatment is dictated by the medical need but immunosuppression is to be minimized.
- Stem cell transplant for the most severe forms can be curative.

Section 5: Special populations
Pregnancy
- Treatment is as usual but with medications approved in pregnancy.

Children
- Treatment is as usual but with medications given based on weight.

Elderly
- Treatment is as usual.

Section 6: Prognosis

BOTTOM LINE/CLINICAL PEARLS
- Patients with phagocytic defects may do well with medical treatment.
- Careful evaluation of any new clinical findings that develop over time is important.

Natural history of untreated disease
• Continued bouts of infections are likely.
• Organ damage may occur.
• Loss of teeth from oral inflammation is common in some of these defects.

Prognosis for treated patients
• Varying with the degree of the genetic defect.

Follow-up tests and monitoring
• Careful follow-up for signs of infection.

Section 7: Reading list

Boxer, LA, How to approach neutropenia. Hematol Am Soc Hematol Educ Program 2012;2012:174–82
Holland SM. Chronic granulomatous disease. Clin Rev Allergy Immunol 2010;38:3–10
Lanza F. Clinical manifestation of myeloperoxidase deficiency. J Mol Med 1998;76:676–81

Suggested websites

NIH. http://rarediseases.info.nih.gov/gard/6100/chronic-granulomatous-disease/resources/1
http://www.aaaai.org/conditions-and-treatments/primary-immunodeficiency-disease/chronic-granulomatous-disease.aspx
http://ghr.nlm.nih.gov/condition/chronic-granulomatous-disease

Section 8: Guidelines
Not applicable for this topic.

Section 9: Evidence
• The genetic defects are rare and for many, medical evidence of treatment plans are not available. For CGD studies on best practices:

Type of evidence	Title, comment	Date
Randomized, double-blind, placebo-controlled study	Itraconazole to prevent fungal infections in chronic granulomatous disease **Comment:** Now routinely adopted	2003 (http://www.ncbi.nlm.nih.gov/pubmed/12802027)
International multicenter randomized prospective placebo-controlled trial	A controlled trial of interferon gamma to prevent infection in chronic granulomatous disease — The International Chronic Granulomatous Disease Cooperative Study Group **Comment:** Used in some centers	1991 (http://www.nejm.org/doi/full/10.1056/NEJM199102213240801)

Section 10: Images

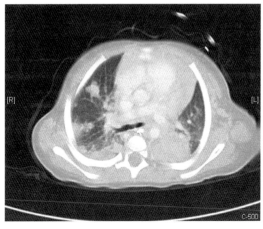

Figure 50.1 Phagocytic defect. A 16-month-old boy with no major past medical history developed fevers 2 weeks prior to admission. A biopsy shows granuloma and *Burkholderia cepacia* was cultured.

Additional material for this chapter can be found online at:
www.mountsinaiexpertguides.com
This includes a case study, multiple choice questions,
and ICD codes

CHAPTER 51

Human Immunodeficiency Virus Infection in Infants, Children, and Adolescents

Gail F. Shust and Roberto Posada

Departments of Pediatrics and Medical Education, Icahn School of Medicine at Mount Sinai, New York, NY, USA

OVERALL BOTTOM LINE

- In the United States, perinatal human immunodeficiency virus (HIV) infection occurs infrequently, and currently most pediatric infections are acquired during adolescence.
- HIV screening should be part of routine adolescent care.
- Acute HIV infection can present as a mononucleosis-like illness. When suspected, an HIV RNA assay is the diagnostic test of choice.
- HIV infection may be asymptomatic for years. Patients with HIV infection can present with an opportunistic infection or with end-organ involvement.
- Treatment of HIV infection involves combination antiretroviral therapy (cART) and results in improved patient outcomes and decreased transmission rates.

Section 1: Background
Definition of disease
- The term pediatric HIV is used to refer to children ≤13 years. Adolescent HIV refers to youth ≥13 years living with HIV.

Disease classification
- Children with current or prior immunologic category 3 classification or category C symptoms (see Disease severity classification in the Clinical diagnosis section) are classified as having AIDS.

Incidence/prevalence
- As of 2011, there were 3.3 million children <15 years living with HIV worldwide.
- In 2011, there were approximately 192 children <13 years and 2293 youth aged 13–19 newly diagnosed with HIV in the United States.
- In 2010, there were 10 798 people with perinatally acquired HIV in the United States. Fifty-three infants were born with HIV in the United States that year.

Economic impact
- CDC estimates that the lifetime treatment cost of a patient with HIV infection is $379 668 (in 2010 dollars). The cost effectiveness of antiretroviral therapy to treat HIV and to prevent mother to infant transmission of the virus has been demonstrated in several studies.

Etiology
- The vast majority of HIV cases in the United States are caused by the HIV-1.

Mount Sinai Expert Guides: Allergy and Clinical Immunology, First Edition. Edited by Hugh A. Sampson.
© 2015 John Wiley & Sons, Ltd. Published 2015 by John Wiley & Sons, Ltd.
Companion website: www.mountsinaiexpertguides.com

Pathology/pathogenesis
- HIV is present in blood, vaginal secretions, and semen of infected individuals and is transmitted through sexual contact, exposure to blood or body fluids, or from an infected woman to her newborn infant.
- HIV infects cells that express the CD4 receptor, and its RNA genome is reverse-transcribed to DNA and integrated into the host DNA.
- Infection is followed by a gradual decline in the function and number of CD4+ lymphocytes and by immune activation and chronic inflammation.

Predictive/risk factors
- Children born to women with HIV, children who are victims of sexual abuse, or adolescents who are sexually active, or use intravenous drugs are at risk for HIV infection. Also at risk are children who have received blood products outside of the United States in countries where the blood supply is not considered safe.

Section 2: Prevention

BOTTOM LINE/CLINICAL PEARLS
- Use of cART during pregnancy combined with zidovudine in the newborn period and avoidance of breastfeeding are highly effective for preventing mother-to-child transmission (PMTCT) of HIV.
- cART also prevents transmission of HIV from infected individuals to their sexual partners and antiretrovirals can be used as pre (PrEP) or post-exposure (PEP) prophylaxis for uninfected individuals.

Screening
- All individuals aged 13–64 should be screened for HIV infection at least once with an HIV antibody immunoassay, with repeat screening at least annually for those considered at risk. All pregnant women should be screened at initiation of prenatal care, and in the third trimester in areas of high HIV prevalence.
- Infants born to women with HIV should be screened for infection with an HIV RNA assay. Two negative RNA assay results, one after 1 month of age and one after 4 months of age, exclude infection.

Primary prevention
- Use of cART for HIV infected women during pregnancy, combined with zidovudine for 6 weeks to the newborn infant and avoidance of breastfeeding, are highly effective for PMTCT of HIV. Cesarean section delivery can further decrease the risk of infant infection when the maternal HIV viral load (VL) is >1000 copies/mL close to the time of delivery.
- The use of cART by HIV infected individuals is associated with decreased transmission rates to sexual partners. Condom use decreases the risk of HIV infection in males and females, and male circumcision decreases the risk of HIV acquisition through vaginal intercourse in males.
- Oral tenofovir or tenofovir/emtricitabine can prevent HIV acquisition when used as PrEP by at-risk HIV-negative individuals.
- PEP can decrease HIV transmission following sexual contact or accidental needle-stick exposures.

Secondary prevention
- Early detection and treatment of HIV infection prevents HIV related complications and decreases the risk of transmission of HIV to others.

Section 3: Diagnosis (Algorithm 51.1)

Algorithm 51.1 Traditional HIV testing

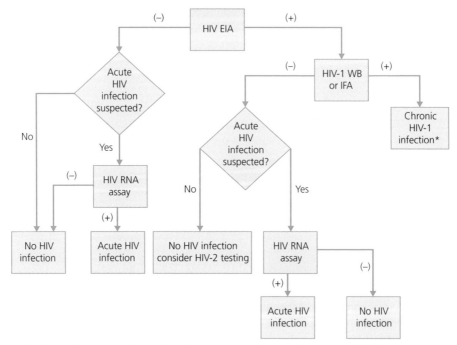

* If <18 months of age positive antibody test results need to be confirmed by an HIV RNA assay.

Algorithm 51.2 New HIV testing

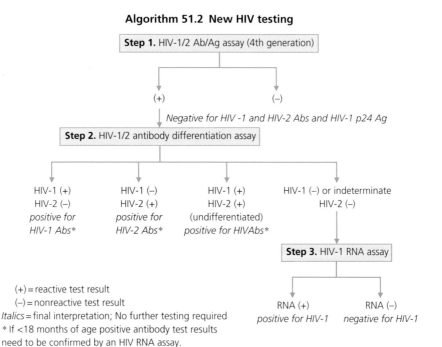

(+) = reactive test result
(–) = nonreactive test result
Italics = final interpretation; No further testing required
* If <18 months of age positive antibody test results
need to be confirmed by an HIV RNA assay.

BOTTOM LINE/CLINICAL PEARLS

- Patients with acute HIV can present with a mononucleosis-like illness.
- Chronic HIV may be asymptomatic or present with opportunistic infections; frequent or more severe manifestations of common infections; wasting, fever, and failure to thrive; or end-organ involvement.
- Acute HIV is diagnosed by a positive HIV RNA assay. The diagnosis of chronic HIV is confirmed by a positive HIV antibody immunoassay.

Differential diagnosis

Differential diagnosis	Features
For chronic HIV infection: primary immunodeficiencies	HIV antibody test
For acute HIV infection: mononucleosis, pharyngitis, influenza	HIV RNA assay positive Negative testing for other diagnoses

Typical presentation

- Acute HIV is often asymptomatic, but may present as a mononucleosis-like illness, with fever and sore throat; a rash may be present. Children with chronic HIV may be asymptomatic or can have varied manifestations with involvement of any organ system. Common presentations include opportunistic infections (e.g. *Pneumocystis* pneumonia) or invasive bacterial infections; failure to thrive; prolonged fever; frequent, persistent, or more severe manifestations of common infections; chronic parotid gland enlargement; chronic dermatitis; complicated varicella; recurrent herpes simplex or herpes zoster; or end-organ involvement such as developmental delay, cardiomyopathy, hepatitis, nephropathy, anemia, thrombocytopenia, or leukopenia.

Clinical diagnosis

History

- A history of prior infections, including frequency, severity, causative pathogen, and response to treatment is important. The clinician should obtain a careful developmental history and enquire about school performance and learning or behavioral problems that may suggest CNS effects of HIV. A complete review of systems should be obtained to identify end-organ involvement. When obtaining the family history it is important to enquire about known maternal HIV or symptoms that suggest undiagnosed infection in the mother. If the patient's mother is known to be HIV infected, details about cART during pregnancy, maternal VL at the time of delivery, mode of delivery, use of neonatal zidovudine prophylaxis, and whether the patient was breastfed should be obtained.

Physical examination

- Height, weight, and head circumference (if <3 years old) should be assessed.
- The dermatologic examination should include an evaluation for atopic dermatitis, diaper rashes, and petechiae or bruising.
- The eyes, ears, nose, and throat examination should include a search for otitis media, thrush, gingivostomatitis, and aphthous ulcers.
- The cervical, axillary, epitrochlear, and inguinal areas should be examined for the presence of enlarged lymph nodes.

- The heart and lungs should be auscultated for possible tachycardia or abnormal breath sounds, and the abdomen should be evaluated for the presence of hepatosplenomegaly.

Useful clinical decision rules and calculators
Not applicable for this topic.

Disease severity classification

CDC classifies pediatric HIV based on clinical and immunological parameters

Category	Symptoms
Category N: non-symptomatic	No symptoms or only one category A symptom
Category A: mildly symptomatic	Two or more of the following: lymphadenopathy, hepatomegaly, splenomegaly, dermatitis, parotitis, recurrent or persistent upper respiratory infections
Category B: moderately symptomatic	Includes persistent oral candidiasis; chronic diarrhea; recurrent herpes simplex virus stomatitis; complicated or recurrent varicella-zoster infections; persistent fever; single episode of serious bacterial infection; and end-organ manifestations of HIV
Category C: severely symptomatic	Includes recurrent serious bacterial infections, opportunistic infections, encephalopathy, and wasting syndrome

CD4$^+$ lymphocyte count/µL (percentage of total lymphocytes)

	>12 months	1–5 years	6–12 years
Immunologic category 1	≥1500 (≥25%)	≥1000 (≥25%)	≥500 (≥25%)
Immunologic category 2	750–1499 (15–24%)	500–999 (15–24%)	200–499 (15–24%)
Immunologic category 3	<750 (<15%)	<500 (<15%)	<200 (<15%)

Laboratory diagnosis
List of diagnostic tests
- When acute HIV infection is suspected, the preferred diagnostic test is an HIV RNA assay because HIV RNA can generally be detected in plasma before antibody tests become positive.
- When chronic HIV infection is suspected, conventional testing with an HIV enzyme immunoassay (EIA) which detects antibodies in plasma against HIV-1 and HIV-2 should be performed. A positive result is automatically confirmed with a Western blot (WB) or immunofluorescent antibody (IFA) assay specific for HIV-1.
- When available, newer "4th generation" HIV-1/2 Antigen/Antibody (Ag/Ab) assays are preferred over conventional EIA assays. These assays may be positive earlier in the window period than traditional EIA. If the result from this test is 'Non-reactive', no further testing is necessary. If the result is 'Reactive', this is considered preliminarily positive, and supplemental testing must be performed, beginning with an HIV-1/HIV-2 antibody differentiation immunoassay. If the result of the differentiation test is positive, the diagnosis is confirmed. If the result of the

differentiation assay is negative or indeterminate, a HIV RNA assay must be performed to rule out acute infection.

- A positive antibody test in an infant <18 months of age may represent infection, or antibody transmitted through the placenta from the mother to the infant in the absence of infection of the child. Therefore, in this age group a positive antibody test result should be confirmed with an HIV RNA assay.
- An alternative to HIV antibody testing in blood samples is oral fluid testing which follows a similar algorithm to conventional testing.
- Rapid HIV antibody tests can provide a result in ≤30 minutes and can be used for point-of-care testing, but positive results must be confirmed with a WB or IFA assay.

List of imaging techniques

Not applicable for this topic.

Potential pitfalls

Antibody HIV testing with EIA may miss acute HIV infection.

Section 4: Treatment

Treatment rationale

- Adherence to cART is critical to prevent development of drug resistance. Therefore, the decision to initiate cART should take into account the ability of the caregiver and child to adhere to the regimen. The goal of treatment is to decrease the HIV plasma VL to undetectable levels and improve immune function.
- Treatment is currently recommended for:
  - All infants <12 months;
  - All children ≥1 year with AIDS or CDC clinical category B or C symptoms;
  - Asymptomatic or mildly symptomatic children in the following categories:
    - ➤ children 1 to <3 years with CD4 cell count <1000 cells/mm³ or CD4 percentage <25%;
    - ➤ children 3 to <5 years with CD4 cell count <750 cells/mm³ or CD4 percentage <25%;
    - ➤ children ≥5 years with CD4 cell count ≤500 cells/mm³.
- Treatment should be considered for asymptomatic or mildly symptomatic children in the following categories:
  - Children 1 to <3 years with CD4 cell count ≥1000 cells/mm³ or CD4 percentage ≥25%;
  - Children 3 to <5 years with CD4 cell count ≥750 cells/mm³ or CD4 percentage ≥25%;
  - Children ≥5 years with CD4 cell count >500 cells/mm³.
- Treatment of adolescents follows the guidelines for treatment of HIV infected adults (see Chapter 52)

When to hospitalize

Patients with HIV infection are generally manged in the outpatient setting. Opportunistic infections or complications due to end organ effects of HIV may require inpatient management.

Managing the hospitalized patient

Management of the hospitalized patient depends on the nature of their complications. Every effort should be made to continue cART without interruption.

Table of treatment

Treatment of HIV generally includes at least three drugs from at least two different classes. Drug resistance testing should be obtained prior to initiating therapy. The following are the preferred regimens for treatment-naïve children

Age	Preferred regimen
Children aged ≥14 days to <3 years	Two nucleoside reverse-transcriptase inhibitors (NRTIs) **plus** lopinavir/ritonavir[a]
Children aged ≥3 years	Two NRTIs **plus** efavirenz[b] Two NRTIs **plus** lopinavir/ritonavir
Children aged ≥6 years	Two NRTIs **plus** atazanavir **plus** low-dose ritonavir Two NRTIs **plus** efavirenz[b] Two NRTIs **plus** lopinavir/ritonavir

Two NRTI options

Abacavir[c] **plus** lamivudine or emtricitabine (children aged ≥3 months)
Tenofovir **plus** lamivudine or emtricitabine (adolescents, Tanner stage 4 or 5)
Zidovudine **plus** lamivudine or emtricitabine

[a] Lopinavir/ritonavir should not be administered to neonates before a post-menstrual age of 42 weeks and a postnatal age of 14 days.
[b] Efavirenz should be used only in children aged ≥3 years with weight ≥10 kg. Unless adequate contraception can be ensured, efavirenz-based therapy is not recommended for females of childbearing age.
[c] Abacavir should only be used in patients who are HLA B*5701 negative.

For treatment-experienced children, resistance testing and prior antiretroviral history should be taken into account when designing cART regimens. Prophylaxis for opportunistic infections is required for children meeting the following criteria

Infection	Indication	Preferred agent
Pneumocystis pneumonia	All infants <12 months Age >1 year and immunologic category C	Trimethoprim-sulfamethoxazole
Mycobacterium avium-complex	Age ≥6 years and CD4 <50 cells/mm^3 Age 2–5 years and CD4 <75 cells/mm^3 Age 1–2 years and CD4 <500 cells/mm^3 Age <1 year and CD4 <750 cells/mm^3	Azithromycin

Prevention/management of complications
- NRTIs can cause lactic acidosis and multi-organ failure. Life-threatening hypersensitivity can be caused by abacavir (in patients with the HLA B*5701 haplotype) or nevirapine (particularly in patients with relatively high CD4 counts). Several antiretroviral drugs are associated with hyeprlipidemia and lipodystrophy.
- Management of treatment complications involves substituting the suspected drug(s) with an alternative agent. For serious complications requiring treatment interruption, all agents should be discontinued simultaneously. Dose reduction is not recommended.

CLINICAL PEARLS
- The decision regarding when to initiate or change cART in children is multifactorial.
- Combination regimens should include at least three drugs from at least two drug classes.
- Drug-resistant virus can develop while on cART due to poor adherence, a regimen that is not potent, or a combination of these factors, resulting in incomplete viral suppression.

Section 5: Special populations

Pregnancy

HIV pregnant women are managed similarly to other adults with HIV infection. Achieving an undetectable VL is associated with decreased transmission of HIV to the newborn infant. See Chapter 52.

Children

Not applicable for this topic.

Elderly

Not applicable for this topic.

Others

- Infants born to HIV-positive mothers
  - Chemoprophylaxis with zidovudine for 6 weeks is recommended for all HIV-exposed infants.
  - HIV-exposed infants whose mothers did not receive antepartum cART should receive zidovudine for 6 weeks plus three doses of nevirapine in the first week of life.
- Adolescents
  - Medication adherence is often poor in this population. A multidisciplinary, motivational team approach may be helpful.
  - Choice of cART for adolescents is complex and dependent upon many factors including body mass, Tanner Stage, and psychosocial factors.
  - Care providers should prepare adolescents over time for transition to the adult care setting.

Section 6: Prognosis

- The risk of disease progression associated with a specific CD4 percentage or count varies with the age of the child.
- Infants ≤12 months old experience higher risks of morbidity and mortality than older children at any CD4 threshold.
- Treatment of HIV-infected children has been associated with enhanced survival, reduction in opportunistic infections and other medical complications, improved growth and neurocognitive function, and improved quality of life.

Follow-up tests and monitoring (see Algorithm 51.3)

Algorithm 51.3 Management of the HIV positive child

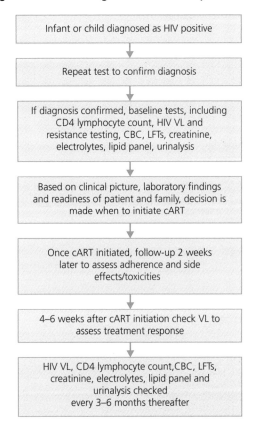

Infant or child diagnosed as HIV positive

↓

Repeat test to confirm diagnosis

↓

If diagnosis confirmed, baseline tests, including CD4 lymphocyte count, HIV VL and resistance testing, CBC, LFTs, creatinine, electrolytes, lipid panel, urinalysis

↓

Based on clinical picture, laboratory findings and readiness of patient and family, decision is made when to initiate cART

↓

Once cART initiated, follow-up 2 weeks later to assess adherence and side effects/toxicities

↓

4–6 weeks after cART initiation check VL to assess treatment response

↓

HIV VL, CD4 lymphocyte count, CBC, LFTs, creatinine, electrolytes, lipid panel and urinalysis checked every 3–6 months thereafter

Section 7: Reading list

Branson BM, Handsfield HH, Lampe MA, Janssen RS, Taylor AW, Clark JE, et al. Revised recommendations for HIV testing of adults, adolescents, and pregnant women in health-care settings. MMWR Recomm Rep 2006;55:1–17; quiz CE1–4

LK, Pickering, CJ Baker, DW Kimberlin (eds). Human immunodeficiency virus infection. Red Book, 29th Edition. Report of the Committee on Infectious Diseases. American Academy of Pediatrics, 2012;418–39.

Suggested websites

http://hivinsite.ucsf.edu/
http://aidsinfo.nih.gov/
www.cdc.gov/hiv/statistics/basics/index.html
www.hivguidelines.org
http://www.unaids.org/en

Section 8: Guidelines
National society guidelines

Guideline title	Guideline source	Date
Guidelines for the use of antiretroviral agents in pediatric HIV infection	Department of Health and Human Services (HHS)	2014 (http://aidsinfo.nih.gov/guidelines/html/2/pediatric-arv-guidelines/0)
Recommendations for use of antiretroviral drugs in pregnant HIV-1-infected women for maternal health and interventions to reduce perinatal HIV transmission in the United States	Department of Health and Human Services (HHS)	2014 (http://aidsinfo.nih.gov/contentfiles/lvguidelines/perinatalgl.pdf)
Guidelines for the prevention and treatment of opportunistic infections among HIV-exposed and HIV-infected children	CDC, National Institutes of Health (NIH); HIV Medicine Association of the Infectious Diseases Society of America (HIVMA/IDSA); the Pediatric Infectious Diseases Society (PIDS); and the American Academy of Pediatrics (AAP)	2013 (http://aidsinfo.nih.gov/contentfiles/lvguidelines/oi_guidelines_pediatrics.pdf)

Section 9: Evidence

Type of evidence	Title	Date
Retrospective cohort study	Decreasing rate of hospitalization for perinatal HIV infection (Clin Infect Dis 2004;39(5): i doi:10.1086/423392	2004 (http://cid.oxfordjournals.org/content/39/5/i.full)
Population surveillance study	Low rates of mother-to-child transmission of HIV following effective pregnancy interventions in the United Kingdom and Ireland, 2000–2006 (AIDS 2008;22(8):973–81)	2004 (http://www.ncbi.nlm.nih.gov/pubmed/18453857)

Additional material for this chapter can be found online at:
www.mountsinaiexpertguides.com
This includes a case study, multiple choice questions, and ICD codes

Section 10: Images

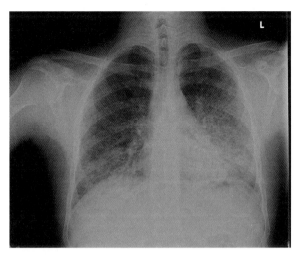

Figure 51.1 Chest X-ray of an 18-year-old man with perinatally acquired HIV and *Pneumocystis* pneumonia showing bilateral reticulonodular densities. The patient's CD4+ lymphocyte count is 18/μL and the percentage CD4 lymphocyte count is 3%. At the time of presentation he had been non-adherent with trimethoprim-sulfamethoxazole which had been prescribed for *Pneumocystis* pneumonia prophylaxis.

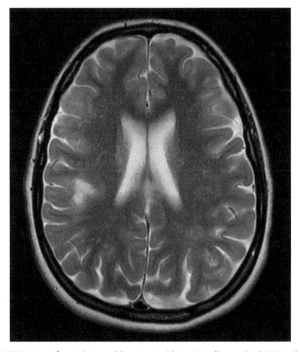

Figure 51.2 Brain MRI image of an 18-year-old woman with perinatally acquired HIV and progressive multifocal leukoencephalopathy. She presented with left hemiparesis and a CD4+ lymphocyte count of 8/μL. The MRI revealed T2 hyperintensities without contrast enhancement. A PCR for JC virus on the cerebrospinal fluid was positive.

CHAPTER 52

Human Immunodeficiency Virus Infection in Adults

Timothy Sullivan and Michael Mullen

Division of Infectious Diseases, Mount Sinai Hospital, New York, NY, USA

OVERALL BOTTOM LINE

- The human immunodeficiency virus (HIV) is a single-stranded RNA virus that causes the acquired immune deficiency syndrome (AIDS)
- HIV infection is typically transmitted via sexual contact, intravenous drug use, other exposure to infected blood products, or via perinatal transmission.
- HIV infection causes the destruction of CD4+ T lymphocytes, which can result in profound immunosuppression, susceptibility to severe infections, and higher rates of certain malignancies, such as non-Hodgkin's lymphoma and cervical cancer.
- HIV infection is also a chronic inflammatory process that may cause cardiac, renal, neurologic, and other comorbidities.
- HIV and AIDS are major causes of morbidity and mortality worldwide; however, antiretroviral therapy (ART) significantly alters the natural history of HIV, suppressing its effects, preserving immune function, and dramatically improving patient survival.

Section 1: Background

Definition of disease

- HIV is a single-stranded RNA retrovirus that causes AIDS. AIDS is defined as HIV infection associated with either a serum CD4+ T-lymphocyte level of <200 cells/μL, or with an "AIDS-defining condition," which includes 24 opportunistic infections, malignancies, and other conditions.

Disease classification

- HIV classification and staging systems have been developed by the CDC and World Health Organization (WHO) for epidemiologic purposes. The CDC system ranges from stage A to C and the WHO system from stage I to IV, with later stages representing more advanced disease.

Incidence/prevalence

- The United Nations estimated that in 2012 there were 35.3 million people living with HIV, 2.3 million new HIV infections, and 1.6 million deaths due to AIDS worldwide.
- The burden of disease is highest in sub-Saharan African, where the prevalence in some countries exceeds 20%.

Mount Sinai Expert Guides: Allergy and Clinical Immunology, First Edition. Edited by Hugh A. Sampson.
© 2015 John Wiley & Sons, Ltd. Published 2015 by John Wiley & Sons, Ltd.
Companion website: www.mountsinaiexpertguides.com

- According to the CDC, in 2010 in the United States there were 1.3 million people aged 13 and older living with HIV, and 47 000 new HIV infections.

Economic impact

- The economic effects of HIV have been devastating, particularly in sub-Saharan Africa and throughout the developing world.
- One study estimated that in the United States in 2002, the lifetime cost of new HIV infections was $36.4 billion, of which $6.7 billion was medical costs and $29.7 billion was due to lost productivity.

Etiology

- HIV is typically transmitted via sexual contact, intravenous drug use, other exposure to infected blood products, or via perinatal transmission.

Pathology/pathogenesis

- The majority of new HIV infections occur by sexual transmission, via the genital or rectal mucosa. Virions typically migrate through intracellular spaces or breaks in the epithelium to infect macrophages, CD4+ T lymphocytes and Langerhans cells. Following transmission, HIV begins replicating in the mucosal, submucosal, and adjacent lymphatic tissues, then typically progresses into the lymphoid tissue of the gut, where it rapidly replicates, causing an exponential rise in the serum HIV viral load and potentially irreversible depletion of CD4+ T lymphocytes. The widespread death of lymphocytes and ongoing viral replication cause the release of inflammatory cytokines, which causes flu-like symptoms. Following the initial innate immune response, there is a cellular and humoral response. CD4+ T-lymphocyte levels typically rise after the acute infection, then steadily decline afterwards.

Predictive/risk factors

These numbers are not clearly defined for HIV/AIDS.

Section 2: Prevention

> **BOTTOM LINE/CLINICAL PEARLS**
> - Several preventive strategies specific to the different modes of HIV transmission have been proven effective. Importantly, for all types of HIV transmission the use of ART in source patients (i.e. "treatment as prevention") has been shown to reduce their infectivity and prevent new infections.

Screening

- In 2013, the US Preventive Services Task Force recommended that all patients aged 15–65, all pregnant women, and all patients younger than 15 or older than 65 and at high risk for HIV be screened. This guideline suggests repeating screening annually in those at very high risk for HIV.
- Available screening tests for established HIV infection are the serum HIV enzyme immunoassay (EIA) in combination with a confirmatory Western blot, as well as rapid HIV antibody testing of both serum and oral fluid. HIV nucleic acid amplification and p24 antigen tests are used to screen for acute HIV.

Primary prevention

- To prevent sexual transmission, abstinence, the use of barrier protection, male circumcision, and both pre- and post-exposure antiretroviral prophylaxis are effective.
- Among intravenous drug users, methadone treatment programs, needle exchange programs, and educational outreach have helped reduce HIV transmission.
- To prevent mother-to-child transmission, perinatal ART and cesarean section delivery in high-risk patients is efficacious.
- For all types of HIV transmission, the use of ART in source patients has been shown to reduce their infectivity and prevent new infections.

Secondary prevention

Not applicable for this topic.

Section 3: Diagnosis (Algorithm 52.1)

> **BOTTOM LINE/CLINICAL PEARLS**
> - When taking a history from a patient with suspected HIV, identifying high-risk behaviors is essential. Additionally, patients who present with acute HIV often complain of viral symptoms, including fever, malaise, myalgias, rash, and lymphadenopathy.
> - On examination, findings in patients with acute HIV are non-specific and include fever, rash, or lymphadenopathy. Patients with advanced HIV/AIDS may present with signs of wasting and chronic illness, chronic skin lesions, signs of acute opportunistic infections, or signs of malignancy.
> - Laboratory testing in patients with suspected HIV should include an HIV antibody test, either via rapid HIV test or serum EIA. In those with suspected acute HIV, a serum HIV RNA PCR or p24 antigen test should be carried out.

Differential diagnosis of acute HIV

Differential diagnosis	Features
Mononucleosis	Very difficult to distinguish clinically, diagnosed on the basis of laboratory testing
Influenza	Very difficult to distinguish clinically, diagnosed on the basis of laboratory testing
Other non-specific viral syndromes	A diagnosis of exclusion

Typical presentation

- Patients with acute HIV infection often present with non-specific symptoms of an acute viral syndrome, including fever, chills, malaise, fatigue, myalgia, and lymphadenopathy. Other presenting complaints include rash, cough, nausea, vomiting, diarrhea, or headache. Rarely, patients with acute HIV may present with an opportunistic infection.
- Patients who are newly diagnosed with AIDS may present with weight loss and signs of chronic illness, or with signs and symptoms of acute opportunistic infections. Given the wide range of opportunistic infections in AIDS patients, presentation at this stage is varied.

Algorithm 52.1 Diagnosis of HIV

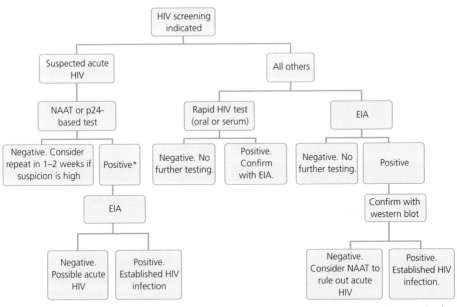

Note: EIA, enzyme immunoassay; NAAT, nucleic acid amplification test. If HIV RNA viral load is used as screening for acute HIV, a cutoff of 10 000 copies/mL is suggested because of the possibility of false positives with lower values.

Clinical diagnosis

History

- When obtaining a history from a patient with suspected HIV, identifying high-risk behaviors such as intravenous drug use, commercial sex work, unprotected intercourse with multiple partners, and men who have sex with men, is essential. Patients who present with acute HIV often complain of viral symptoms including fever, chills, malaise, fatigue, myalgia, and lymphadenopathy. Other presenting complaints include rash, cough, nausea, vomiting, diarrhea, or headache. It is important to gauge the acuity of these symptoms, especially in relation to recent high-risk behaviors.
- When interviewing a patient with suspected long-term HIV infection or AIDS, it is important to assess for complaints consistent with active opportunistic infections, as well as signs of prolonged immunosuppression, such as recurrent infections or other unexplained illnesses. Additionally, patients with AIDS may complain of cognitive decline or other neurologic deficits.

Physical examination

- The initial physical examination of a patient with suspected HIV infection or AIDS should be comprehensive, because of the varied, non-specific, and sometimes subtle examination findings.
- When examining patients with suspected acute HIV, the clinician should include a search for rash, lymphadenopathy, signs of intravenous drug use, and signs of other concurrent sexually transmitted infections.
- The examination of a patient with suspected AIDS, in addition to the above, should include a meticulous search for opportunistic infections and other sequelae of AIDS, including but not limited to: general wasting, ocular infections, oropharyngeal lesions, chronic skin lesions (especially those suggestive of Kaposi's sarcoma), signs of pneumonia, gastrointestinal infection, hepatosplenomegaly, peripheral neuropathy, or central nervous system pathology.

Useful clinical decision rules and calculators
Not applicable for this topic.

Disease severity classification
Not applicable for this topic.

Laboratory diagnosis
List of diagnostic tests
- *HIV serum EIA:* indicated for screening for established HIV infection. Highly sensitive. The current, "third generation" test typically becomes positive about 3 weeks after HIV infection.
- *p24 antigen test:* used for the detection of acute HIV. Typically becomes positive about 2 weeks after acute infection and 1 week before the EIA. Currently available in combination with EIA as the "fourth generation" HIV test.
- *HIV Western blot:* used to confirm a positive EIA. Highly specific, but less sensitive. May remain negative for up to 3 weeks after EIA becomes positive in early HIV infection.
- *Rapid HIV tests:* antibody tests that are performed on serum or oral fluid. Results may be returned in minutes. Sensitivity has been reported as similar to the serum EIA, although sensitivity may be lower in early HIV infection.
- *HIV nucleic acid amplification tests:* HIV RNA and DNA PCR testing is the recommended screening test for suspected acute HIV infection. Its use is limited by high cost and slow turn-around time (about 2 days)

Lists of imaging techniques
- The use of imaging studies in newly diagnosed HIV or AIDS patients should be guided by clinical suspicion of opportunistic infections or malignancies.

Potential pitfalls/common errors made regarding diagnosis of disease
- Acute HIV infection is commonly mistaken for a non-specific viral syndrome. Additionally, even when clinicians suspect acute HIV, often the correct diagnostic test (either a nucleic acid amplification or p24 test) is not performed.
- Screening for asymptomatic HIV infection may be overlooked in high-risk patients until they become symptomatic with an AIDS-defining illness.

Section 4: Treatment
Treatment rationale
- ART has revolutionized the care of patients with HIV, resulting in preserved immune function, reduced rates of opportunistic infections and other complications, and significantly improved survival for millions of patients.
- Antiretroviral agents and the recommendations for their use are continually evolving. Early guidelines suggested initiating ART only in patients with AIDS or otherwise low CD4 levels. However, given the enhanced efficacy and improved tolerability of current regimens, as well as recent evidence indicating that starting treatment earlier may be beneficial, recent guidelines recommend starting ART sooner. The 2013 WHO guidelines recommend starting ART in patients with AIDS or CD4 counts of 500 cells/μL or less, while the most recent guidelines from the US Department of Health and Human Services recommend initiating ART for all patients with HIV.
- The general approach when initiating ART is to start three active antiretroviral agents from at least two different medication classes. Classes include nucleoside analog reverse transcriptase

inhibitors, non-nucleoside reverse transcriptase inhibitors, protease inhibitors, integrase strand transfer inhibitors, and entry inhibitors. Recent guidelines from the US Department of Health and Human Services include recommendations for preferred and alternative regimens. Second line and salvage regimen choices are typically guided by HIV resistance testing or other contraindications to first line medications.

When to hospitalize
Not applicable for this topic.

Managing the hospitalized patient
Not applicable for this topic.

Table of treatment
Preferred and alternative regimens for the initial treatment of HIV

Treatment	Comment

Medical
• Preferred regimens:
  1. Efavirenz/tenofovir/emtricitabine
  2. Ritonavir-boosted atazanavir + tenofovir/
    emtricitabine
  3. Ritonavir-boosted darunavir + tenofovir/
    emtricitabine
  4. Raltegravir + tenofovir/emtricitabine
	Efavirenz: may cause significant neuropsychiatric side effects
	Tenofovir: may cause renal toxicity and a reduction in bone mineral density
	Protease inhibitors: potent inhibitors of the cytochrome p450 enzymes, resulting in numerous drug–drug interactions. May also cause severe gastrointestinal and metabolic side effects

• Alternative regimens:
  1. Rilpivirine/tenofovir/emtricitabine
  2. Efavirenz + abacavir/lamivudine
  3. Rilpivirine + abacavir/lamivudine
  4. Ritonavir-boosted atazanavir, darunavir, lopinavir or fosamprenavir + abacavir/lamivudine
  5. Ritonavir-boosted lopinavir or fosamprenavir + tenofovir/emtricitabine
  6. Raltegravir + abacavir/lamivudine
  7. Elvitegravir/cobicistat/tenofovir/emtricitabine
	Atazanavir: may cause indirect hyperbilirubinemia that does not reflect liver damage
	Abacavir: may cause a fatal hypersensitivity reaction. Contraindicated in patients who are positive for HLA-B*5701
	Cobicistat: CYP 3A inhibitor, numerous drug–drug interactions

All medications that are joined by a forward slash (e.g. tenofovir/emtricitabine) are available in co-formulated fixed-dose combinations. Treatment recommendations are likely to change as new drugs become available.

Prevention/management of complications
• Older ART regimens were associated with several severe, debilitating and potentially fatal adverse reactions, including lactic acidosis, hepatic steatosis, anemia, renal failure, lipodystrophy, peripheral neuropathy, and chronic diarrhea. In addition to managing associated symptoms, the cornerstone of managing these adverse effects in the modern ART era is changing the patient's treatment to a better-tolerated regimen.

Section 5: Special populations

Pregnancy

- The care of pregnant women with HIV presents several challenges, given the imperative need to prevent the spread of HIV from mother to child, as well as the potential teratogenicity of certain antiretrovirals.
- All pregnant women should be started on ART.
- Pregnant women with HIV should be managed with close coordination between obstetrics and HIV specialists.

Children

- There are several distinct challenges to treating a child with HIV, including overcoming barriers to ART adherence and managing social and psychological stressors, especially among victims of sexual abuse.

Elderly

- As a result of the efficacy of modern ART, patients with HIV are living longer, and the number of elderly HIV patients is rising.
- The care of elderly patients with HIV must incorporate consideration of the long-term effects of HIV infection, including cardiac, renal, and neurologic disease, and the potential for long-term side effects of ART.

Others

Not applicable for this topic.

Section 6: Prognosis

Natural history of untreated disease

- In the absence of ART, following the initial infection and widespread destruction of CD4+ T lymphocytes, HIV causes a gradual decline in CD4 cell levels. The rate of decline of CD4 cells and the time until the development of AIDS is highly variable.
- A small subset of patients, called "long-term non-progressors," exhibit minimal reductions in CD4 levels despite HIV infection. Another minority of patients, called "elite controllers" maintain undetectable serum levels of HIV without ART.
- Without treatment, most patients eventually develop profound immunosuppression, which may result in opportunistic infections and death.

Prognosis for treated patients

- The outcomes of patients who begin treatment early in the course of HIV infection, are adherent to ART, and have few comorbid medical conditions are generally excellent.
- Recent studies have shown that the survival of patients with well-controlled HIV may be similar to that of the general population.

Follow-up tests and monitoring

- Patients being treated with ART require life-long regular follow-up to ensure treatment efficacy, and monitor for adverse effects.

Section 7: Reading list

Cohen MS, Chen YQ, McCauley M, Gamble T, Hosseinipour MC, Kumarasamy N, et al. Prevention of HIV-1 infection with early antiretroviral therapy. N Engl J Med 2011;365:493–505

Global report: UNAIDS report on the global AIDS epidemic 2013. Geneva, Switzerland: 2013

HIV Surveillance Report. Centers for Disease Control and Prevention. 2011; vol. 23

Hutchinson AB, Farnham PG, Dean HD, Ekwueme DU, del Rio C, Kamimoto L, et al. The economic burden of HIV in the United States in the era of highly active antiretroviral therapy: evidence of continuing racial and ethnic differences. J Acquir Immune Defic Syndr 2006;43:451–7

Kitahata MM, Gange SJ, Abraham AG, Merriman B, Saag MS, Justice AC, et al. Effect of early versus deferred antiretroviral therapy for HIV on survival. N Engl J Med 2009;360:1815–26

Panel on Antiretroviral Guidelines for Adults and Adolescents. Guidelines for the use of antiretroviral agents in HIV-1-infected adults and adolescents. Department of Health and Human Services, 2013

Ray M, Logan R, Sterne JA, Hernandez-Diaz S, Robins JM, Sabin C, et al. The effect of combined antiretroviral therapy on the overall mortality of HIV-infected individuals. AIDS (London, England). 2010;24:123–37

Rodger AJ, Lodwick R, Schechter M, Deeks S, Amin J, Gilson R, et al. Mortality in well controlled HIV in the continuous antiretroviral therapy arms of the SMART and ESPRIT trials compared with the general population. AIDS (London, England). 2013;27:973–9

Schneider E, Whitmore S, Glynn KM, Dominguez K, Mitsch A, McKenna MT. Revised surveillance case definitions for HIV infection among adults, adolescents, and children aged <18 months and for HIV infection and AIDS among children aged 18 months to <13 years – United States, 2008. MMWR Recomm Rep 2008;57:1–12

Screening for HIV: Final Recommendation Statement. AHRQ Publication No. 12-05173-EF-3. US Preventive Services Task Force, 2013

World Health Organization. Consolidated guidelines on general HIV care and the use of antiretroviral drugs for treating and preventing HIV infection: recommendations for a public health approach. 2013 9241505729

Suggested websites

aidsinfo.nih.gov

hivinsite.ucsf.edu

www.cdc.gov/hiv

www.who.int/hiv

Section 8: Guidelines
National society guidelines

Guideline title	Guideline source	Date
Panel on Antiretroviral Guidelines for Adults and Adolescents. Guidelines for the use of antiretroviral agents in HIV-1-infected adults and adolescents	Department of Health and Human Services (DHHS)	2014 (http://aidsinfo.nih.gov/contentfiles/lvguidelines/adultandadolescentgl.pdf)
Screening for HIV: Final Recommendation Statement. AHRQ Publication	US Preventive Services Task Force (USPSTF)	2013 (Ann Intern Med 2005;143:32–7)
Guidelines for the Prevention and Treatment of Opportunistic Infections in HIV-Infected Adults and Adolescents	Department of Health and Human Services (DHHS)	2013 (http://aidsinfo.nih.gov/contentfiles/adult_oi.pdf)

International society guidelines

Guideline title	Guideline source	Date
Consolidated guidelines on general HIV care and the use of antiretroviral drugs for treating and preventing HIV infection: recommendations for a public health approach	World Health Organization (WHO)	2013 (http://www.who.int/hiv/pub/guidelines/arv2013/en/)

Section 9: Evidence
Too numerous to list here.

Section 10: Images
Not applicable for this topic.

Additional material for this chapter can be found online at:
www.mountsinaiexpertguides.com
This includes a case study, multiple choice questions, and ICD codes

CHAPTER 53

Infections in the Compromised Host

Charlotte Cunningham-Rundles
Departments of Medicine and Pediatrics, The Immunology Institute, Icahn School of Medicine at Mount Sinai, New York, NY, USA

OVERALL BOTTOM LINE
- Patients with severe unusual or recurrent infections may have defects in the immune system from non-genetic causes.
- These are called secondary immune defects.
- The underlying causes are likely to be anatomic obstruction, previous organ damage, untreated allergy, immunosuppression given for other diseases, viral infections, malignancy, or malnutrition.
- The type of infections experienced will be based on the location of the organ damage, and type of immunosuppression, viral infection, or cancer.
- Subjects may be either sex, and of any age, but are more likely to be adults.
- Careful microbiologic cultures are important.
- The goal of treatment is to define the type of infection, the cause of the illness, and evaluate if protective measures can be instituted.

Section 1: Background

Definition of disease

- The immune system is composed of a large network of cells and organs working together. As a strong immunity is so important for heath, nature has provided a number of overlapping immune systems to cope with an entire range of microbes. However, in a number of medical conditions, the immune system is not able to protect against infections due to underlying causes. Depending on the type and size of the immune defect, the infections that may develop can vary widely.

Disease classification

- The first objective is to determine the nature of the underlying cause and attempt correction or amelioration of this condition. For example, the use of steroids or immunosuppressants for allergic or autoimmune disease is likely to impair the number and/or function of these immune cells.
- To define the type of immune defect underlying various infections, immunologists use a classification system based on the components of the immune network:
  - *T cells:* arise in the thymus and help control viruses, and aid in antibody production;
  - *B cells:* develop into plasma cells and produce long-lasting antibodies;

Mount Sinai Expert Guides: Allergy and Clinical Immunology, First Edition. Edited by Hugh A. Sampson.
© 2015 John Wiley & Sons, Ltd. Published 2015 by John Wiley & Sons, Ltd.
Companion website: www.mountsinaiexpertguides.com

- *Combined defects:* in which both T and B cells are defective;
- *Phagocytic cells:* neutrophils go to the site of infection and engulf and digest bacteria;
- *Complement:* a system of proteins that interact to aid the function of antibodies but also control immune reactions;
- *Innate immunity:* a group of cells that do not need to be primed to work.

Incidence/prevalence
- The incidence of secondary immune defects is unknown but is likely to be common.
- Secondary immune defects may be due to drugs such as steroids, chemotherapy, chronic leukemias (chronic lymphocytic leukemia), or a viral infection (such as Epstein–Barr virus or HIV). In these cases, immune defects can lead to a variety of infections and also inflammatory/autoimmune disease.

Economic impact
- Unrecognized secondary immune defects lead to both morbidity and mortality.

Etiology
- Secondary immune defects result from loss or abnormality of one or more of the many components of the immune system.
- The mechanisms for this loss may be due to many causes, the main ones being the use of medications, presence of unrecognized malignancy, or viral infections.

Pathology/pathogenesis
- Immune defects may also be secondary to other causes.
- Genetics: complex inheritance patterns may obscure any genetic contributions.
- Pathology: as the immune system contains many components and various members of this network are found in all organs, the pathology of immune defects is based on the organ itself:
  - Acute bacterial infections of the lungs, blood, or solid organs;
  - Inflammatory disease of the joints, lung, liver, and so on;
  - Autoimmunity, in particular immune thrombocytopenia or hemolytic anemia;
  - Chronic gastrointestinal inflammation with loss of absorptive surfaces leading to diarrhea, malnutrition, iron deficiency anemia, hypoalbuminemia, and so on.

Predictive/risk factors
Not applicable for this topic.

Section 2: Prevention
Screening
- Patients with medical histories suggestive of immune defects (e.g. recurrent infections, autoimmunity, enlarged spleen, lymphadenopathy) can be tested with screening tests to determine if serum immunoglobulins are normal, if vaccines have led to the production of antibodies, and if the cells of the immune system are found in normal proportions.

Primary prevention
There are no primary preventive measures.

Secondary prevention
There are no secondary preventive measures.

Section 3: Diagnosis

- Immune defects generally lead to acute or recurrent bacterial infections, infections with unusual organisms, or infections that prove difficult to eliminate.
- In some cases, significant infections have not occurred but various forms of inflammatory or auto-immune disease have occurred (e.g. interstitial lung disease, arthritis, hematologic cytopenias, gastrointestinal infections, or inflammation).
- The clinical examination can be normal or show non-specific signs such as lung abnormalities (rales, rhonchi) or lymphadenopathy, splenomegaly, pallor, or evidence of malnutrition or gastrointestinal disease is present.

Differential diagnosis

Differential diagnosis	Features
Allergy/asthma	Recurrent infections; pneumonias
Chronic viral/parasitic infection	Infections, weight loss
Malignancy/lymphoma	Weight loss, fever
Medications	Rash, fever

Typical presentation

- The typical scenario is an adult who has a significant medical history of asthma and has been treated with steroids for some time, who now has had several episodes of pneumonia. Laboratory testing shows somewhat low serum IgG and antibody production to the pneumococcal vaccine shows a blunted response. The immune defect may be due to steroid use in this case. In other cases, the antibody response may be poor when the underlying cause is an expansion of clonal B cells, characteristic of chronic lymphocytic leukemia (CLL). Here, in early stages, CLL may not lead to a high lymphocyte count but antibody functions are not normal.

Clinical diagnosis

History

- Symptoms are as heterogeneous as the organs and systems affected, and depend on the nature of the immune defect. In 80% of cases, lung infections occur, specifically pneumonia or chronic bronchitis. A history of difficult-to-treat chronic sinusitis is very common; a history of having one or more previous sinus surgeries is often found. Gastrointestinal disease is seen in some. Details sought in the clinical history should include duration and onset of symptoms, fatigue, fever, weight loss, shortness of breath. Weight loss is common. Obtaining a detailed family history is always important, as well as questions about smoking, drug use, and the medications tried.

Physical examination

- Physical examination should start with evaluation for signs of systemic illness, including weight loss.
- Fever may be present with acute infections, otherwise chronic fever would be uncommon.
- Patients with lung disease may be short of breath, have a productive or non-productive cough, and may have pulmonary signs such as rhonchi or rales on examinination.
- Lymphadenopathy is common, and enlarged spleen may be detected.
- Skin changes include scarring from previous herpes zoster; vitiligo appears to be common.

- Chronic conjunctivitis, iritis, or episcleritis, may be observed.
- Joint complaints include changes due to previous joint infections, or autoimmune, chronic arthritis.

Laboratory diagnosis
List of diagnostic tests
- Complete blood count (anemia, moderate leukocytosis, thrombocytosis).
- Serum IgG, IgA, IgM.
- Tests for functional antibody (e.g. tetanus, diphtheria).
- CRP and sedimentation rate.
- Microbial cultures where applicable.
- Liver function tests, renal function, and electrolytes.
- Serum iron, folate and vitamin B$_{12}$ if malabsorption is suspected.
- Microbiologic studies to exclude infectious etiologies.

Lists of imaging techniques
- Chest X-ray.
- Complete lung functions (spirometry and diffusion capacity).
- High resolution CT of the chest.
- Ultrasound for question of splenomegaly.
- CT of the abdomen to examine organ size, lymphadenopathy.
- MRI may be preferred to minimize exposure to ionizing radiation.

Potential pitfalls/common errors made regarding diagnosis of disease
- Failing to diagnose immune defects in adults leads to excess morbidity.
- Over-diagnosis can lead to excess medical costs as therapies can be expensive.

Section 4: Treatment
Treatment rationale
- The goals of therapy are to provide protection against infections and, where possible, to use any available therapy to enhance the immune system.
  - *Antibiotics:* when an immune deficiency has been documented, antibiotics should be started immediately for fevers and other manifestations of infection after appropriate cultures have been obtained. These cultures are important to direct further therapy if the infection does not respond to the initial antibiotic chosen. Prophylactic antibiotics can be of benefit, especially for subjects with chronic lung disease. A satisfactory combination of antibiotics includes amoxicillin-clavulanate, erythromycin, trimethoprim-sulfamethoxazole, or a cephalosporin. In adults, amoxicillin-clavulanate, trimethoprim-sulfamethoxazole, tetracyclines, or a cephalosporin are useful. Quinolones are best saved to treat acute infections.
  - *Immunoglobulin:* when significant loss of antibody production has occurred and this has been fully documented, the optimum treatment is immunoglobulin replacement. The usual starting dosage for the intravenous forms is 400–600 mg/kg/month; IVIg can be given at home. Subcutaneous treatment is also quite effective; smaller doses are given once a week.
  - *Specific treatment for T-cell deficiency:* there are few specific treatments for T-cell immune deficiencies aside from bone marrow and stem cell transplants for the most severe forms (SCID). Other therapies, such as cytokines, remain investigational.
  - *Specific treatment of phagocytic disorders:* there are very few treatments for the phagocytic disorders, aside from the use of antibiotics as needed, or G-CFS to raise the neutrophil count.

- *Specific treatment for complement deficiency:* fresh frozen plasma from healthy donors can transiently replace specific complement components in patients with isolated complement component defects and severe infections. However, this is not clinically shown to be of use.

Table of treatment

Treatment	Comments
Conservative	Antibiotics for acute care as needed Prophylactic antibiotics for some
Medical	Immunoglobulin replacement when loss of antibody documented; 400–600 mg/kg, IV or SC Antibiotics as above
Surgical	Biopsies if pathology suspected
Radiological	To examine lungs or other organs as needed
Complementary	Vitamins and nutrients as needed
Other	Enforce normal activities, schooling, work, etc.

Prevention/management of complications
Not applicable for this topic.

> **CLINICAL PEARLS**
> - Steroids and other immunosuppressants are to be avoided when the immune system is impaired.
> - Smoking is a risk factor for progressive lung disease.
> - Do not start immunoglobulin therapy unless a complete evaluation of antibody production has been carried out.

Section 5: Special populations
Pregnancy
- Treatment is as usual but with medications approved in pregnancy.

Children
- Treatment is as usual but with medications given based on weight.

Elderly
- Treatment is as usual but with medications given based on weight.

Section 6: Prognosis

> **BOTTOM LINE/CLINICAL PEARLS**
> - Most adults with immune defects will do well if the correct therapy is initiated.
> - Careful evaluation of any new clinical findings that develop over time is important.
> - Using antibiotics according to the requirements of the disease is essential; these choices are based on published data.

Natural history of untreated disease

• Continued infections and possibly unregulated inflammatory disease may occur.

Prognosis for treated patients

• Varying with the disease, but clearly improved with treatment.

Follow-up tests and monitoring

• Careful follow-up for signs of new infections not adequately treated is important. For patients on immunoglobulin therapy, attention to trough values (the IgG at the lowest points before retreatment) is essential.

Section 7: Reading list

Primary Immune Deficiency Disease: Cecil Medicine 22nd edition, Elsevier
Ocampo CJ, Peters AT. Antibody deficiency in chronic rhinosinusitis: epidemiology and burden of illness. Am J Rhinol Allergy 2013;27:34–8

Suggested websites

American Associate of Asthma Allergy and Immune Deficiency. http://www.aaaai.org/conditions-and-treatments/primary-immunodeficiency-disease.aspx
Immune Deficiency Foundation. www.primaryimmune.org
Jeffrey Modell Foundation. www.info4pi.org
NIH. http://www.niaid.nih.gov/topics/immunedeficiency/

Section 8: Guidelines
National society guidelines

Guideline title	Guideline source	Date
Practice parameter for the diagnosis and management of primary immunodeficiency	American Academy of Allergy, Asthma and Immunology (AAAAI)	2005 (https://www.aaaai.org/Aaaai/media/MediaLibrary/PDF%20Documents/Practice%20and%20Parameters/immunodeficiency2005.pdf)

Section 9: Evidence
Not applicable for this topic.

Section 10: Images
Not applicable for this topic.

Additional material for this chapter can be found online at:
www.mountsinaiexpertguides.com
This includes a case study, multiple choice questions, and ICD codes

Index

Page numbers in *italic* refer to figures. Page numbers in **bold** refer to tables.

Mount Sinai Expert Guides: Allergy and Clinical Immunology, First Edition. Edited by Hugh A. Sampson.
© 2015 John Wiley & Sons, Ltd. Published 2015 by John Wiley & Sons, Ltd.
Companion website: www.mountsinaiexpertguides.com